Lessons in Immunity: From Single-Cell Organisms to Mammals

Lessons in Immunity: From Single-Cell Organisms to Mammals

Edited by

Loriano Ballarin
University of Padova, Padova, Italy

Matteo Cammarata
University of Palermo, Palermo, Italy

AMSTERDAM • BOSTON • HEIDELBERG • LONDON
NEW YORK • OXFORD • PARIS • SAN DIEGO
SAN FRANCISCO • SINGAPORE • SYDNEY • TOKYO

Academic Press is an imprint of Elsevier

Academic Press is an imprint of Elsevier
125 London Wall, London EC2Y 5AS, UK
525 B Street, Suite 1800, San Diego, CA 92101-4495, USA
50 Hampshire Street, 5th Floor, Cambridge, MA 02139, USA
The Boulevard, Langford Lane, Kidlington, Oxford OX5 1GB, UK

Notices
Knowledge and best practice in this field are constantly changing. As new research and experience broaden our understanding, changes in research methods, professional practices, or medical treatment may become necessary.

Practitioners and researchers must always rely on their own experience and knowledge in evaluating and using any information, methods, compounds, or experiments described herein. In using such information or methods they should be mindful of their own safety and the safety of others, including parties for whom they have a professional responsibility.

To the fullest extent of the law, neither the Publisher nor the authors, contributors, or editors, assume any liability for any injury and/or damage to persons or property as a matter of products liability, negligence or otherwise, or from any use or operation of any methods, products, instructions, or ideas contained in the material herein.

The cover image for this book was inspired by the Italian Association of Developmental and Comparative Immunobiology (IADCI) logo.

British Library Cataloguing-in-Publication Data
A catalogue record for this book is available from the British Library

Library of Congress Cataloging-in-Publication Data
A catalog record for this book is available from the Library of Congress

ISBN: 978-0-12-803252-7

For information on all Academic Press publications
visit our website at https://www.elsevier.com/

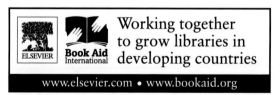

Working together
to grow libraries in
developing countries

www.elsevier.com • www.bookaid.org

Typeset by TNQ Books and Journals
www.tnq.co.in

Contents

7. Immune-Related Signaling in Mussel and Bivalves

Paola Venier, Stefania Domeneghetti, Nidhi Sharma,
Alberto Pallavicini and Marco Gerdol

8. Crustacean Immunity: The Modulation of Stress Responses

Chiara Manfrin, Alberto Pallavicini, Silvia Battistella,
Simonetta Lorenzon and Piero G. Giulianini

9. How Insects Combat Infections

Małgorzata Cytryńska, Iwona Wojda and Teresa Jakubowicz

10. *Aedes aegypti* Immune Responses to Dengue Virus

Cole Schonhofer, Heather Coatsworth, Paola Caicedo,
Clara Ocampo and Carl Lowenberger

11.   Protective Responses in Invertebrates

Magda de Eguileor, Annalisa Grimaldi and Gianluca Tettamanti

12.   Echinoderm Antimicrobial Peptides: The Ancient Arms of the Deuterostome Innate Immune System

Vincenzo Arizza and Domenico Schillaci

13.   Inflammatory Response of the Ascidian *Ciona intestinalis*

*Parrinello Nicolò, Cammarata Matteo,
Parrinello Daniela and Vizzini Aiti*

List of Contributors

Luigi Abelli University of Ferrara, Ferrara, Italy

Vizzini Aiti University of Palermo, Palermo, Italy

Claudio Alimenti University of Camerino, Camerino, Macerata, Italy

Vincenzo Arizza University of Palermo, Palermo, Italy

Loriano Ballarin University of Padova, Padova, Italy

Silvia Battistella University of Trieste, Trieste, Italy

Kornélia Bodó University of Pécs, Pécs, Hungary

Francesco Buonocore University of Tuscia, Viterbo, Italy

Paola Caicedo CIDEIM, Cali, Valle del Cauca, Colombia

Matteo Cammarata University of Palermo, Palermo, Italy

Laura Canesi University of Genova, Genova, Italy

Heather Coatsworth Simon Fraser University, Burnaby, BC, Canada

Maria R. Coscia Institute of Protein Biochemistry, National Research Council of Italy, Naples, Italy

Małgorzata Cytryńska Maria Curie-Sklodowska University, Lublin, Poland

Parrinello Daniela University of Palermo, Palermo, Italy

Magda de Eguileor University of Insubria, Varese, Italy

Stefania Domeneghetti University of Padova, Padova, Italy

Francesco Drago University of Lille – Science and Technology, Villeneuve D'Ascq, France

Péter Engelmann University of Pécs, Pécs, Hungary

Antonella Franchini Modena and Reggio Emilia University, Modena, Italy

Nicola Franchi University of Padova, Padova, Italy

Michela Furlan University of Trieste, Trieste, Italy

François Gagné Emerging Methods Section, Aquatic Contaminants Research Division, Environment Canada, Montréal, QC, Canada

Marco Gerdol University of Trieste, Trieste, Italy

Stefano Giacomelli Institute of Protein Biochemistry, National Research Council of Italy, Naples, Italy

Piero G. Giulianini University of Trieste, Trieste, Italy

Annalisa Grimaldi University of Insubria, Varese, Italy

Yuya Hayashi Aarhus University, Aarhus, Denmark; Karlsruhe Institute of Technology (KIT), Karlsruhe, Germany

Teresa Jakubowicz Maria Curie-Sklodowska University, Lublin, Poland

Christophe Lefebvre University of Lille – Science and Technology, Villeneuve D'Ascq, France

Simonetta Lorenzon OGS (National Institute of Oceanography and Experimental Geophysics), Sgonico (TS), Italy

Carl Lowenberger Simon Fraser University, Burnaby, BC, Canada

Pierangelo Luporini University of Camerino, Camerino, Macerata, Italy

Davide Malagoli University of Modena and Reggio Emilia, Modena, Italy

Annalaura Mancia University of Ferrara, Ferrara, Italy

Chiara Manfrin University of Trieste, Trieste, Italy

Valerio Matozzo University of Padova, Padova, Italy

Cammarata Matteo University of Palermo, Palermo, Italy

László Molnár University of Pécs, Pécs, Hungary

Parrinello Nicolò University of Palermo, Palermo, Italy

Clara Ocampo CIDEIM, Cali, Valle del Cauca, Colombia

Umberto Oreste Institute of Protein Biochemistry, National Research Council of Italy, Naples, Italy

Enzo Ottaviani University of Modena and Reggio Emilia, Modena, Italy

Alberto Pallavicini University of Trieste, Trieste, Italy

Maria G. Parisi University of Palermo, Palermo, Italy

Carla Pruzzo University of Genova, Genova, Italy

Giuseppe Scapigliati University of Tuscia, Viterbo, Italy

Domenico Schillaci University of Palermo, Palermo, Italy

Cole Schonhofer Simon Fraser University, Burnaby, BC, Canada

Marco Scocchi University of Trieste, Trieste, Italy

Nidhi Sharma University of Padova, Padova, Italy

Gianluca Tettamanti University of Insubria, Varese, Italy

Adriana Vallesi University of Camerino, Camerino, Macerata, Italy

Gerardo R. Vasta University of Maryland School of Medicine, Baltimore, MD, United States

Paola Venier University of Padova, Padova, Italy

Jacopo Vizioli University of Lille – Science and Technology, Villeneuve D'Ascq, France

Iwona Wojda Maria Curie-Sklodowska University, Lublin, Poland

Preface

Animals constitute the greatest part of eukaryotic biodiversity, with more than 2 million known species grouped in approximately 35 phyla.

The exploitation of only a limited part of this great variety of species was fundamental for the advancement of immunobiology, starting with the original experiments of Elie Metchnikoff with sea star larvae, which posed the basis for the phagocytosis theory, up to the recent studies on Toll receptors in Drosophila by Jules A. Hoffmann, which led to comprehension of the role of Toll-like receptors in innate immunity.

Animals have evolved a wide range of approaches to cope with foreign, potentially pathogenic organisms, and today, the increasing need to extend our knowledge of immune responses requires new, suitable, and simple model organisms for the study of the variety of defense strategies present in metazoans, besides the few species investigated so far. This is of general biological interest and might reveal new adaptive solutions and unknown recognition and effector mechanisms, useful for further progresses in immunology. It also has an applied interest, as a solid knowledge of invertebrate immunity is fundamental for setting up biological methods to control invertebrates, which are vectors of diseases or pests for crops. In addition, a better knowledge of the immune system of farmed species can be of great help in the optimization of the rearing strategies in cattle breeding and aquaculture. Furthermore, focusing on mammals only, as most immunologists do, does not allow for the study of the evolution of immune defense and host–parasites coevolution.

This book stems from the activity of the Italian Association of Developmental and Comparative Immunobiology, born in 1997, which coordinates the activity of many research teams on the common theme of immune responses in *no mouse, no man* models through periodic scientific meetings. We invited part of its members and other international collaborators with consolidated competence in their respective fields to write on specific aspects of their research. The outcome is a series of short chapters (lessons), in the form of overviews, in which a wealth of new and reviewed information, concerning many aspects of immunity in invertebrates and vertebrates, can be found. The aim is to provide scientists and teachers with an easy and updated tool reporting, in an evolutionary perspective, the state of the art in relevant fields of immunobiology.

We thank all the authors and reviewers for their important contributions and their patience with the process that, finally, brought this book to fruition.

Matteo and Loriano

Chapter 1

Ciliate Pheromones: Primordial Self-/Nonself-Recognition Signals

Adriana Vallesi, Claudio Alimenti, Pierangelo Luporini
University of Camerino, Camerino, Macerata, Italy

INTRODUCTION

Independently of their prokaryotic or eukaryotic nature, cells are evolutionarily driven to socialize to acquire the temporary or stable multicellular organization necessary to increase their size and engage in functional specialization and partition of labor.[1] This ancient impulse to socialize implies a very early evolution of the cell's ability to discriminate between self and nonself, which is a sine qua non condition for pursuing effective cell–cell communication, cooperation, and structure–function integration. In its most basic aspects, this ability is primarily directed to the recognition of self-signaling molecules, as exemplified by the quorum-sensing phenomena in which bacteria perceive their environmental population densities and activities and, consistently, vary their behavior and metabolism.[2,3] It then undergoes vast functional diversification among the unicellular eukaryotes in which it governs impressive phenomena of cell aggregation based on kin discrimination in social amoebas.[4,5] Its maximal complexity is eventually shown by animals with the evolution of innate and adaptive immunity systems that are primarily directed to recognizing and processing nonself molecules for the defense of body integrity.[6,7]

This chapter focuses on the biology and structure of diffusible protein signals, nowadays known as pheromones and earlier as mating-type factors/ substances or gamones, that control self/nonself recognition in protist ciliates. Together with Dinoflagellates and Apicomplexa, ciliates (Ciliophora) form the group of Alveolata, which clusters with those of Stramenopiles (diatoms) and Rhizaria (foraminifers and radiolarians) into the so-called SAR supergroup.[8]

Lessons in Immunity: From Single-Cell Organisms to Mammals
http://dx.doi.org/10.1016/B978-0-12-803252-7.00001-1

PHEROMONE IDENTIFICATION

Ciliate pheromones are the chemical markers of genetically distinct vegetative cell classes—only two of the same sex in some species or multiple with indefinite numbers in others[9,10]—that have been described as mating types because their mixing determines a ciliate-specific mating phenomenon of conjugation. Ciliate conjugation is a sexual phenomenon as it involves a temporary union in mating pairs between cells, which mutually exchange gamete nuclei, undergo fertilization, and develop new micro- and macronuclei from the synkarya. However, it has nothing to do with the general phenomena of fertilization between gametes of opposite sexes. One major reason for opposing this parallelism is that many species of ciliates may form mating pairs between genetically different cells (heterotypic pairs), as well as between genetically alike (clonal) cells (homotypic mating pairs). Although destined to generate self-fertilization, these homotypic pairs are fully fertile (the *Blepharisma* case excepted) just like the heterotypic ones.

It is precisely by virtue of this unique capability of ciliates to form homotypic (intraclonal or selfing) mating pairs that ciliate pheromones were identified more than half a century ago.[11] By investigating mating interactions in *Euplotes patella*—the first *Euplotes* species used to study the Mendelian genetics of ciliate multiple mating systems controlled by a series of alleles codominantly expressed at a single genetic locus (annotated as *mat* locus)—Kimball[11] observed that an experimental condition sufficient to induce the formation of homotypic mating pairs was the simple suspension of cell cultures with cell-free filtrates from other cultures of different mating types. From this observation it became evident that in *E. patella*, and ciliates in general, the mating-type factors (pheromones) can be freely released into the extracellular environment and that the presence of these molecules in solution can be promptly detected by assaying the mating-induction activity of cell-free filtrates.

By applying this mating-induction assay to cell-free filtrates, pheromones have been identified in species of *Blepharisma*, *Dileptus*, *Oxytricha*, *Ephelota*, and *Tokophrya* in addition to other *Euplotes* species (Refs 12, 13, as reviews). However, studies of structure–function characterization have been carried out to varying degrees of complexity only on pheromones isolated from *Blepharisma japonicum*, *Euplotes raikovi*, *Euplotes octocarinatus*, *Euplotes nobilii*, and *Euplotes crassus*. These studies are reviewed in this chapter with particular attention to the cross-reactions that some *Euplotes* pheromones show with the signaling system components of more modern organisms.

PHEROMONE STRUCTURES

The first two pheromones to be purified and structurally characterized belong to the pink-colored freshwater ciliate, *B. japonicum*. Although they are of two mating types (I and II) defined as "complementary," of which nothing is known about their genetic determination, their molecular structures are chemically unrelated. The pheromone isolated from the type-I cells (originally designated as gamone 1 or blepharmone) is an unstable glycoprotein of 272 amino acids and 6 *N*-linked sugars.[14] It is particularly rich in polar and aromatic amino acids (Asn 10.3%, Ser 10.3%, Tyr 8.1%, Trp 5.1%), synthesized in the form of a cytoplasmic precursor, and active in inducing mating between type-II cells at picogram concentrations. In contrast, the second pheromone distinctive of type-II cells (also designated as gamone 2 or blepharismone) is a very stable tryptophan derivative, namely a calcium-3-(2′-formyl-amino-5′-hydroxybenzoyl) lactate.[15] This has also been obtained by chemical synthesis and is active at nanomolar concentrations in attracting type-I cells besides those for inducing their mate.[16]

Quite different is the picture that emerges for the pheromone structures determined in four species of *Euplotes*, namely *E. raikovi*, *E. nobilii*, *E. octocarinatus*, and *E. crassus*. In all these species, pheromones have been shown to form species-specific families of structurally homologous proteins. Among these pheromone families, a more in-depth structural knowledge has been obtained for *E. raikovi* and *E. nobilii*, which secrete comparatively larger amounts of pheromones. Up to 200 µg of pure protein per liter can be recovered from *E. raikovi* cell-free filtrates.[17] This has greatly facilitated chemical and genetic approaches to the determination of significant numbers of pheromone primary amino acid sequences. It subsequently opened up the way to NMR and crystallographic analyses of the pheromone three-dimensional structures based on the use of proteins at a natural isotope composition purified from cell-free filtrate preparations.

In *E. raikovi*, nine distinct amino acid pheromone sequences in their form of cytoplasmic precursors (pre/propheromones) and six three-dimensional structures of the secreted molecules are known[18–24] (Fig. 1.1). In contrast to the tight structural conservation of the strongly hydrophobic presegment (or signal peptide) of 19 amino acids and (to a slightly lesser extent) of the prosegment of 16–18 amino acids, the secreted pheromones of 37–40 amino acids (51 only in pheromone E*r*-23) show minimal sequence conservation. Only the positions of six cysteines are fully conserved, and the sequence dissimilarity between any two pheromones may be as high as 74%. In any case, despite this wide variability in the amino acid sequence, all the pheromones (pheromone E*r*-23 in part excepted) mimic one another in their three-dimensional conformation. This is based on a fold of three nearly parallel, right-handed α helices (increased to five with the addition of two single-turn helices in E*r*-23) that remain tightly associated with each other by the close proximity and strategic disposition of their disulfide bonds. As is usually required for waterborne signaling molecules that must maintain long-term activity in the environment, the stability of the globular conformation of *E. raikovi* pheromones is such that even heating these proteins up to 95°C does not cause unfolding and disruption of their secondary structures.[25] However, in spite of showing closely comparable molecular architectures and equivalent stabilities, each pheromone has its own unmistakable cell type structural earmarks that are likely deputed to confer specificity to its

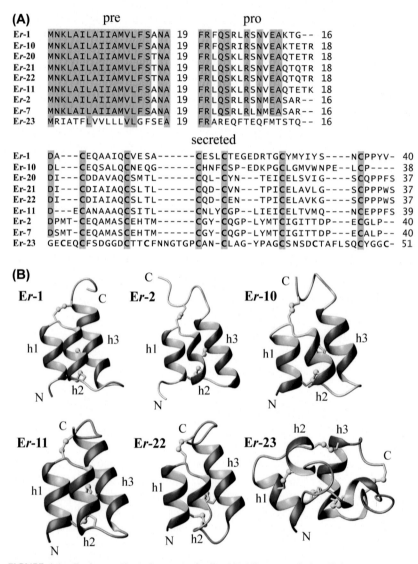

FIGURE 1.1 *Euplotes raikovi* pheromone family. (A) Alignment of nine distinct sequences of pheromone precursors, as deduced from their DNA-coding sequences. Sequence alignment is based on the Clustal W algorithm and optimized manually by gap insertions. Residues conserved among all sequences, or all but one sequence, are shadowed. The positions of the cysteine residues are highlighted in bold. The numbers of residues of the pre, pro, and secreted regions are reported on the right of the sequences. (B) Ribbon presentations (as visualized by the program MOLMOL) of the six pheromone structures (side view) that have been determined by NMR analysis of native protein preparations. The Protein Data Bank codes are as follows: 1erc (E*r*-1), 1erd (E*r*-2), 1erp (E*r*-10), 1ery (E*r*-11), 1hd6 (E*r*-22), and 1ha8 (E*r*-23). The amino and carboxyl termini of each molecule are labeled N and C, respectively, and the sulfur atoms involved in the disulfide bonds are indicated as spheres. The three more regular α-helices common to all six molecules are labeled h1–h3 starting from the *N*-terminus.

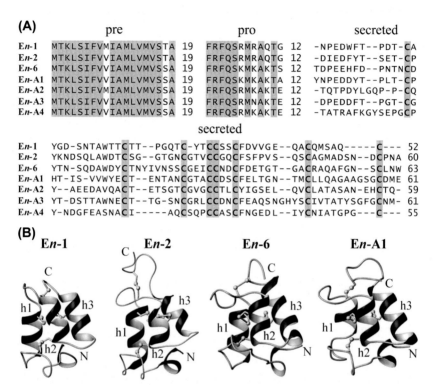

(A)

	pre		pro		secreted
E*n*-1	MTKLSIFVMIAMLVMVSTA	19	FRFQSRMRAQTG	12	-NPEDWFT--PDT-CA
E*n*-2	MTKLSIFVVIAMLVMVSTA	19	FRFQSRMRAQTG	12	-DIEDFYT--SET-CP
E*n*-6	MTKLSIFVVIAMLVMVSSA	19	FRFQSKMKAKTS	12	TDPEEHFD--PNTNCD
E*n*-A1	MTKLSIFVVIAMLVMVSSA	19	FRFQSKMKAKTA	12	YNPEDDYT--PLT-CP
E*n*-A2	MTKLSIFVMIAMLVMVSSA	19	FRFQSRMKAKTE	12	-TQTPDYLGQP-P-CQ
E*n*-A3	MTKLSIFVVIAMLVMVSSA	19	FRFQSRMNAKTE	12	-DPEDDFT--PGT-CG
E*n*-A4	MTKLSIFVVIAMLVMVSSA	19	FRFQSRMKAKTE	12	-TATRAFKGYSEPGCP

secreted

E*n*-1	YGD-SNTAWTTCTT--PGQTC-YTCCSSCFDVVGE--QACQMSAQ-----C---	52
E*n*-2	YKNDSQLAWDTCSG--GTGNCGTVCCGQCFSFPVS--QSCAGMADSN--DCPNA	60
E*n*-6	YTN-SQDAWDYCTNYIVNSSCGEICCNDCFDETGT--GACRAQAFGN--SCLNW	63
E*n*-A1	HT-IS-VVWYECT--ENTANCGTACCDSCFELTGN--TMCLLQAGAAGSGCDME	61
E*n*-A2	Y--AEEDAVQACT--ETSGTCGVGCCTLCYIGSEL--QVCLATASAN-EHCTQ-	59
E*n*-A3	YT-DSTTAWNECT--TG-SNCGRLCCDNCFEAQSNGHYSCIVTATYSGFGCNM-	61
E*n*-A4	Y-NDGFEASNACI-----AQCSQPCCASCFNGEDL--IYCNIATGPG---C---	55

(B)

E*n*-1   E*n*-2   E*n*-6   E*n*-A1

FIGURE 1.2   *Euplotes nobilii* pheromone family. (A) Alignment of seven distinct sequences of pheromone precursors, as deduced from their DNA-coding sequences. (B) Ribbon presentations (as visualized by the program MOLMOL) of the four pheromone structures that have been determined by NMR analysis of native protein preparations. The Protein Data Bank codes are as follows: 2nsv (E*n*-1), 2nsw (E*n*-2), 2jms (En-6), and 2kk2 (En-A1). Indications and symbols as in Fig. 1.1.

signaling activity. These earmarks are imposed by the evolution of variations that are most apparent for the shape, extension, and spatial arrangement of the carboxy-terminal domain, as well as for the geometry of the interhelix loops of the molecules.

The overall structural organization of *E. nobilii* pheromones strictly matches the *E. raikovi* pheromone organization with the close phylogenetic kinship that links these two species.[26,27] Nevertheless, *E. nobilii* pheromones, for which seven amino acid sequences of the precursor forms[28] and four NMR structures have been determined[29–31] (Fig. 1.2), have longer sequences (from 52 to 63 amino acids), include eight instead of six cysteines, and, more importantly, show structural specificities that appear closely correlated with the different ecology that distinguishes *E. nobilii* from *E. raikovi*. While *E. raikovi* thrives in temperate waters, *E. nobilii* has colonized the Antarctic and Arctic seas.[32,33] Hence, *E. nobilii* pheromones are cold-adapted, psychrophilic proteins. With respect to *E. raikovi* pheromones, their overall contents of polar and hydrophobic amino acids are markedly different, most likely in functional correlation with their improved interactions with the solvent.[34] They are much richer in Thr (11.7% vs 5.7%), Asn (7.7% vs 4.2%), and Ser (8.6% vs 5.7%) residues and poorer in Leu (1.1% vs 7.3%), Pro (4.7% vs 8.9%), and Ile (1.6% vs 5.7%). Structurally more apparent are, however, the reduced extensions that *E. nobilii* pheromones show for the three helices of the molecular architecture with respect to *E. raikovi* pheromones. These reductions determine a spatial preponderance of regions devoid of a regular secondary organization, implying that the activity of *E. nobilii* pheromones in the thermodynamically adverse environment of the polar waters is facilitated by an improved flexibility of their molecular backbones. Indeed, *E. nobilii* pheromones have been measured to be much less thermostable than *E. raikovi* pheromones, unfolding upon heating to only 55–70°C.[25–35]

Much less information is available on the structures of *E. octocarinatus* and *E. crassus* pheromones for which only the amino acid sequences are known on the basis of their respective DNA-coding sequences. The determination of three-dimensional conformations of these pheromones has been made impractical by the very low concentrations in which they are secreted: 0.5 µg of pure protein per liter of cell-free filtrate are usually obtained in *E. octocarinatus* and 15–20 µg in *E. crassus*.[36,37]

Nine distinct pheromone amino acid sequences have been determined in *E. octocarinatus* (Fig. 1.3). They are twice as long as the *E. raikovi* and *E. nobilii* pheromone sequences, extending from 85 to 109 amino acids with 10 cysteines (8 in the pheromone Phr4).[38,39] The positions of only 4 of the 10 cysteines have counterparts in *E. raikovi* and *E. nobilii* pheromones, implying that the *E. octocarinatus* pheromones have only two disulfide bonds and few structural motifs in common with those of *E. raikovi* and *E. nobilii*. They also appear to be unique among *Euplotes* pheromones in functioning as chemoattractants between cells of different mating types.[40]

In *E. crassus*, pheromones have been thought to be represented by insoluble membrane-bound proteins[37,41] and as such are difficult to extract and characterize from cell membrane preparations. Evidence that *E. crassus* pheromones are, instead, constitutively secreted into the extracellular environment as in other *Euplotes* species was obtained from interspecific mating-induction assays,[37] suggested by the notion that cross-mating reactions are relatively frequent between *Euplotes* species in correlation with their high-multiple (virtually open) mating systems.[9,42] The genetic control of these *E. crassus* pheromones appears not to conform with the general *Euplotes* pattern provided by multiple series of alleles at a single *mat* locus. Results from molecular approaches have been found to be more consistently explained by assuming that this control involves a phenomenon of *mat* gene duplication responsible for the production of two distinct *E. crassus* pheromone subfamilies. One includes the cell type-specific pheromones, and the other

```
                pre                                  pro
Phr1     MKAIFIILAILMVTQA 16   FKMTSKVNTKLQSQIQSKFQSKNKQASTFQTSSKLK 36
Phr1*    MKAIFIILAILMVTQA 16   FKMTSKVNTKLQSQIQSKFQSKNKLASTFQTSSQLK 36
Phr2     MKAIFIILAILMVTQA 16   FKMTSKVNTKLQSQIQSKFQSKNKLASTFQTSSQLK 36
Phr2*    MKAIFIILAILMVTQA 16   FKMTSKVNTKLQSQIQSKFQSKNKLASTFQTSSQLK 36
Phr3     MKAIFIILAILMVTQA 16   FKMTSKVNTKLQSQIQSKFQSKNKLASTFQTSSQLK 36
Phr3*    MKAIFIILAILMVTQA 16   FKMTSKVNTKLQSQIQSKFQSKNKLASTFQTSSQLK 36
Phr5-1   MKAIFIILAILMVTQA 16   FKMTSKVNTKLQSQIQSKFQSKNKLASTFMTNLKTK 36
Phr5-2   MKAIFIILAILMVTQA 16   FKMTSKVNTKLQSQIQSKFQSKNKLASTFMTNLKTK 36
Phr4     MKAIFIILAILMVTQA 16   FKMTSKV--K--SMNMSRNMSKN--TSTLGT----K 26

                                  secreted
Phr1     --GECDTIIPD---FTGCNAND-DCPLSFT-CSATGNDKELCD-------AIGQNVVDMIF
Phr1*    --GECDTIIPD---FTGCNAND-ACPLSFT-CSATGNDEQLCN-------AAGQNVIDMIF
Phr2     --DSCLNDPEQRFYITGCSNNP-VCGDAFD-CSATGDDEEKCD-------AVGHNVIDLFY
Phr2*    --DSCLNDPEQRFYITGCSNNP-VCGDAFD-CSATGDDEEKCD-------AVGQNVIDLFY
Phr3     --YYCWEEPYTS-SITGCSTSL-ACYEASD-CSVTGNDQDKCN-------NVGQNMIDKFF
Phr3*    --YYCWEEPYTS-SITGCSTSL-ACYEASD-CSVTGDDTDKCN-------DVGYNMYYKFN
Phr5-1   DAPDCYSQTY----LTGCNTNPDKCWYNSNGCGSTNGSTDMLYYMTRKS-CVGDNIAQVIF
Phr5-2   DAPDCYSQTY----LTGCNTNPDKCWYNSNGCGSTDGSLGECYTNDPENPGVGDNIAQVIF
Phr4     YTYGC---P-Q----TNTPTQQ-DCYDAMY-YTFMA----MCD--------LYPDPEHPMF

Phr1     AHWS-TCWNTPLNCESFAYQTYAIYNAPELCGCD-H---VDEETWLEILDSVCPDID-  99
Phr1*    AHWS-TCWNTYGNCIEFARQTYAIYNAPELCGCD-Y---VDEETWINTLESVCPYV--  98
Phr2     YFWG-TCVNDYASCIMFAATTYNMYNGPENCGCT-Y---VDYEDWLDYF--DCPSFSG 101
Phr2*    YFWG-TCVNDYASCIMFAATTYNMYSGPENCGCINQ---VSYADWLDYF--DCPSFSG 102
Phr3     ELWG-VCINDYETCLQYVDRAWIHYSDSEFCGCTNP---EQESAFRDAMD--CLQF--  99
Phr3*    SLWG-NC-NDYETCLQYVDRAWIHYNESGFCGCTNQ---ALESQFRELFD--CWQFS-  99
Phr5-1   DRWMLGCYEDVSNCVVDAGAMYAIFSSQYLCNCG-----YEFGNVNDFTYGFCGVYP- 108
Phr5-2   DRWMLGCYEDVSNCVVDAGAMYAIFSSQYLCNCG-----YEFGNVNDFTYGFCGVYP- 109
Phr4     PSYD--------SCQEESDSADEFYTN--QCGCGGYGMAAAHDQVCLLALGVCIPE--  85
```

FIGURE 1.3 *Euplotes octocarinatus* pheromone family. Alignment of nine distinct sequences of pheromone precursors, as deduced from the determination of their DNA-coding sequences. Indications as in Fig. 1.1.

includes a new pheromone species that appears to be synthesized in common among cells of compatible mating types.[37,41] The functions of this "shared" pheromone, of which only a single 56 amino acid sequence with eight cysteines (designated E*c*-α) has been determined, are still obscure. Preliminary evidence suggests that it may behave like an adaptor or scaffold protein that selectively interacts with the cell type-specific pheromones to mediate and/or reinforce their receptor-binding reactions.[41] This possibility is supported by an unusually strong propensity of the E*c*-α pheromone to oligomerize when it is purified by chromatographic separation and is reinforced by the comparison of its sequence with the three 45 amino acid sequences with 10 cysteines (designated E*c*-1, E*c*-2, and E*c*-3) that have been determined for the subfamily of the cell type-specific pheromones (Fig. 1.4). This comparison makes it evident that a major distinctive structural trait of the E*c*-α pheromone is the evolution of an unusually extended hydrophilic domain lying centrally in the molecule. This domain lacks Cys residues, abounds in Gly residues, and likely takes a random-coil conformation, which is presumptive for a specific capability of the E*c*-α pheromone to interact with the other proteins.

	pre		pro	
Ec-1	MKTYFLIALAMMLISAAFA	19	EKEVSPVVKELLASDADLLT	20
Ec-2	MKTYFLIALAMMLISAAFA	19	EKEVSPVVKELLASDADLLT	20
Ec-3	MKTYFLIALAMMLISAAFA	19	EKEVSPVVKELLASDADLLT	20
Ec-α	MNAKALLIMTLLLFTCTMA	19	FRAKSRSKLMTSSQLG----	16

secreted

Ec-1	--GCFGCAPTICQFCEAIVNP-NPDVY---CGDSQQYCHCCSECVG-----HMDCP	45
Ec-2	--GCFDCATNICQFCEAIVNP-NPDMW---CKEAQEYCHCCSECVG-----HMDCP	45
Ec-3	--LCPGCAPNICQLCTYVVNP-NPDVY---CGDSQEYCHCCSGCVG-----HMDCP	45
Ec-α	DDHCPTDVLMTCGYLQGRYNQGNYEEVGGLCNMSAEFCHCCSACDEPEVSPYSNCE	56

FIGURE 1.4 *Euplotes crassus* pheromones. Multiple alignments of four distinct sequences of pheromone precursors, as deduced from their DNA-coding sequences. Three sequences (Ec-1, Ec-2, and Ec-4) are cell type specific and one (Ec-α) is shared identically among different cell types. Indications as in Fig. 1.1.

PHEROMONE ACTIVITY

As outlined earlier, it is essentially due to the application of mating-induction assays that ciliate pheromones have been identified. This application has thus decisively contributed to supporting the generalization that ciliate pheromones function exclusively as "sexual factors" committed to stimulating cell mating by binding in paracrine (or heterologous) fashion only to cells other than those from which they are synthesized and secreted.[12] However, observations on the physiology of pheromone secretion in *E. raikovi* turned out to counter this view, because cells were shown to secrete their pheromones throughout their life cycle independently of their inability to mate during the immaturity stage to vary their rates of pheromone secretion in relation to the environmental concentrations of their pheromone and to refrain from forming homotypic mating pairs in the presence of environmental excess of their pheromone.[43] A more coherent view with these observations thus appeared to be one predicting that ciliate pheromones, in addition to acting as nonself-mating signals, also (and most likely, primarily) act as self-signals committed to promoting the vegetative proliferation (mitotic growth) of their same source cells to which they bind in autocrine (or autologous) fashion.[43,44]

A decisive support for an autocrine, cell growth-promoting activity of ciliate pheromones was provided by the finding that *E. raikovi* cells bind their pheromones to membrane-bound isoforms that arise by a splicing mechanism of intron-like sequences from the same genes encoding the pheromones in the transcriptionally active cell macronucleus.[45,46] These isoforms (functionally regarded as pheromone receptors) incorporate the full sequence of the cytoplasmic pheromone precursor and, using the signal (pre) peptide (normally expected to be proteolytically removed before the pheromone secretion) as transmembrane-anchoring domain, take a spatial orientation typical of membrane proteins of type-II, which have the C-terminal end directed to the cell outside and the N-terminal end directed to the cell inside. Given this structural equivalence between pheromones and extracellular binding domains of the twin receptor molecules, the way pheromones interact with their receptors on the cell

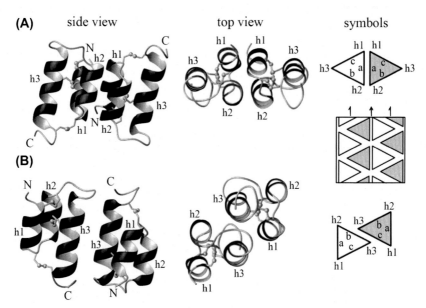

FIGURE 1.5 Intermolecular helix–helix interactions in the crystal structure of the *Euplotes raikovi* pheromone Er-1. (A) Structure of the symmetrical dimer 1 in which two molecules are related by a twofold axis (→). Each monomer involves helices 1 and 2, delimiting face *a*, in the formation of a four-helix bundle. (B) Structure of the asymmetrical dimer 2 in which two molecules are related by a twofold screw axis (⌒). Each monomer stacks helix 3, and its adjacent faces *b* and *c*, in an antiparallel fashion to form a linear structure without symmetrical contacts. The Er-1 molecule packing into the crystal lattice is shown in the boxed diagrammatic presentation. Shadowed molecules mimic ligand-binding (pheromone receptor) molecules oriented with their C-terminus toward the cell outside, while light molecules mimic soluble pheromone molecules oriented with their C-terminus toward the cell inside. *After Weiss MS, Anderson DH, Raffioni S, Bradshaw RA, Ortenzi C, Luporini P, et al. A cooperative model for ligand recognition and cell adhesion: evidence from the molecular packing in the 1.6 Å crystal structure of the pheromone Er-1 from the ciliate protozoan* Euplotes raikovi. Proc Natl Acad Sci USA *1995;92:10172–6.*

surface has been thought to be fully mimicked by the protein–protein interactions that determine the molecular packing of the *E. raikovi* pheromone Er-1 into crystals.[22] In the bidimensional plane of the crystal, the Er-1 molecules (that may be figured as pyramids with a triangular base) associate with one another by means of all three of their faces (*a*, *b*, and *c* delimited by helices 1 and 2, 2 and 3, and 1 and 3, respectively) through the cooperative utilization of initially weak interactions that arise from the formation of two distinct types of dimer. One of these involves face *a* of each monomer and is symmetrical with the two monomers related by a twofold axis; the other involves faces *b* and *c* and is asymmetrical with the two monomers related by a twofold screw axis (Fig. 1.5). This association is such that half of the molecules direct their carboxy-terminus to one side of the plane and may thus reflect the spatial orientation of the pheromone receptors on the cell surface. The second half of the molecules, instead, direct their amino-terminus to the opposite side of the plane and may thus be regarded as free pheromone molecules that bind to their receptors. In line with a cooperative model of protein–protein interactions, the homotypic pheromone/pheromone receptor complexes formed by cells, which grow suspended with their own (self) pheromone, have been observed to undergo clustering and internalization via endocytotic vesicles, whereas the heterotypic complexes formed by cells that have been suspended with a nonself-pheromone for being induced to mate are not internalized and are believed to be in some way involved in bridging cells into mating pairs.[47]

PHEROMONE STRUCTURE–FUNCTION RELATIONSHIPS WITH OTHER SIGNALING PROTEINS

Evolutionary relationships of proteins are commonly inferred using traditional automatic sequence/structure comparison methods such as PSI-BLAST and Dali. The reliability of these methods is, however, generally regarded as sound only for globular proteins that are larger than 100 residues, which is not the case of *Euplotes* pheromones characterized by quite short polypeptide chains. To assess small globular proteins for their evolutionary relationships, an alternative method has been provided by a comparative analysis of the variety of structural folds that functionally diverse proteins (encompassing growth factors, toxins, enzyme inhibitors, and others) have adopted for their small (an average of 57 ± 29 residues) disulfide-rich (an average of 3 ± 1) domains, which are either individual or included within larger polypeptide chains and characterized by global folds that are stabilized primarily by disulfide bonds and, in second place, by secondary structure elements and hydrophobic interactions.[48] In this analysis, and with the exception of pheromone Er-23 that presents a unique five-helix globular array, *Euplotes* pheromones have been classified together with disulfide-rich domains of other four-protein families represented by anaphylatoxins (C5a), oncogene-encoded proteins (p8^{MTCPI}), sea anemone toxins K, and cysteine-rich secretory proteins within a fold group identified by a disulfide-bonded three-helix bundle with right-handed connections between the α-helices. While classified within the same fold group, these protein families, however, show quite disparate functions and mechanisms of action with respect to *Euplotes* pheromones, and lacking a functional analogy their structural relationships with *Euplotes* pheromones thus appear to be better interpreted as a result of phenomena of convergent evolution rather than of homology.

More significantly, structure–function relationships have been observed between the *E. raikovi* pheromone family and another family of long-distance waterborne protein pheromones that various species of the common marine mollusk *Aplysia* freely release from their yolk gland into the environment and use in the phenomena of intra- and interspecific attraction of sexually mature individuals toward their egg cordons.[49] In their active form, these 56–58 amino acid proteins, designated as attractins in relation to their activity, have a compact, folded structure (annotated as "α-hairpin" in the above classification of protein fold groups) that is stabilized by three tightly conserved disulfide bonds and dominated by two antiparallel helices, the second of which is essentially formed by the heptapeptide Ile-Glu-Glu-Cys-Lys-Thr-Ser.[50] This building block is common to all attractins of the different species of *Aplysia* (which well accounts for attractin interspecific attractiveness) and finds a close counterpart in the third helix of *E. raikovi* pheromones in terms of both the conformation of its helical backbone and the orientation of its side chains. In addition, it is likely directly involved in receptor-binding interactions, as is shown to be the case for the third helix of *E. raikovi* pheromones, since the attractin activity is abolished by mutating the charged residues that are exposed on its surface.[51]

A last intriguing point on the relationships of *Euplotes* pheromones with other signaling proteins has been quite fortuitously revealed by experiments in which some prototypic animal growth factors and cytokines were used to competitively inhibit the autocrine cell-binding interactions of the *E. raikovi* pheromone Er-1.[52] Human interleukin-2 (hIL-2) and, to a lesser extent, epidermal growth factor were surprisingly observed to exert strong inhibitory activity. At a 50-fold molar excess, hIL-2 appeared able to inhibit almost completely the pheromone binding to its target cell surface receptors. Considering the disparity in molecular dimensions that separates hIL-2 and Er-1 and precludes reliable comparisons between the two protein families, a possible explanation for this hIL-2 competitive activity has tentatively been identified with some degree of the sequence similarity that hIL-2 and Er-1 bear at the level of two in their sequence segments, one extended for five amino acids (Leu_{56}-Gln-Cys-Leu-Glu_{60} in hIL-2 and Iso_8-Gln-Cys-Val-Glu_{12} in Er-1) and the other for seven (Thr_{102}-Phe-Met-Cys-Glu-Tyr-Ala_{108} in hIL-2 and Arg_{25}-Thr-Gly-Cys-Tyr-Met-Tyr_{31} in Er-1). The Cys residue included in each of the two segments is involved in the formation of a disulfide bond known to be essential for the hIL-2 biological activity,[53] and the shorter segment represents a substantially conserved motif within both the hIL-2 and Er-1 protein families in addition to being well exposed on the molecular surface.

Cross-reactions between the IL-2 and *E. raikovi* pheromone systems have supported a possible functional significance of these common sequence motifs. It has initially been shown[54] that Er-1 binds specifically to the IL-2 receptor on the surface of CTLL-2 cells that are a mouse T lymphocyte line totally dependent on IL-2 for survival and proliferation. The binding involves the α and β subunits of the trimeric IL-2 receptor in particular and occurs with an appreciable higher affinity to the α subunit that has a leading role in the ligand-binding activity of the IL-2 receptor being the first subunit that interacts with extracellular IL-2. More recently, it has been observed that the pheromone Er-1 also exerts strong effects on some cellular functions that IL-2 regulates in the human lymphoid T cells of the Jurkat line.[55] These cells, suspended in a low serum–containing medium enriched with the addition of Er-1 nanomolar concentrations, were initially reported to significantly increase their proliferation and

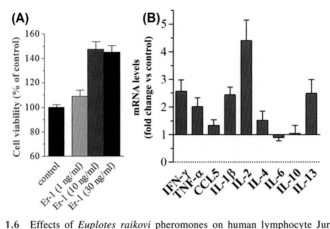

FIGURE 1.6 Effects of *Euplotes raikovi* pheromones on human lymphocyte Jurkat cells. (A) Viability of Jurkat cells cultured for 48h in the absence (control) or in the presence of increasing concentrations of pheromone Er-1. Histograms represent the mean±SEM of data from at least four independent experiments. Data are expressed by setting the control samples as 100%. (B) Measurements by quantitative PCR of the mRNA levels of different cytokines in Jurkat cells grown in the presence of 10ng/ml Er-1 for 48h in restrictive culture conditions. Each histogram represents the mean±SEM of data from at least three independent experiments. Quantitative changes were determined putting equal to 1 the mRNA levels in cells grown in the absence of Er-1 (control). *After Cervia D, Catalani E, Belardinelli MC, Perrotta C, Picchietti S, Alimenti C, et al. The protein pheromone Er-1 of the ciliate* Euplotes raikovi *stimulates human T-cell activity: involvement of interleukin-2 system.* Exp Cell Res *2013;319:56–67.*

secretion rates, beside that of IL-2, of a wide spectrum of cytokines including IFN-γ, TNF-α, IL-1β, and IL-13 (Fig. 1.6). They were later observed to undergo a significant decrease in the expression of the α subunit of the IL-2 receptor due to the reversible and time-dependent endocytosis of this receptor and activate the transduction pathway that is regulated by the protein kinases Erk1 and Erk2.

CONCLUSIONS

Significant numbers of molecular structures of ciliate pheromones have been determined from distinct species of *Euplotes*. This determination has made manifest that these waterborne signaling molecules form species-specific families of small, disulfide-rich globular proteins in full accord with their genetic determination at a single multiallelic locus. Within each family the global pheromone structure has been shown to acquire virtually unlimited polymorphisms from variations in shape and geometry that interest individual structural elements. The varying degrees of intra- and interspecific relationships of structural homology that link *Euplotes* pheromones to one another closely recall the relationships of homology which exist within and between families of signal proteins of higher life forms. In these families, each component can compete and cross-react with its family members to elicit multiple and context-dependent cell responses. Similarly, *Euplotes* pheromones have been shown to be fully able to bind cells in mutual competition[56] and to carry out a spectrum of activities that is not exclusively limited to eliciting cell mating as hypothesized for the eccentric case of the structurally unrelated glycoprotein and tryptophan-derivative pheromones of *B. japonicum*.[12] In addition to including a paracrine-like (nonself) activity, this spectrum also includes an autocrine (self) activity, which is probably primary and directed to promoting the vegetative proliferation of the same cells from which pheromones are constitutively synthesized and secreted throughout the life cycle.[44] The similarities of structure that some *Euplotes* pheromones have revealed with *Aplysia* attractins and the mammalian cytokine IL-2 most likely represent fortuitous instances of convergent molecular evolution. Nevertheless, they provide evidence that functionally important sequence motifs may be evolutionarily conserved from ancient to more modern cell signaling proteins and stimulate investigations on their potential into biotechnological and finalized perspectives.

REFERENCES

1. Grosberg RK, Strathmann RR. The evolution of multicellularity: a minor major transition? *Ann Rev Ecol Evol Syst* 2007;**38**:621–54.
2. Waters CM, Bassler BL. Quorum sensing: cell-to-cell communication in bacteria. *Ann Rev Cell Dev Biol* 2005;**21**:319–46.
3. Gibbs KA, Urbanowski ML, Greenberg EP. Genetic determinants of self identity and social recognition in bacteria. *Science* 2008;**321**:256–9.
4. Benabentos R, Hirose S, Sucgang R, Curk T, Katoh M, Ostrowski EA, et al. Polymorphic members of the *lag* gene family mediate kin discrimination in *Dictyostelium*. *Curr Biol* 2009;**19**:567–72.
5. Hirose S, Benabentos R, Ho HI, Kuspa A, Shaulsky G. Self-recognition in social amoebae is mediated by allelic pairs of *Tiger* genes. *Science* 2011;**333**:467–70.
6. Cooper MD, Alder MN. The evolution of adaptive immune systems. *Cell* 2006;**124**:815–22.
7. Rosengarten RD, Nicotra ML. Model systems of invertebrate allorecognition. *Curr Biol* 2011;**21**:R82–92.
8. Adl SM, Simpson AGB, Lane CE, Lukes J, Bass D, Bowser SS, et al. The revised classification of eukaryotes. *J Eukaryot Microbiol* 2012;**59**:429–93.
9. Valbonesi A, Ortenzi C, Luporini P. The species problem in a ciliate with a high-multiple mating type system, *Euplotes crassus*. *J Protozool* 1992;**39**:45–54.
10. Phadke SS, Zufall RA. Rapid diversification of mating systems in ciliates. *Biol J Linn Soc* 2009;**98**:187–97.
11. Kimball RF. The nature and inheritance of mating types in *Euplotes patella*. *Genetics* 1942;**27**:269–85.
12. Miyake A. Fertilization and sexuality in ciliates. In: Hausmann K, Bradbury PC, editors. *Ciliates, cells as organisms*. Stuttgart: Gustav Fisher; 1996. p. 243–90.
13. Luporini P, Alimenti C, Vallesi A. Ciliate pheromone structures and activity: a review. *Ital J Zool* 2015;**82**:3–15.
14. Sugiura M, Harumoto T. Identification, characterization, and complete amino acid sequence of the conjugation-inducing glycoprotein (blepharmone) in the ciliate *Blepharisma japonicum*. *Proc Natl Acad Sci USA* 2001;**98**:14446–51.

15. Kubota T, Tokoroyama T, Tsukuda J, Koyama H, Miyake A. Isolation and structure determination of blepharismin, a conjugation initiating gamone in the ciliate *Blepharisma*. *Science* 1973;**179**:400–2.

16. Sugiura M, Shiotani H, Suzaki T, Harumoto T. Behavioural changes induced by the conjugation-inducing pheromones, gamones 1 and 2, in the ciliate *Blepharisma japonicum*. *Eur J Protistol* 2010;**46**:143–9.

17. Raffioni S, Miceli C, Vallesi A, Chowdhury SK, Chait BT, Luporini P, et al. Primary structures of *Euplotes raikovi* pheromones from cells with variable mating interactions. *Proc Natl Acad Sci USA* 1992;**89**:2071–5.

18. Brown LR, Mronga S, Bradshaw RA, Ortenzi C, Luporini P, Wüthrich K. Nuclear magnetic resonance solution structure of the pheromone Er-10 from the ciliated protozoan *Euplotes raikovi*. *J Mol Biol* 1993;**231**:800–16.

19. Mronga S, Luginbühl P, Brown LR, Ortenzi C, Luporini P, Bradshaw RA, et al. The NMR solution structure of the pheromone Er-1 from the ciliated protozoan *Euplotes raikovi*. *Prot Sci* 1994;**3**:1527–36.

20. Ottiger M, Szyperski T, Luginbühl P, Ortenzi C, Luporini P, Bradshaw RA, et al. The NMR solution structure of the pheromone Er-2 from the ciliated protozoan *Euplotes raikovi*. *Prot Sci* 1994;**3**:1515–26.

21. Luginbühl P, Ottiger M, Mronga S, Wüthrich K. Structure comparison of the NMR structures of the pheromones Er-1, Er-10, and Er-2 from *Euplotes raikovi*. *Prot Sci* 1994;**3**:1537–46.

22. Weiss MS, Anderson DH, Raffioni S, Bradshaw RA, Ortenzi C, Luporini P, et al. A cooperative model for ligand recognition and cell adhesion: evidence from the molecular packing in the 1.6 Å crystal structure of the pheromone Er-1 from the ciliate protozoan *Euplotes raikovi*. *Proc Natl Acad Sci USA* 1995;**92**:10172–6.

23. Liu A, Luginbühl P, Zerbe O, Ortenzi C, Luporini P, Wüthrich K. NMR structure of the pheromone Er-22 from *Euplotes raikovi*. *J Biomol NMR* 2001;**19**:75–8.

24. Zahn R, Damberger F, Ortenzi C, Luporini P, Wüthrich K. NMR structure of the *Euplotes raikovi* pheromone Er-23 and identification of its five disulfide bonds. *J Mol Biol* 2001;**313**:923–31.

25. Geralt M, Alimenti C, Vallesi A, Luporini P, Wüthrich K. Thermodynamic stability of psychrophilic and mesophilic pheromones of the protozoan ciliate *Euplotes*. *Biology* 2013;**2**:142–50.

26. Jiang J, Zhang Q, Warren A, Al-Rasheid KAS, Song W. Morphology and SSU rRNA gene based phylogeny of two marine *Euplotes* species, *E. orientalis* spec. nov. and *E. raikovi* Agamaliev, 1966 (Ciliophora, Euplotida). *Eur J Protistol* 2010;**46**:121–32.

27. Di Giuseppe G, Erra F, Frontini FP, Dini F, Vallesi A, Luporini P. Improved description of the bipolar ciliate, *Euplotes petzi*, and definition of its basal position in the *Euplotes* phylogenetic tree. *Eur J Protistol* 2014;**50**:402–11.

28. Vallesi A, Alimenti C, Pedrini B, Di Giuseppe G, Dini F, Wüthrich K, et al. Coding genes and molecular structures of the diffusible signalling proteins (pheromones) of the polar ciliate, *Euplotes nobilii*. *Mar Genomics* 2012;**8**:9–13.

29. Pedrini B, Placzek WJ, Koculi E, Alimenti C, La Terza A, Luporini P, et al. Cold-adaptation in sea-water-borne signal proteins: sequence and NMR structure of the pheromone En-6 from the Antarctic ciliate *Euplotes nobilii*. *J Mol Biol* 2007;**372**:277–86.

30. Placzek WJ, Etezady-Esfarjani T, Herrmann T, Pedrini B, Peti W, Alimenti C, et al. Cold-adapted signal proteins: NMR structures from the Antarctic ciliate *Euplotes nobilii*. *IUBMB Life* 2007;**59**:578–85.

31. Di Giuseppe G, Erra F, Dini F, Alimenti C, Vallesi A, Pedrini B, et al. Antarctic and Arctic populations of the ciliate *Euplotes nobilii* show common pheromone-mediated cell-cell signalling and cross-mating. *Proc Natl Acad Sci USA* 2011;**108**:3181–6.

32. Valbonesi A, Luporini P. Description of two new species of *Euplotes* and *Euplotes rariseta* from Antarctica. *Polar Biol* 1990;**11**:47–53.
33. Di Giuseppe G, Barbieri M, Vallesi A, Luporini P, Dini F. Phylogeographical pattern of *Euplotes nobilii*, a protist ciliate with a bipolar biogeographical distribution. *Mol Ecol* 2013;**22**:4029–37.
34. Alimenti C, Vallesi A, Pedrini B, Wüthrich K, Luporini P. Molecular cold-adaptation: comparative analysis of two homologous families of psychrophilic and mesophilic signal proteins of the protozoan ciliate, *Euplotes*. *IUBMB Life* 2009;**61**:838–45.
35. Cazzolli G, Skrbic T, Guella G, Faccioli P. Unfolding thermodynamics of cysteine-rich proteins and molecular thermal-adaptation of marine ciliates. *Biomolecules* 2013;**3**:967–85.
36. Schulze Dieckhoff H, Freiburg M, Heckmann K. The isolation of gamones 3 and 4 of *Euplotes octocarinatus*. *Eur J Biochem* 1987;**168**:89–94.
37. Alimenti C, Vallesi A, Federici S, Di Giuseppe G, Dini F, Carratore V, et al. Isolation and structural characterization of two water-borne pheromones from *Euplotes crassus*, a ciliate commonly known to carry membrane-bound pheromones. *J Eukaryot Microbiol* 2011;**58**:234–41.
38. Brünen-Nieveler C, Weiligmann JC, Hansen B, Kuhlmann HW, Möllenbeck M, Heckmann K. The pheromones and pheromone genes of new stocks of the *Euplotes octocarinatus* species complex. *Eur J Protistol* 1998;**34**:124–32.
39. Möllenbeck M, Heckmann K. Characterization of two genes encoding a fifth so far unknown pheromone of *Euplotes octocarinatus*. *Eur J Protistol* 1999;**35**:225–30.
40. Kuhlmann HW, Brünen-Nieveler C, Heckmann K. Pheromones of the ciliate *Euplotes octocarinatus* not only induce conjugation but also function as chemoattractants. *J Exp Zool* 1997;**277**:38–48.
41. Vallesi A, Alimenti C, Federici S, Di Giuseppe G, Dini F, Guella G, et al. Evidence for gene duplication and allelic codominance (not hierarchical dominance) at the mating type locus of the ciliate, *Euplotes crassus*. *J Eukaryot Microbiol* 2014;**61**:620–9.
42. Nobili R, Luporini P, Dini F. Breeding system, species relationships and evolutionary trends in some marine species of Euplotidae (Ciliata Hypotrichida). In: Battaglia B, Beardmore J, editors. *Marine organisms: genetics, ecology and evolution*. New York: Plenum Press; 1978. p. 591–616.
43. Luporini P, Miceli C. Mating pheromones. In: Gall JG, editor. *The molecular biology of ciliated protozoa*. New York: Academic Press; 1986. p. 263–99.
44. Vallesi A, Giuli G, Bradshaw RA, Luporini P. Autocrine mitogenic activity of pheromones produced by the protozoan ciliate *Euplotes raikovi*. *Nature* 1995;**376**:522–4.
45. Miceli C, La Terza A, Bradshaw RA, Luporini P. Identification and structural characterization of a cDNA clone encoding a membrane-bound form of the polypeptide pheromone Er-1 in the ciliate protozoan *Euplotes raikovi*. *Proc Natl Acad Sci USA* 1992;**89**:1988–92.
46. Ortenzi C, Alimenti C, Vallesi A, Di Pretoro B, La Terza A, Luporini P. The autocrine mitogenic loop of the ciliate *Euplotes raikovi*: the pheromone membrane-bound forms are the cell binding sites and potential signaling receptors of soluble pheromones. *Mol Biol Cell* 2000;**11**:1445–55.
47. Luporini P, Alimenti C, Ortenzi C, Vallesi A. Ciliate mating types and their specific protein pheromones. *Acta Protozool* 2005;**44**:89–101.
48. Cheek S, Krishna SS, Grishin NV. Structural classification of small, disulfide-rich protein domains. *J Mol Biol* 2006;**359**:215–37.
49. Painter SD, Chong MG, Wong MA, Gray A, Cormier JG, Nagle GT. Relative contributions of the egg layer and egg cordon to pheromonal attraction and the induction of mating and egg-laying behavior in *Aplysia*. *Biol Bull* 1991;**181**:81–94.
50. Schein CH, Nagle GT, Page JS, Sweedler JV, Xu Y, Painter SD, et al. *Aplysia* attractin: biophysical characterization and modeling of a water-borne pheromone. *Biophys J* 2001;**81**:463–72.

51. Painter SD, Cummuns SF, Nichols AE, Akalal DBG, Schein CH, Braun W, et al. Structural and functional analysis of *Aplysia* attractins, a family of water-borne protein pheromones with interspecific attractiveness. *Proc Natl Acad Sci USA* 2004;**101**:6929–33.

52. Ortenzi C, Miceli C, Bradshaw RA, Luporini P. Identification and initial characterization of an autocrine pheromone receptor in the protozoan ciliate *Euplotes raikovi*. *J Cell Biol* 1990;**111**:607–14.

53. Wang X, Rickert M, Garcia KC. Structure of the quaternary complex of interleukin-2 with its alpha, beta, and gamma receptors. *Science* 2005;**310**:1159–63.

54. Vallesi A, Giuli G, Ghiara P, Scapigliati G, Luporini P. Structure-function relationships of pheromones of the ciliate *Euplotes raikovi* with mammalian growth factors: cross-reactivity between Er-1 and IL-2 systems. *Exp Cell Res* 1998;**241**:253–9.

55. Cervia D, Catalani E, Belardinelli MC, Perrotta C, Picchietti S, Alimenti C, et al. The protein pheromone Er-1 of the ciliate *Euplotes raikovi* stimulates human T-cell activity: involvement of interleukin-2 system. *Exp Cell Res* 2013;**319**:56–67.

56. Ortenzi C, Luporini P. Competition among homologous polypeptide pheromones of the ciliated *Euplotes raikovi* for binding to each other's cell receptor. *J Eukaryot Microbiol* 1995;**42**:242–8.

Chapter 2

Cell Death Pathways in an Unconventional Invertebrate Model

Enzo Ottaviani, Davide Malagoli
University of Modena and Reggio Emilia, Modena, Italy

INTRODUCTION

Apoptosis, autophagy-mediated cell death, and necrosis are the three best characterized typologies of cell death.[1] Twenty years ago, Majno and Joris[2] suggested that necrosis is not a form of cell death, but rather it is a postmortal state common to all the typologies of cell death. The principle division of cell death processes proposed by Majno and Joris was between active processes, like apoptosis, and passive cell death processes, like oncosis. In this view, apoptosis and oncosis must be considered two premortal processes. While apoptosis requires energy and leads to cell shrinkage and nuclear fragmentation, oncosis is an ATP-independent process characterized by marked cell swelling, progressive cytoplasmic vacuolization, increased plasma membrane permeability, and DNA breakdown in a nonspecific manner. This classification did not include autophagy as a mechanism leading a cell to death.[2] This distinction among cell death modalities has been overcome by the observation of several other different typologies of cell death, like programmed necrosis,[3] mitotic catastrophe, anoikis, entosis,[1] and other nonapoptotic cell death modalities.[4] An additional biological process involved in cell death is autophagy. Autophagy is usually defined as a prosurvival mechanism, thus its role as an active effector of cell death is still controversial.[5–7] The themes that stemmed from cell death processes are numerous and have been reviewed several times.[1,8,9] Pioneering studies on oxidative stress and cell death put the mitochondrion under the spotlight of studies on programmed cell death,[10,11] and recent advances also confirmed that mitochondrion is a fundamental player of this finely regulated process.[9]

In this chapter, we will examine the effect of three drugs on the induction of cell death-related pathways in the IPLB-LdFB insect cell line. The

Lessons in Immunity: From Single-Cell Organisms to Mammals
http://dx.doi.org/10.1016/B978-0-12-803252-7.00002-3

17

molecules whose effects were investigated are the reducing sugar 2-deoxy-D-ribose (dRib), the nitric oxide (NO) donor sodium nitroprusside (SNP), and the ATP synthase inhibitor oligomycin A. All these molecules target the IPLB-LdFB cells at the mitochondrial level, sorting different effects. While the largest part of the articles dealing with cell death in invertebrates has the fruit fly *Drosophila melanogaster* or the nematode *Caenorhabditis elegans* as models, here we will focus on a cell line that has been derived from the larvae of the pest moth *Lymantria dispar*. Despite the limited information available about their genomes and transcriptomes, the unconventional animal models are fundamental to filling the numerous gaps that the well-established models leave in the knowledge of complex mechanisms such as immune response, stress, and cell death.[12] The IPLB-LdFB cell line is derived from the larval fat body of the gypsy moth *L. dispar*.[13] The larval fat body of insects can be considered a function analogous of the vertebrate liver, and it intervenes in numerous activities, including regulation of nutrients and immune response.[14,15] In consideration of the deep rearrangements occurring during metamorphosis, the insect fat body is a frequent subject for studies on cell death processes, especially apoptosis and autophagy.[16–18]

SIGNALING PATHWAYS IN APOPTOTIC CELL DEATH OF THE IPLB-LdFB INSECT CELL LINE

Apoptosis is an ancestral type of cell death, and its basis is well preserved during evolution.[19,20] Similarly to the Toll-like receptors in vertebrate immunity, which were discovered after the isolation of the Toll receptor in *D. melanogaster*,[14] the discovery of the apoptotic machinery in mammals stemmed from the isolation of the first caspase in *C. elegans*.[21] Several genes, whose products are involved in apoptosis in vertebrates, have a functionally conserved counterpart in invertebrates. Just as examples, the genes *mcd.1*, *mcd.2*, *eya*, *rox8*, and *ceds* were found in *D. melanogaster* and *C. elegans*.[22–29] The degree of conservation of the apoptotic machinery prompted the studies in other invertebrate models, assuming that the mechanisms conserved in *D. melanogaster* and humans may be similar in other insects.

dRib induces apoptosis in human peripheral blood mononuclear cells and human fibroblasts. The real mechanism of action of dRib is still unknown,[30] but its addition to the culture medium results in an increased oxidative stress for the cells likely due to the depletion of the intracellular levels of reduced glutathione, a key molecule for antioxidant protection. Accordingly, the proapoptotic action of dRib is blocked by antioxidants, such as N-acetyl cysteine (NAC), a precursor of glutathione.[31–33]

Studies on the IPLB-LdFB insect cell line have shown that dRib was able to cause cell death in this model. The proapoptotic action of dRib was evident after 48 h, and it was completely reverted by the concomitant incubation with NAC.[33] The central role of the mitochondrion in the dRib-mediated cell death was suggested by the observation that anti-Bcl-2 antibody prevented dRib-mediated cell death and contemporaneously elicited the depolarization of the mitochondrial membrane. A similar effect on the mitochondrial membrane was observed with the K^+ ionophore valinomycin.[33,34] Unfortunately, the anti-Bcl-2 solution contained sodium azide, and there is no information on the sequence of a potential IPLB-LdFB homologue for Buffy, the *Drosophila* counterpart of Bcl-2.[35] This limited the experiments with the anti-Bcl-2 antibody. However, further observations confirmed the central role of the mitochondrion in the dRib-mediated apoptosis in the IPLB-LdFB cell line. Similarly to the intrinsic apoptotic pathway described in mammals, dRib-mediated cell death is associated with the release of cytochrome c from mitochondria. Moreover, apoptotic activity in IPLB-LdFB cells is an active process that requires ATP, and it occurs in concomitance with the increase of a caspase-3-like activity and the oligonucleosomal DNA fragmentation.[36] The presence of cytochrome c in the cytoplasm of apoptotic IPLB-LdFB cells was shown by western blot, but a mechanistic connection between the release of cytochrome c and the occurrence of apoptosis was not demonstrated. In nematodes and insects other than *L. dispar*, cytochrome c does not appear to be involved in either the apoptotic pathway or the caspase activation.[37] In mollusks the apoptotic pathways are highly conserved;[38] they include a caspase-3-like activity activated by cytochrome c[39] and may represent a general response of circulating hemocytes to xenobiotics.[40] Independently from the role of cytochrome c in mediating dRib proapoptotic effects on IPLB-LdFB cells, it is clear that the mitochondrion plays a fundamental role in regulating the onset of apoptosis in *L. dispar* fat body. This may represent a further contribution in favor of the hypothesis describing the mitochondrion as the determinant of the response of the cells in a suicidal or adaptive way.[9] In mammalian models, cell death might indeed represent a plastic and dynamic cell response to exogenous stimuli. For instance, in many vertebrate cell types, growth factors act as prosurvival players by regulating cell death.[41] Similarly, the response of IPLB-LdFB cells to the reducing sugar dRib may be modified by exogenous factors. In the presence of the mammalian growth factors, platelet-derived growth factor (PDGF)-AB or transforming growth factor (TGF)-β1, the effects of dRib were significantly reduced.[42] The receptors able to bind these heterologous proteins were not identified, but the signaling pathway involved in their actions was assessed by means of specific inhibitors. The prosurvival effects of mammalian growth factors on IPLB-LdFB require the activation of several signaling kinases, such as the phosphatidylinositol 3-kinase (PI 3-kinase), the protein kinase A (PKA), and protein kinase C (PKC). In the presence of the respective inhibitors, wortmannin for PI 3-kinase,[43] H89 for PKA,[44] and calphostin C for PKC,[45] the prosurvival effects of PDGF-AB and TGF-β1 are significantly impaired, and they do not prevent the apoptosis induced by dRib[46] (Fig. 2.1).

Further evidence of the effects of oxidative stress on apoptotic cell death in IPLB-LdFB cells was obtained with the NO donors, SNP, and S-nitroso-N-acetylpenicillamine. SNP is known to release NO spontaneously in aqueous

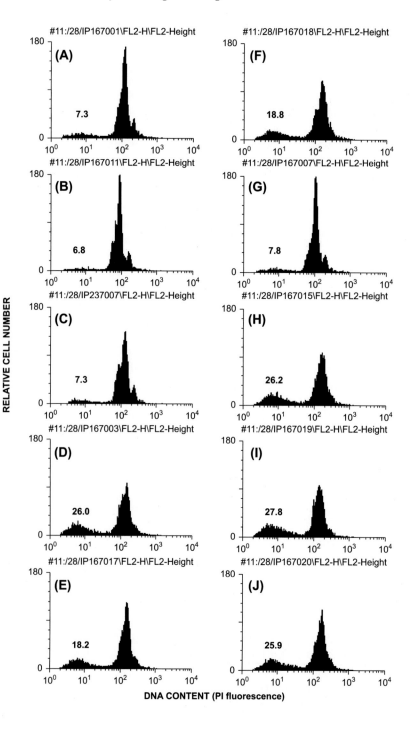

solution, acting as a source of oxidative stress and stimulating the activity of inducible NO synthase (iNOS).[47] Our immunocytochemical observations demonstrated that the NO donor induced the synthesis of iNOS within 18 h of incubation. Cytofluorimetric analysis showed that SNP also provoked apoptosis in the IPLB-LdFB cell line after 48 h of incubation, a time comparable with that reported for the pentose dRib.[33,47] The hypothesis that SNP proapoptotic effects were mediated by the activity of iNOS was excluded because the NOS inhibitors N^ω-nitro-L-arginine methyl ester (L-NAME) and N-(3-(aminomethyl)-benzyl)acetamide (1400W) were both unable to block the SNP-induced apoposis. However, the mechanisms by which NO promotes cell death may be numerous and include direct damage of DNA, the destabilization of mito-chondrial membrane potential, or the activation of specific signaling pathways. We investigated the effects of NO as a chemical stressor by using the scavenger NAC, as it was already done for preventing the effects of dRib.[33,42,47] Unfor-tunately, NAC boosted the effects of SNP, increasing the number of apoptotic cells and accelerating their death.[47] One potential explanation for our observa-tion could be that the NO released by SNP reacted with NAC, forming active and more stable intermediates, such as S-nitrosothiols, resulting in a subsequent increase in the bioavailability of NO.[48,49] We then explored the potential signal-ing pathways activated by SNP in apoptotic IPLB-LdFB.[50] By using the protein kinase inhibitors H89, calphostin C, and wortmannin (which acts upstream of the activation of PKB), we have obtained evidence for the activation of multiple signaling pathways. The PKA inhibitor, H89, significantly reduced the effects of SNP, suggesting a positive role for PKA in NO-mediated apoptosis in IPLB-LdFB. Conversely, calphostin C and wortmannin potentiated the effects of SNP, indicating that PKC and PKB may act by reducing, or at least slowing down, the rate of cell demise after SNP treatment.[50] The proapoptotic role played by PKA in the SNP-mediated apoptosis is different from the protective role played by the same kinase in mediating the effects of the growth factors PDGF-AB and TGF-β1. This observation evidences the complexity of the signaling pathways in the control of cell death and makes it difficult to find a single and specific activity for the majority of the mediators playing a role in the apoptotic process.

FIGURE 2.1 Original output of the cytofluorimetric analysis of the IPLB-LdFB cell line after 48 h of incubation with different molecules. (A) Ex-cell 405 medium *(JRH Biosciences, KS, USA)* (control); (B) 20 ng/ml PDGF-AB; (C) 5 pg/ml TGF-β1; (D) 50 mM dRib; (E) 20 ng/ml PDGF-AB + 50 mM dRib; (F) 5 pg/ml TGF-β1 + 50 mM dRib; (G) 100 nM wortmannin; (H) 100 nM wortman-nin + 50 mM dRib; (I) 100 nM wortmannin + 50 mM dRib + 20 ng/ml PDGF-AB; (J) 100 nM wort-mannin + 50 mM dRib + 5 pg/ml TGF-β1. Cytofluorimetric readings were taken using a FACScan *(Becton–Dickinson, Mountain View, CA, USA)* equipped with a single 488-nm argon laser. A total of 10,000 events was acquired in list mode and analyzed with the "Lysys II" software program. The numbers in each panel indicate the percentage of apoptotic cells. *Modified from Ottaviani E, Barbieri D, Malagoli D, Kletsas D. Involvement of PI 3-kinase, PKA and PKC in PDGF- and TGF-β-mediated prevention of 2-deoxy-D-ribose-induced apoptosis in the insect cell line, IPLB-LdFB.* Cell Biol Int *2001;25:171–7.*

Even if the molecular details of the pathways activated by NO donors in *L. dispar* cells have not been determined, it is worth mentioning that we had indications of the release of cytochrome c from the mitochondria.[50] As it was suggested for the experiments with dRib, the mitochondrion may have represented the main target of a complex response, involving numerous pathways simultaneously.

AUTOPHAGY-MEDIATED CELL DEATH IN IPLB-LdFB

Since its first morphological descriptions in the late 1950s[51] and after the pioneering experiments of the 1960s and the 1970s,[52,53] autophagy garnered progressively increasing attention until the end of the 20th century.[54] Then, after the first molecular information on the autophagic machinery in yeast became available,[55] interest in autophagy accelerated, and a search on available public databases identified autophagy among the most studied cellular processes (see for instance the "Results per year" in PubMed at http://www.ncbi.nlm.nih.gov/pubmed). Three main types of autophagy are described, on the basis of the size and the type of the material involved: macroautophagy, microautophagy, and chaperone-mediated autophagy.[55–59] As many other authors, hereafter, we will refer only to macroautophagy using the term autophagy. Today, the modalities of the process of autophagy are well known, and they have been reviewed several times.[60–65] The crucial subcellular element in which autophagy takes place is the autophagosome, which forms directly from, or in close proximity with, the endoplasmic reticulum.[66,67]

The amount of morphological and molecular evidence concerning autophagy increased so quickly and is so varied that the adoption of specific guidelines for the interpretation of results concerning the experiments on autophagy became necessary.[8] The relationships between autophagy and cell death have been noticed almost immediately,[68] but the true role of autophagy as a process finalized to cell death in vertebrates and invertebrates is still debated.[6] In several occasions, the simultaneous activity of mediators usually involved in either apoptotic or autophagy-mediated cell death has been displayed.[69,70] Tsujimoto and Shimizu[63] proposed that the balance in the expression of the programmed cell death-related molecules Bcl-2 or Bcl-xL, and of the autophagy-related (Atg) mediators Atg5 and Atg6, is the cause of the final outcome of a process that can lead to either autophagy (survival) or autophagic death. In humans, Bcl-2 and Bcl-xL are pro-survival proteins involved in the prevention of cytochrome c exiting from the mitochondria, whereas Atg 6 and Atg 5 are yeast proteins involved in autophagosome formation and elongation, respectively.[63] Gordy and He[71] reported the involvement of Beclin 1 (the mammalian ortholog of the yeast Atg 6) in apoptosis. Both Beclin 1 and Atg 5 are cleaved by caspases and calpain 1 and 2, respectively, inducing apoptosis enhancement. This seems to be due to the cleavage products targeted to mitochondria provoking a direct cytochrome c release.[71] The experiments that tried to disentangle the apoptosis–autophagy relationship encountered several difficulties, and important recommendations have been provided to help scientists distinguish between a natural response of living organisms and artifacts due to the experimental settings.[72]

In the IPLB-LdFB cell line we have observed autophagic cell death after incubation with oligomycin A[73] that we were using to understand the role and the importance of ATP in apoptosis.[74] Oligomycin A, an inhibitor of mitochondrial ATP synthase, lowers ATP levels to about one-third within 30 min in the IPLB-LdFB cells. This important destabilization in the energy balance of the cells elicits different responses, with a minority of cells undergoing apoptosis and a large majority activating an autophagic process.[73] As it was observed for dRib- and SNP-mediated apoptosis, the mitochondrion seems to play a relevant role in this case. We have observed that, after a short treatment with oligomycin A and a successive incubation in oligomycin A-free medium, the IPLB-LdFB cells underwent a massive reorganization of cytoskeletal filaments and a significant mitochondrial injury. This latter phenomenon was associated with the increase of reactive oxygen species (ROS) in the cytoplasm of dying IPLB-LdFB cells, which presented a highly vacuolated cytoplasm and the morphology associated with an intense autophagic process. We therefore hypothesized that the cytoskeletal reorganization and the subsequent autophagic process might represent prosurvival processes finalized to protect the cells from the increased production of ROS by the damaged mitochondria. However, since the mitochondrial damage is too wide to be recovered, the intense autophagic process and the increased ROS concentrations led the IPLB-LdFB cells to death.[75] Further experiments demonstrated the existence of one or more mediators released in the medium by oligomycin A-treated IPLB-LdFB cells.[74] These mediators can induce an intense autophagic cell death in oligomycin A-untreated insect cells. Interestingly, in this case, the ATP levels of cells dying for autophagy-mediated cell death are comparable to those of control cells, suggesting the existence of a specific pathway that can start autophagy in the absence of a real deficit in ATP levels and in the presence of undamaged mitochondria.[74]

CONCLUDING REMARKS

Several studies have demonstrated a close connection between mitochondrial activity and the balancing between cell survival and cell death. The same stimulus can result in different outcomes, and at least in mammals it has been suggested that this may be related to a specific metabolic state.[9] The transitory importance of specific organs during the animal lifetime is well known and has led to suggestive theories, such as that of the disposable soma theory of aging.[76] The resources available to an organism are limited and exhaustible. This may lead to investing a considerable amount of energy in some organs in juveniles, eg, the thymus in mammals, and then to dismantling those very organs during aging. The same might be true at the cellular level, where usually protective pathways may be subverted toward cell death in the presence of specific conditions that make cell death unavoidable or advantageous.[9] These considerations, which derived mainly from studies in mammals, have been extended to other organisms, like holometabolous insects, which undergo a complete metamorphosis and deeply rearrange their organisms by developing some organs and reducing, or disposing of, others.[16] Our experiments on an unconventional insect model demonstrated that chemical stressors targeting mitochondria may result in the activation of different pathways and can promote different modalities of cell death. In some cases, the same kinase played different roles under diverse conditions. For instance, PKA exerted a protective and antiapoptotic role when activated via PDGF-AB or TGF-β1, while it promoted the proapoptotic effects of the NO donor, SNP.[47,50] Our results suggest that the mitochondria may play a major role in eliciting different responses, which include apoptosis and autophagic-mediated cell death. This strengthens recent theories, mainly based on experiments performed in mammals, which pose the mitochondria at the intersection of the suicidal or adaptive response versus different stressors.[9]

REFERENCES

1. Galluzzi L, Vitale I, Abrams JM, Alnemri ES, Baehrecke EH, Blagosklonny MV, et al. Molecular definitions of cell death subroutines: recommendations of the Nomenclature Committee on Cell Death 2012. *Cell Death Differ* 2012;**19**:107–20.
2. Majno G, Joris I. Apoptosis, oncosis, and necrosis. An overview of cell death. *Am J Pathol* 1995;**146**:3–15.
3. Jain MV, Paczulla AM, Klonisch T, Dimgba FN, Rao SB, Roberg K, et al. Interconnections between apoptotic, autophagic and necrotic pathways: implications for cancer therapy development. *J Cell Mol Med* 2013;**17**:12–29.
4. Tait SW, Ichim G, Green DR. Die another way–non-apoptotic mechanisms of cell death. *J Cell Sci* 2014;**127**:2135–44.
5. Ambjørn M, Ejlerskov P, Liu Y, Lees M, Jäättelä M, Issazadeh-Navikas S. IFNB1/interferon-β-induced autophagy in MCF-7 breast cancer cells counteracts its proapoptotic function. *Autophagy* 2013;**9**:287–302.
6. Nelson C, Baehrecke EH. Eaten to death. *FEBS J* 2014;**281**:5411–7.
7. Descloux C, Ginet V, Clarke PG, Puyal J, Truttmann AC. Neuronal death after perinatal cerebral hypoxia-ischemia: focus on autophagy-mediated cell death. *Int J Dev Neurosci* 2015;**45**:75–85.
8. Klionsky DJ, Abdalla FC, Abeliovich H, Abraham RT, Acevedo-Arozena A, Adeli K, et al. Guidelines for the use and interpretation of assays for monitoring autophagy. *Autophagy* 2012;**8**:445–544.
9. Green DR, Galluzzi L, Kroemer G. Cell biology. Metabolic control of cell death. *Science* 2014;**345**:1250256.
10. Liu X, Kim CN, Yang J, Jemmerson R, Wang X. Induction of apoptotic program in cell-free extracts: requirement for dATP and cytochrome c. *Cell* 1996;**86**:147–57.
11. Green D, Kroemer G. The central executioners of apoptosis: caspases or mitochondria? *Trends Cell Biol* 1998;**8**:267–71.

12. Conti F, Abnave P, Ghigo E. Unconventional animal models: a booster for new advances in host-pathogen interactions. *Front Cell Infect Microbiol* 2014;**4**:142.
13. Lynn DE, Dougherty EM, McClintock JT, Loeb M. Development of cell lines from various tissues of Lepidoptera. In: Kuroda Y, Kurstak E, Maramorosch K, editors. *Invertebrate and fish tissue culture.* Tokyo: Japan Scientific Societies Press; 1988. p. 239–42.
14. Lemaitre B, Hoffmann J. The host defense of *Drosophila melanogaster. Annu Rev Immunol* 2007;**25**:697–743.
15. Nässel DR, Kubrak OI, Liu Y, Luo J, Lushchak OV. Factors that regulate insulin producing cells and their output in *Drosophila. Front Physiol* 2013;**4**:252.
16. Malagoli D. Cell death in the IPLB-LdFB insect cell line: facts and implications. *Curr Pharm Des* 2008;**14**:126–30.
17. Tian L, Liu S, Liu H, Li S. 20-hydroxyecdysone upregulates apoptotic genes and induces apoptosis in the *Bombyx* fat body. *Arch Insect Biochem Physiol* 2012;**79**:207–19.
18. Mauvezin C, Ayala C, Braden CR, Kim J, Neufeld TP. Assays to monitor autophagy in *Drosophila. Methods* 2014;**68**:134–9.
19. Golstein P, Kroemer G. Redundant cell death mechanisms as relics and backups. *Cell Death Differ* 2005;**12**(Suppl. 2):1490–6.
20. Romero A, Novoa B, Figueras A. The complexity of apoptotic cell death in mollusks: an update. *Fish Shellfish Immunol* 2015;**46**:79–87.
21. Yuan J, Shaham S, Ledoux S, Ellis HM, Horvitz HR. The *C. elegans* cell death gene *ced-3* encodes a protein similar to mammalian interleukin-1β-converting enzyme. *Cell* 1993;**75**:641–52.
22. Kimura KI, Truman JW. Postmetamorphic cell death in the nervous and muscular systems of *Drosophila melanogaster. J Neurosci* 1990;**10**:403–11.
23. Wolff T, Ready DF. Cell death in normal and rough eye mutants of *Drosophila. Development* 1991;**113**:825–39.
24. Hengartner MO, Ellis RE, Horvitz HR. *Caenorhabditis elegans* gene ced-9 protects cells from programmed cell death. *Nature* 1992;**356**:494–9.
25. Vaux DL, Weissman IL, Kim SK. Prevention of programmed cell death in *Caenorhabditis elegans* by human bcl-2. *Science* 1992;**258**:1955–7.
26. Brand S, Bourbon HM. The developmentally-regulated *Drosophila* gene *rox8* encodes an RRM-type RNA binding protein structurally related to human TIA-1-type nucleolysins. *Nucleic Acids Res* 1993;**21**:3699–704.
27. Sugimoto A, Friesen PD, Rothman JH. Baculovirus p35 prevents developmentally programmed cell death and rescues a *ced-9* mutant in the nematode *Caenorhabditis elegans. EMBO J* 1994;**13**:2023–8.
28. Steller H. Mechanisms and genes of cellular suicide. *Science* 1995;**267**:1445–9.
29. White E. Life, death, and the pursuit of apoptosis. *Genes Dev* 1996;**10**:1–15.
30. Nakajima Y, Madhyastha R, Maruyama M. 2-Deoxy-D-ribose, a downstream mediator of thymidine phosphorylase, regulates tumor angiogenesis and progression. *Anticancer Agents Med Chem* 2009;**9**:239–45.
31. Staal FJ, Ela SW, Roederer M, Anderson MT, Herzenberg LA, Herzenberg LA. Glutathione deficiency and human immunodeficiency virus infection. *Lancet* 1992;**339**:909–12.
32. Barbieri D, Grassilli E, Monti D, Salvioli S, Franceschini MG, Franchini A, et al. D-ribose and deoxy-D-ribose induce apoptosis in human quiescent peripheral blood mononuclear cells. *Biochem Biophys Res Commun* 1994;**201**:1109–16.
33. Barbieri D, Malagoli D, Cuoghi B, Ottaviani E. An anti-Bcl-2 antibody prevents 2-deoxy-D-ribose-induced apoptosis in the IPLB-LdFB insect cell line. *Cell Mol Life Sci* 2001;**58**:653–9.

34. Kletsas D, Barbieri D, Stathakos D, Botti B, Bergamini S, Tomasi A, et al. The highly reducing sugar 2-deoxy-D-ribose induces apoptosis in human fibroblasts by reduced glutathione depletion and cytoskeletal disruption. *Biochem Biophys Res Commun* 1998;**243**:416–25.
35. Quinn L, Coombe M, Mills K, Daish T, Colussi P, Kumar S, et al. Buffy, a *Drosophila* Bcl-2 protein, has anti-apoptotic and cell cycle inhibitory functions. *EMBO J* 2003;**22**:3568–79.
36. Malagoli D, Iacconi I, Marchesini E, Ottaviani E. Cell-death mechanisms in the IPLB-LdFB insect cell line: a nuclear located Bcl-2-like molecule as a possible controller of 2-deoxy-D-ribose-mediated DNA fragmentation. *Cell Tissue Res* 2005;**320**:337–43.
37. Blackstone NW, Green DR. The evolution of a mechanism of cell suicide. *Bioessays* 1999;**21**:84–8.
38. Sokolova IM. Apoptosis in molluscan immune defense. *Inv Surv J* 2009;**6**:49–58.
39. Sokolova IM, Evans S, Hughes FM. Cadmium-induced apoptosis in oyster hemocytes involves disturbance of cellular energy balance but no mitochondrial permeability transition. *J Exp Biol* 2004;**207**(Pt 19):3369–80.
40. Russo J, Madec L. Haemocyte apoptosis as a general cellular immune response of the snail, *Lymnaea stagnalis*, to a toxicant. *Cell Tissue Res* 2007;**328**:431–41.
41. Collins MK, Perkins GR, Rodriguez-Tarduchy G, Nieto MA, López-Rivas A. Growth factors as survival factors: regulation of apoptosis. *Bioessays* 1994;**16**:133–8.
42. Ottaviani E, Barbieri D, Franchini A, Kletsas D. PDGF and TGF-β partially prevent 2-deoxy-D-ribose-induced apoptosis in the fat body cell line IPLB-LdFB from the insect *Lymantria dispar*. *J Insect Physiol* 2000;**46**:81–7.
43. Arcaro A, Wymann MP. Wortmannin is a potent phosphatidylinositol 3-kinase inhibitor: the role of phosphatidylinositol 3,4,5-trisphosphate in neutrophil responses. *Biochem J* 1993;**296** (Pt 2):297–301.
44. Wieprecht M, Wieder T, Geilen CC. N-[2-bromocinnamyl(amino)ethyl]-5-isoquinolinesulphonamide (H-89) inhibits incorporation of choline into phosphatidylcholine via inhibition of choline kinase and has no effect on the phosphorylation of CTP: phosphocholine cytidylyltransferase. *Biochem J* 1994;**297**(Pt 1):241–7.
45. Tamaoki T. Use and specificity of staurosporine, UCN-01, and calphostin C as protein kinase inhibitors. *Methods Enzymol* 1991;**201**:340–7.
46. Ottaviani E, Barbieri D, Malagoli D, Kletsas D. Involvement of PI 3-kinase, PKA and PKC in PDGF- and TGF-β-mediated prevention of 2-deoxy-D-ribose-induced apoptosis in the insect cell line, IPLB-LdFB. *Cell Biol Int* 2001;**25**:171–7.
47. Ottaviani E, Barbieri D, Malagoli D, Franchini A. Nitric oxide induces apoptosis in the fat body cell line IPLB-LdFB from the insect *Lymantria dispar*. *Comp Biochem Physiol* 2001;**128B**:247–54.
48. Ignarro LJ, Edwards JC, Gruetter DY, Barry BK, Gruetter CA. Possible involvement of S-nitrosothiols in the activation of guanylate cyclase by nitroso compounds. *FEBS Lett* 1980;**110**:275–8.
49. Ignarro LJ, Lippton H, Edwards JC, Baricos WH, Hyman AL, Kadowitz PJ, et al. Mechanism of vascular smooth muscle relaxation by organic nitrates, nitrites, nitroprusside and nitric oxide: evidence for the involvement of S-nitrosothiols as active intermediates. *J Pharmacol Exp Ther* 1981;**218**:739–49.
50. Malagoli D, Conte A, Ottaviani E. Protein kinases mediate nitric oxide-induced apoptosis in the insect cell line IPLB-LdFB. *Cell Mol Life Sci* 2002;**59**:894–901.
51. Clark SL. Cellular differentiation in the kidneys of newborn mice studied with the electron microscope. *J Biophys Biochem Cytol* 1957;**3**:349.
52. Deter RL, De Duve C. Influence of glucagon, an inducer of cellular autophagy, on some physical properties of rat liver lysosomes. *J Cell Biol* 1967;**33**:437–49.

53. Kovács J, Réz G. Autophagocytosis. *Acta Biol Acad Sci Hung* 1979;**30**:177–99.
54. Lockshin RA, Osborne B, Zakeri Z. Cell death in the third millennium. *Cell Death Differ* 2000;**7**:2–7.
55. Huang WP, Klionsky DJ. Autophagy in yeast: a review of the molecular machinery. *Cell Struct Funct* 2002;**27**:409–20.
56. Reggiori F, Klionsky DJ. Autophagy in the eukaryotic cell. *Eukaryot Cell* 2002;**1**:11–21.
57. Wang CW, Klionsky DJ. The molecular mechanism of autophagy. *Mol Med* 2003;**9**:65–76.
58. Klionsky DJ. Autophagy: from phenomenology to molecular understanding in less than a decade. *Nat Rev Mol Cell Biol* 2007;**8**:931–7.
59. Xie Z, Klionsky DJ. Autophagosome formation: core machinery and adaptations. *Nat Cell Biol* 2007;**9**:1102–9.
60. Bursch W. The autophagosomal-lysosomal compartment in programmed cell death. *Cell Death Differ* 2001;**8**:569–81.
61. Cuervo AM. Autophagy: in sickness and in health. *Trends Cell Biol* 2004;**14**:70–7.
62. Levine B, Klionsky DJ. Development by self-digestion: molecular mechanisms and biological functions of autophagy. *Dev Cell* 2004;**6**:463–77.
63. Tsujimoto Y, Shimizu S. Another way to die: autophagic programmed cell death. *Cell Death Differ* 2005;**12**:1528–34.
64. Vabulas RM, Hartl FU. Protein synthesis upon acute nutrient restriction relies on proteasome function. *Science* 2005;**310**:1960–3.
65. Mizushima N, Komatsu M. Autophagy: renovation of cells and tissues. *Cell* 2011;**147**:728–41.
66. Tooze SA, Yoshimori T. The origin of the autophagosomal membrane. *Nat Cell Biol* 2010;**12**:831–5.
67. Mizushima N, Yoshimori T, Ohsumi Y. The role of Atg proteins in autophagosome formation. *Annu Rev Cell Dev Biol* 2011;**27**:107–32.
68. Clarke PG. Developmental cell death: morphological diversity and multiple mechanisms. *Anat Embryol Berl* 1990;**181**:195–213.
69. Shimizu S, Kanaseki T, Mizushima N, Mizuta T, Arakawa-Kobayashi S, Thompson CB, et al. Role of Bcl-2 family proteins in a non-apoptotic programmed cell death dependent on autophagy genes. *Nat Cell Biol* 2004;**6**:1221–8.
70. Yu L, Alva A, Su H, Dutt P, Freundt E, Welsh S, et al. Regulation of an ATG7-beclin 1 program of autophagic cell death by caspase-8. *Science* 2004;**304**:1500–2.
71. Gordy C, He YW. The crosstalk between autophagy and apoptosis: where does this lead? *Protein Cell* 2012;**3**:17–27.
72. Galluzzi L, Bravo-San Pedro JM, Vitale I, Aaronson SA, Abrams JM, Adam D, et al. Essential versus accessory aspects of cell death: recommendations of the NCCD 2015. *Cell Death Differ* 2015;**22**:58–73.
73. Tettamanti G, Malagoli D, Marchesini E, Congiu T, de Eguileor M, Ottaviani E. Oligomycin A induces autophagy in the IPLB-LdFB insect cell line. *Cell Tissue Res* 2006;**326**:179–86.
74. Malagoli D, Boraldi F, Annovi G, Quaglino D, Ottaviani E. New insights into autophagic cell death in the gypsy moth *Lymantria dispar*: a proteomic approach. *Cell Tissue Res* 2009;**336**:107–18.
75. Tettamanti G, Malagoli D, Ottaviani E, de Eguileor M. Oligomycin A and the IPLB-LdFB insect cell line: actin and mitochondrial responses. *Cell Biol Int* 2008;**32**:287–92.
76. Kirkwood TB. Evolution of ageing. *Nature* 1977;**270**:301–4.

Chapter 3

Immunotoxicology Approaches in Ecotoxicology: Lessons From Mollusks

Valerio Matozzo
University of Padova, Padova, Italy

François Gagné
Emerging Methods Section, Aquatic Contaminants Research Division, Environment Canada, Montréal, QC, Canada

MOLLUSK HEMOCYTES: TYPES AND FUNCTIONS

In mollusks, hemocytes circulate freely in the circulatory system where they are involved in various biological processes, such as wound and tissue repair, shell production and repair, and nutrition. However, these cells have also been extensively studied for their ability to interact with foreign materials and to develop immune responses. For these reasons, hemocytes are generically called "immunocytes."

In the scientific literature, mollusk hemocyte characterization is one of the most debated problems, mainly due to different classification criteria that have been adopted to classify circulating cells. Regarding bivalves, hemocytes have formerly been indicated by various terms, such as lymphocytes, amoebocytes, agranular and granular leukocytes, macrophages, and fibrocytes.[1–4] In a number of studies, the presence of two circulating hemocyte types, granulocytes and hyalinocytes, has been suggested in bivalves. Granulocytes generally contain cytoplasmic granules, whereas hyalinocytes have few or no granules.[5,6] Although the percentage of granulocytes and hyalinocytes can vary markedly among species, the two hemocyte types have been identified in *Mya arenaria*,[7] *Mytilus edulis*,[8] *Mytilus galloprovincialis*,[9,10] *Mercenaria mercenaria*,[11] *Crassostrea virginica*,[12] *Ruditapes decussatus*,[13] *Tapes (Ruditapes) philippinarum*,[14] *Cerastoderma glaucum*,[15] *Chamelea gallina*,[16] *Meretrix lusoria*,[17] *Saccostrea kegaki*, *Ostrea circumpicta*, and *Hyotissa hyotis*.[18] However, some authors have suggested that not all hemocyte types are present in each bivalve species. For example, Ottaviani et al.[19] suggested that in *M. galloprovincialis*, there is only one type of hemocyte that undergoes two

Lessons in Immunity: From Single-Cell Organisms to Mammals
http://dx.doi.org/10.1016/B978-0-12-803252-7.00003-5

29

different aging-related stages: hyalinocytes represent a proliferative stage, and they mature to become granulocytes. In the sunray venus clam, *Macrocallista nimbosa*, Jauzein et al.[20] have identified a unique hemocyte population, which exhibits distinct morphological characteristics and intracellular parameters. In *Crassostrea rhizophorae*, various techniques (flow cytometry, histological evaluation, histochemical detection, and transmission electron microscopy (TEM)) have been used to classify hemocytes, and the different hemocyte subpopulations have been indicated as different stages of one cell type only.[21] In that case, it has been suggested that hemocytes initially accumulate granules and then lose their complexity (with no reduction in size) as they degranulate in response to environmental stress.[21]

In gastropods, there is no consensus about the classification criteria for hemocytes, and one or two types of hemocytes have generally been described.[22] Like bivalves, gastropod hyalinocytes (or agranular cells) have a high nuclear/cytoplasmic ratio and few cytoplasmic granules, whereas granulocytes contain cytoplasmic granules and have a low nuclear/cytoplasmic ratio. Using light microscopy and TEM and differential centrifugation and staining reactions, a single type of circulating hemocyte (agranular) has been identified in the blood of *Aplysia californica* and *Megathura crenulata*.[23] In the freshwater gastropod *Pomacea canaliculata*, flow cytometry analysis identified two populations of hemocytes on the basis of differences in size and internal organization.[24] The first population contains small and agranular cells, and the second one displays a larger size and a more articulated internal organization.[24] In the European *Haliotis tuberculata*, flow cytometry, phase contrast observation, and TEM were able to detect only agranular cells, both large and small.[25] In *Biomphalaria glabrata*, three distinct types of hemocytes have been described: large cells with numerous mitochondria and large aggregates of glycogen particles; medium-size cells with few organelles and glycogen; and small cells with organelles and few secretory granules.[26] Conversely, in the blood of *Lymnaea stagnalis*, only one type of cell—the amoebocyte—has been identified.[27] In the hemolymph of *Haliotis asinina* both hyalinocytes and granulocytes (described by TEM) circulate, even if the shape and size of the granules are different from those observed in other mollusk species.[28] In *Oncomelania hupensis*, two types of hemocyte cell categories—type I (macrophage-like) and type II (lymphocyte-like)—have been distinguished based on cell shape, size, surface structure, internal structure, functions, structure of cytoplasm, and the processes of spikelike filopodia.[29] The nucleus diameter/cell diameter ratio and morphological characteristics were studied to classify hemocytes of the snail *Babylonia areolata*. The results revealed the presence of two main types of hemocytes, namely granulocytes and hyalinocytes; the latter were smaller than the former.[30] Ottaviani[31] identified only one cell type—the spreading hemocyte—in the freshwater snail *Viviparus ater*. The author suggested that these cells are similar to the spreading cells found in other gastropods and represent the ancestral cell responsible for defense mechanisms.[31] Conversely, in the blood of the freshwater snail *Planorbarius corneus*, spreading and round cells were observed; the former showed abundant cytoplasm, pseudopods, and irregular nuclei, whereas the latter had electron-dense granules in the mitochondria matrix.[32] Summarizing, two important aspects about mollusk hemocyte classification remain to be clarified:

1. Do different hemocyte types represent distinct cell lineages or different maturation stages?
2. Can the different techniques used to classify hemocytes produce controversial results?

Despite these unresolved aspects, it has been demonstrated that mollusk hemocytes are remarkably competent cells in nonspecific immunity. Mollusks rely on an innate, nonlymphoid immune system that includes both cellular and humoral components. Hemocyte-mediated reactions include the recognition of nonself particles, chemotaxis, opsonization, phagocytosis, encapsulation, intracellular digestion, degranulation with a release of cytotoxic substances, and the production of antimicrobial peptides, reactive oxygen species (ROS), and nitric oxide (NO).

The body of data on immunocompetence comes from bivalves as animal models in the study of interactions between chemicals or toxins and innate immunity. Bivalves are sedentary and accumulate large quantities of suspended particles during feeding. Consequently, they can accumulate many xenobiotics, in addition to a plethora of microorganisms, at concentrations that could far exceed the concentration found in the water column and sediments.[33] This is especially the case with the advent of nanotechnology: bivalves can readily accumulate aggregates of nanoparticles (NPs), leading to inflammatory responses, making this species at risk to this growing industry.[34,35] Bivalves are amenable to both in vitro and in vivo experiments. The hemolymph could be retrieved in a nondestructive manner, which makes bivalves ethical from the animal-care perspective (Fig. 3.1). Hemolymph also permits studies on endangered species or species at risk. Bivalves

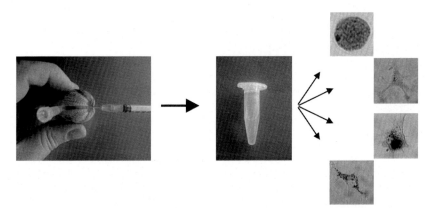

FIGURE 3.1   Hemolymph collection and hemocyte types in a clam species (*Ruditapes philippinarum*).

could be exposed in situ using experimental cages at sites of concern, if animals are not found locally, or they can be exposed in the laboratory. These invertebrates are therefore constantly exposed to foreign agents and bodies. Although vertebrates possess an acquired or adaptive immunity based on the complement component (antibody production), mollusks and other invertebrates rely solely on innate or natural immunity.[36] However, a primitive immunoglobulin is seemingly present in invertebrates: the molluskan defense molecule (MDM).[37] MDM is preferentially expressed in hemocytes and involved in the agglutination of foreign microparticles in snails. However, the exposure of snails to surface waters contaminated by municipal effluents failed to influence MDM gene expression.[38] Nevertheless, the role of Ig-mediated immunity in snails (and perhaps in other invertebrates) is not well understood presently, and more research is required to understand these new fundamental functions in invertebrates. The allograft inflammatory factor-1 (AIF-1) has also been identified in sponges and abalones.[39,40] This cytokine is involved in the recognition and rejection of allografts. In bivalves, the hemocytes are responsible for both the production of various cytokines and phagocytosis of foreign particles. It is important to highlight that the site of hemopoiesis has yet to be identified in this group, but some evidence suggests that the cells mature in the hemolymph, given the cellular diversity in this compartment. Regarding clams, analysis of the hemocyte cytoskeleton revealed mitotic spindles radiating from the microtubule-organizing centers located at the spindle poles (centrosomes) of undifferentiated cells (hemoblasts), suggesting that hemoblasts are able to divide in the hemolymph.[41] In oysters, it has been demonstrated that stem-like cells located in the irregularly folded structures of gills are precursors of hemocytes.[42] These progenitor cells expressed SRY (sex-determining region Y)-box 2 (also called SOX2), which is involved in the self-renewal and maintenance of pluripotent stem cells, and superoxide dismutase (SOD), which are hemocyte specific and not expressed in the gill epithelium.

INTERACTION BETWEEN HEMOCYTES AND TOXICANTS: THE IMMUNOMARKER APPROACH

Environmental factors, such as temperature, salinity, oxygen, pH, nutrients, and pollutants, can affect immune parameters in mollusks, potentially increasing their susceptibility to pathogens. The hemocyte parameters that have been selected as immunomarkers include mainly the total hemocyte count (THC), hemocyte viability, hemocyte morphology and size, hemocyte adhesion capability, phagocytic activity, hydrolytic and oxidative enzyme activities, lysosomal membrane stability, and ROS and NO production. Most of the studies have been focused on the evaluation of the immunotoxic effects of "traditional" pollutants (eg, heavy metals and various organic pollutants) in mollusks. Currently, there is increasing concern for the potential environmental risk posed by "emerging contaminants." These are man-made or naturally occurring chemicals or materials that have the potential to enter the environment, but the risks to human health and the environment are not well known. Emerging contaminants include, for example, pharmaceuticals and personal care products (PPCPs), phytoestrogens, synthetic musks, brominated compounds, chlorinated paraffins, fluorinated compounds, nonhalogenated compounds, phthalates, and nanomaterials.

In this context, various immunomarkers have been used in ecotoxicological studies, both in vitro and in vivo, to assess the effects of this class of pollutants in mollusks. Among emerging contaminants, PPCPs are a large group of chemicals used either by humans for personal health or by agribusiness to enhance the growth and health of livestock. These compounds raise concerns due to their continuous release into aquatic ecosystems where they can affect nontarget organisms. An exhaustive list of the immunomarkers that have been used to evaluate the negative effects of PPCPs on the hemocyte parameters of mollusks is provided in Table 3.1. In snails, an immunotoxicogenomic investigation of *L. stagnalis*, which was exposed to environmentally relevant concentrations of four mixtures of representative therapeutic classes (antibiotics, psychoactives, antihypertensives, and hypolipemics), was performed to determine if these mixtures—individually and as a global mixture—could influence immune-related gene expression.[38] The effects caused by pharmaceutical mixtures were then compared with those induced by a treated municipal effluent known for its contamination. The study revealed that snail immunocompetence was differently affected by the therapeutic class mixtures compared to the global mixture. Toll-like receptor 4 (TLR4), AIF-1, catalase (CAT), and glutathione reductase (GR) gene expression were highly influenced by psychiatric, antibiotic, hypolipemic, and antihypertensive therapeutic classes.[38] However, the effects of antibiotic mixtures (composed of ciprofloxacine, erythromycin, novobiocin, oxytetracycline, sulfamethoxazole, and trimethoprim) were dominant over the other classes. Moreover, the GR, CAT, and AIF-1 genes were significantly correlated with immunocompetence, as determined by phagocytosis, hemocyte viability, and density. The study revealed that changes in immune responses caused by the municipal effluent were similar to those induced by the global pharmaceutical mixture, and the latter shared similarities with the antibiotic mixture. Overall, results suggested that pharmaceutical mixtures in municipal effluents represent a risk for gastropod immunocompetence, and the antibiotics could represent a model therapeutic class for municipal effluent toxicity studies in *L. stagnalis*.

It is noteworthy that the strongest signals in gene expression in snails exposed to either municipal effluents or selected PPCPs are the Toll receptors and selenium-dependent glutathione peroxidase (SeGPx).[63] Indeed, TLR4 and SeGPx were expressed sixfold and fourfold, respectively, compared to snails exposed to upstream surface waters from the effluent discharge. TLR4 is a protein involved in both the recognition of liposaccharides from gram-negative

TABLE 3.1 Examples of Hemocyte Parameters That Have Been Used to Evaluate the Effects of Pharmaceuticals and Personal Care Products in Mollusks

PPCPs	Mollusk Species (Exposure Type)	Hemocyte Parameters	References
Antibiotics			
Mixture of ciprofloxacine, erythromycine, novobiocin, oxytetracycline, sulfamethoxazole, trimethoprim	*Lymnaea stagnalis* (in vivo exposure)	Hemocyte viability	38
		Hemocyte count	
		Phagocytic activity	
		Thiol levels	
		ROS levels	
		NOS1, NOS2	
		MDM	
		TLR4	
		AIF-1	
Trimethoprim	*Dreissena polymorpha* (in vitro exposure)	DNA damage	43
		Apoptosis	
		Lysosomal membrane stability	
Ciprofloxacin, erythromycin, novobiocin, oxytetracycline, sulfamethoxazole, trimethoprim (alone or as a mixture)	*Elliptio complanata* (in vitro exposure)	Hemocyte viability	44
		ROS levels	
		Thiol levels	
		Phagocytosis	
		Lysozyme activity	
		NO production	
		COX activity	

NSAIDs

Drug	Species	Immunomarker	Ref
Ibuprofen	*Ruditapes philippinarum* (in vivo exposure)	THC Hemocyte diameter Hemocyte volume Cell proliferation NR uptake LDH activity DNA fragmentation	45
Ibuprofen	*R. philippinarum* (in vivo exposure)	Lysosomal membrane stability	46
Ibuprofen	*D. polymorpha* (in vivo exposure)	DNA damage Apoptosis Micronuclei Lysosomal membrane stability	47
Diclofenac	*D. polymorpha* (in vivo exposure)	DNA damage Apoptosis Micronuclei Lysosomal membrane stability	48

Continued

TABLE 3.1 Examples of Hemocyte Parameters That Have Been Used to Evaluate the Effects of Pharmaceuticals and Personal Care Products in Mollusks—cont'd

PPCPs	Mollusk Species (Exposure Type)	Hemocyte Parameters	References
Paracetamol	*D. polymorpha* (in vivo exposure)	DNA damage	49
		Apoptosis	
		Micronuclei	
		Lysosomal membrane stability	
Diclofenac + Paracetamol + Ibuprofen	*D. polymorpha* (in vivo exposure)	DNA damage	50
		Apoptosis	
		Micronuclei	
		Lysosomal membrane stability	
Ibuprofen + Diuron + Isoturon	*Crassostrea gigas* (in vivo exposure)	Cell mortality	51
		Phagocytosis	
		Catecholase-type phenoloxidase activity	
Anticancer Agents			
Cyclophosphamide	*Mytilus edulis* (in vivo exposure)	Lysosomal membrane stability	52
		Micronuclei	
		DNA damage	

Lipid Regulators

Mixture of atorvastatin, gemfibrozil, bezafibrate	*L. stagnalis* (in vivo exposure)	Hemocyte viability Hemocyte count Phagocytic activity Thiol levels ROS levels NOS1, NOS2 MDM TLR4 AIF-1	38
Bezafibrate, gemfibrozil	*Mytilus galloprovincialis* (in vitro exposure)	Lysozyme release NO levels Phagocytosis Lysosomal membrane stability	53
Bezafibrate, gemfibrozil	*M. galloprovincialis* (injection)	Lysosomal membrane stability Lysozyme release Phagocytosis	53

Continued

TABLE 3.1 Examples of Hemocyte Parameters That Have Been Used to Evaluate the Effects of Pharmaceuticals and Personal Care Products in Mollusks—cont'd

PPCPs	Mollusk Species (Exposure Type)	Hemocyte Parameters	References
Antihypertensive Drugs			
Mixture of atenolol, furosemide, hydrochlorothiazide, lisinopril	*L. stagnalis* (in vivo exposure)	Hemocyte viability	38
		Hemocyte count	
		Phagocytic activity	
		Thiol levels	
		ROS levels	
		NOS1, NOS2	
		MDM	
		TLR4	
		AIF-1	
Atenolol	*D. polymorpha* (in vitro exposure)	Hemocyte viability	54
Antidepressant Agents			
Fluoxetine	*M. galloprovincialis* (in vivo exposure)	cAMP/PKA activity ABCB mRNA	55
Fluoxetine	*Venerupis philippinarum* (in vivo exposure)	THC	56
		Hemocyte diameter	
		Hemocyte volume	
		Cell proliferation	
		NR uptake	

Compound	Species	Immunomarkers	Reference
Carbamazepine	E. complanata (in vitro exposure)	Phagocytosis; Cell adherence; Esterase activity; Lipid peroxidation	57
Carbamazepine	M. galloprovincialis (in vivo exposure)	Lysosomal membrane permeability	58
Mixture of venlafaxine, carbamazepine, diazepam	L. stagnalis (in vivo exposure)	Hemocyte viability; Hemocyte count; Phagocytic activity; Thiol levels; ROS levels; NOS1, NOS2; MDM; TLR4; AIF-1	38
Amitriptyline, clomipramine, citalopram, paroxetine	Haliotis tuberculata (in vitro exposure)	Phagocytosis; ROS; Esterase activity; Lysosomal membrane stability	59

Continued

TABLE 3.1 Examples of Hemocyte Parameters That Have Been Used to Evaluate the Effects of Pharmaceuticals and Personal Care Products in Mollusks—cont'd

PPCPs	Mollusk Species (Exposure Type)	Hemocyte Parameters	References
Antibacterial agents			
Triclosan, methyl-triclosan	*H. tuberculata* (in vitro exposure)	Hemocyte morphology and density	60
		Hemocyte metabolism	
Triclosan	*R. philippinarum* (in vivo exposure)	THC	61
		Hemocyte diameter and volume	
		Pinocytotic activity	
		Lysozyme activity	
		Hemocyte proliferation	
		Cytotoxicity	
		DNA fragmentation	
Triclosan	*D. polymorpha* (in vivo exposure)	DNA fragmentation	62
		Apoptosis	
		Micronuclei	
		Lysosomal membrane stability	

AIF-1, allograft inflammatory factor-1; *cAMP/PKA*, cAMP-dependent protein kinase; *CAT*, catalase; *COX*, cyclooxygenase; *CR*, glutathione reductase; *HSP70*, heat-shock protein 70; *LDH*, lactate dehydrogenase; *MDM*, molluskan defensive molecule; *NO*, nitric oxide; *NOS1*, nitric oxide synthetase isoform 1; *NOS2*, nitric oxide synthetase isoform 2; *NR*, Neutral Red; *NSAIDs*, nonsteroidal antiinflammatory drugs; *PPCPs*, pharmaceuticals and personal care products; *ROS*, reactive oxygen species; *SeGPx*, selenium-dependent glutathione peroxidase; *SOD*, superoxide dismutase; *THC*, total hemocyte count; *TLR4*, Toll-like receptor 4.

bacteria and the activation of the innate immune system. They can serve as complementary immunomarkers of the lysozyme that is involved in the hydrolysis of peptidoglycans of gram-positive bacteria. TLR4 recognizes pathogen-associated molecular patterns that are found in infectious agents and mediates the production of cytokines for immune protection. The interaction of xenobiotics with this receptor warrants more investigations to better understand the interaction of xenobiotics and the microorganisms in respect to the immune system. SeGPx is involved in the elimination of lipid peroxides in membranes that are produced in phagosomes during oxidative burst to destroy the ingested bacteria. In this respect, SeGPx is an indicator of inflammation. Hence, snails exposed to municipal effluents recognized gram-negative bacteria and produced inflammation.

The growing development of nanotechnologies can have, as a negative consequence, the release into the environment of NPs, whose toxic effects on nontarget species are largely unknown. NPs are particles with a size ranging between 1 and 100 nm and include, for instance, metallic particles, fullerenes, oxides, nanocomposites, and quantum dots. NPs are widely used in many products and in many applications, including medical treatments, food packaging, cosmetics, paints, sportswear, renewable energy, electronic devices, and environmental remediation. This is mainly due to the peculiar physicochemical properties of NPs. Various studies have focused on the evaluation of NP toxicity in nontarget organisms, such as mollusks. Regarding these invertebrates, there is a broad consensus that the immune system is a target for NP toxicity.[64] Table 3.2 summarizes the main immunomarkers that have been used to assess the immunotoxic effects of NPs in mollusks. Regarding NPs, immunotoxicogenomic studies in invertebrates are scarce. In nematodes exposed to silver NPs, increased expression of SOD-3 and abnormal dauer formation protein (daf-12) genes, which are involved in development and longevity, suggest that oxidative stress and inflammation were induced in exposed animals.[75]

MOLLUSK IMMUNOMARKERS: THE ROLE OF CONFOUNDING FACTORS

Although the results presented in this chapter indicate clearly that the immune system of mollusks is an important target for pollutants and suggest that hemocytes are useful cell models for assessing the impact of various substances in these invertebrates, the interpretation of the results obtained in laboratory-controlled conditions is often difficult because of the lack of a clear relationship between experimental conditions and immunomarker responses. In some studies, a nonlinear variation pattern of the immunomarker responses has been observed in mollusks exposed to pollutants, low concentrations stimulating hemocyte parameters, while high levels inhibit them. For example, in clams (*Venerupis philippinarum*) exposed to fluoxetine (an antidepressant), THC values increased significantly at the lowest concentration tested but decreased at the

TABLE 3.2 Examples of Hemocyte Parameters That Have Been Used to Evaluate the Effects of Nanoparticles in Mollusks

NPs	Mollusk Species (Exposure Type)	Hemocyte Parameters	References
n-TiO$_2$ (alone or in combination with 2,3,7,8-TCDD)	*Mytilus galloprovincialis* (in vitro exposure)	Phagocytosis	64
		Lysosomal membrane stability	
n-TiO$_2$	*Ruditapes philippinarum* (in vivo exposure)	Phagocytic activity	65
n-TiO$_2$	*M. galloprovincialis* (in vivo exposure)	THC	66
		Phagocytosis	
		Lysosomal membrane stability	
		ROS and NO	
		Preapoptosis	
		Immune-related gene transcription	
n-TiO$_2$, n-Ag	*Crassostrea virginica* (in vitro exposure)	Phagocytosis	67
n-TiO$_2$, n-SiO$_2$, n-ZnO, n-CeO$_2$	*M. galloprovincialis* (in vitro exposure)	Hemocyte viability	68
		Lysosomal membrane stability	
		Phagocytosis	
		Lysozyme release	
		ROS and NO	
		Mitochondrial parameters	
n-TiO$_2$	*Dreissena polymorpha* (in vivo exposure)	Viability	69
		Phagocytosis	
		ERK1/2 and p38 MAPKs	
n-Ag	*Elliptio complanata* (in vivo exposure)	Hemocyte viability	34
		Phagocytosis	
		Cytotoxicity	

TABLE 3.2 Examples of Hemocyte Parameters That Have Been Used to Evaluate the Effects of Nanoparticles in Mollusks—cont'd

NPs	Mollusk Species (Exposure Type)	Hemocyte Parameters	References
CdS QDs	*M. galloprovincialis* (in vitro exposure)	Cell viability	70
		ROS	
		CAT activity	
		DNA damage	
		Acid phosphatase activity	
		MXR transport activity	
		Phagocytosis	
		Actin cytoskeleton	
CdS QDs	*M. galloprovincialis* (in vivo exposure)	Hemocyte density	71
		Differential cell counts	
		Cell viability	
		Lysosomal membrane stability	
		DNA damage	
CdTe QDs	*E. complanata* (in vivo exposure)	THC	72
		Hemocyte viability	
		Phagocytosis	
		Cytotoxicity	
CdS QDs Ag₂S NP	*Mytilus edulis* (in vitro exposure)	DNA integrity	73
n-CuO n-Ag	*M. galloprovincialis* (in vivo exposure)	DNA damage	74

Ag₂S NP, silver sulfide nanoparticles; *CAT*, catalase; *CdS QDs*, cadmium-based quantum dots; *CdTe QDs*, cadmium–telluride quantum dots; *CeO₂*, cerium oxide; *ERK1/2* and *p38 MAPKs*, mitogen-activated protein kinase ERK1/2 and p38; *MXR*, multixenobiotic resistance; *NO*, nitric oxide; *ROS*, reactive oxygen species; *SiO₂*, silicon dioxide; *n-Ag*, silver nanoparticles; *2,3,7,8-TCDD*, 2,3,7,8-tetrachlorodibenzo-p-dioxins; *THC*, total hemocyte count; *n-TiO₂*, titanium dioxide; *ZnO*, zinc oxide.

highest concentrations tested, suggesting a biphasic response of clams to fluoxetine exposure. This peculiar dose response is known as hormesis, a phenomenon characterized by low-dose stimulation and high-dose inhibition. An in vitro study demonstrated that the exposure of abalone (*H. tuberculata*) hemocytes to four common antidepressants (amitriptyline, clomipramine, citalopram, and paroxetine) for 48 h induced a biphasic response of different immunological end points (phagocytosis, levels of ROS, esterase activity, and lysosomal membrane destabilization), with an increase at the lowest concentration and a decrease at higher concentrations.[59] An opposite biphasic response was observed in mussels (*M. edulis*) exposed to North Sea produced water: cell viability, phagocytosis, and cytotoxicity were inhibited after exposure to low concentrations of oil well-produced water, while higher concentrations caused significant increases in immunomarkers.[76] These results indicate that experiments under laboratory-controlled conditions did not always produce obvious outcomes in hemocyte parameters. To explain this inconsistency, it has been suggested that (1) hemocyte parameters measured, methods used, and experimental timing might not be the most relevant; (2) high-interindividual variation might hide potential effects, therefore not allowing demonstration of statistically significant contrasts; and (3) because hemocytes maintain organism homeostasis and integrity, they might not be as sensitive to environmental variations.[77] An additional hyphotesis— related to the ecological history of the organisms—has been proposed to explain the unexpected results. Indeed, it has been demonstrated that animals experiencing different environmental conditions in the field can respond differently to contaminant exposure under laboratory-controlled conditions.[78] Consequently, attention should be addressed in selecting experimental animals for ecotoxicological surveys, taking animal origin into account.

Various laboratory and field studies have demonstrated that the immune responses of mollusks (bivalves in particular) can be modulated by factors (both biotic and abiotic) different from environmental pollutants, which should be taken into account as confounding factors. For example, seasonal and gender-related differences in phagocytic activity have been observed in bivalves.[79] In particular, the phagocytic activity in female mussels (*M. edulis*) was significantly reduced when the cells were exposed to 10^{-5} M of mercuric chloride, while a significant reduction for males was also observed for exposure levels that were 10-fold higher (10^{-4} M). In clams (*R. philippinarum*) collected during the prespawning phase, various hemocyte parameters (THC, hemocyte size frequency distribution, endocytotic activity, lysozyme, acid phosphatase, SOD, and CAT activities) were measured to ascertain whether the two sexes reach the stressful spawning period with different degrees of immunosurveillance.[80] The results demonstrated that gender-related differences in immune parameters occur in clams and highlight that females had more active hemocytes than males during the prespawning period. During mollusk spawning, important physiological functions can be modulated, including immune responses. A relationship between decreased phagocytic activity and the spawning phase has been demonstrated in mussels (*M. edulis*).[81] The phagocytic activity of mussel hemocytes during the spawning period can be 60% lower than that of mussels after the spawning period.[82] In addition, spawning can decrease the phagocytic capacity of mussel hemocytes exposed to metal (Cd).[82] Tides can also affect hemocyte parameters of mollusks. Indeed, hemocytes from soft-shell clams (*M. arenaria*) exposed for a long period to air (low tide) are more sensitive to the toxic effects of metals.[83] Similarly, the spatial distribution of animals on the shore (upper, middle, and lower) can influence mollusk immunocompetence. In the soft-shell clam *M. arenaria*, bivalves that are located in upper and middle ranges have phagocytic activity significantly lower than those from the lower range.[84] The distance from the shore also influences the number of circulating hemocytes: mollusks collected closer to the shore can have a higher number of cells than clams from beds further offshore.[85] A multibiomarker approach has been used to assess the effects of different environmental conditions in the clam *R. philippinarum*.[86] Bivalves were collected monthly in two sites of the Lagoon of Venice (Italy) that were differently influenced by both anthropogenic impact and natural conditions: a seaward site, close to a Lagoon inlet, characterized by high hydrodynamism and influenced by the intense passage of ships, and a landward site characterized by low hydrodynamism and influenced by both riverine inputs and agricultural wastewaters. Immunomarkers highlighted an overall better condition for clams from the seaward site. Interestingly, no significant differences in sediment contamination levels were observed between the two sampling sites, suggesting once again that environmental factors different from environmental pollutants—such as salinity, total chlorophyll, sediment grain size, and organic matter—can strongly influence hemocyte parameters in mollusks.

Biomarkers that not only provide mechanistic information on the mode of action of xenobiotics and infective agents but are also predictive of impacts at higher levels of biological organization are of value in ecological risk assessment.[87] An investigation of wild clam (*M. arenaria*) populations revealed that sites with low clam numbers and a reduced growth index had significantly higher levels of lipid peroxidation and metallothioneins.[88] A closer examination of these sites revealed that lower recruitment of young clams occurred, suggesting important changes in population structure. In a follow-up study, clams found at polluted sites had increased immunoactivity and inflammation in respect to clams at pristine sites.[89] The study revealed that clam density corrected for salinity differences (estuary) were significantly correlated with hemocyte activity, phagocytosis, and cellular energy expenses. The clams were also more sensitive to temperature changes in respect to energy expense (ie, clams spend more energy per temperature changes). Hence, immunocompetence and energy expense biomarkers were strongly associated with clam population metrics and could serve as predictive biomarkers, not only for clam health but also for population health. Hence, many environmental variables—such as clam bed distance from the shoreline, salinity, reproductive status (spawning), site quality, and temperature—have to be taken into account for immunocompetence biomarkers in the prediction of population health in estuaries. The development of immunotoxicogenomics will also lead to a better understanding of cumulative environmental stressors, especially for immunocompetence responses that are sensitive to the physiological state of the organisms and the concomitant presence of biological and chemical agents. High-throughput tools, such as toxicogenomics and other omics strategies, such as proteomics and metabolomics, hold promise to increase the understanding of the fundamental processes that underlie the interaction of microorganisms and the effects of exposure to xenobiotics on the immune system.

REFERENCES

1. Nakahara H, Bevelander G. An electron microscope study of ingestion of thorotrast by amoebocytes of *Pinctada radiata*. *Tex Rep Biol Med* 1969;**27**:101–9.
2. Cheng TC, Rifkin E. Cellular reactions in marine molluscs in response to helminth parasitism. In: Snieszko SF, editor. *Diseases of fish and shellfish. American Fisheries Society Symposium*, vol. **5**. 1970. p. 443–96.
3. Feng SY, Feng JS, Burke CN, Khairallah LH. Light and electron microscopy of the leucocytes of *Crassostrea virginica* (Mollusca: Pelecypoda). *Z Zellforsch Mikrosk Anat* 1971;**120**:222–45.
4. Foley DA, Cheng TC. Morphology, hematologic parameters, and behavior of hemolymph cells of the quahaug clam, *Mercenaria mercenaria*. *Biol Bull* 1974;**146**:343–56.
5. Cheng TC. Bivalves. In: Ratcliffe NA, Rowley AF, editors. *Invertebrate blood cells*. London: Academic Press; 1981. p. 233–300.
6. Hine PM. The inter-relationships of bivalve haemocytes. *Fish Shellfish Immunol* 1999;**9**:367–85.
7. Huffman JE, Tripp MR. Cell types and hydrolytic enzymes of soft shell clam (*Mya arenaria*) hemocytes. *J Invertebr Pathol* 1982;**40**:68–74.
8. Pipe RK. Hydrolytic enzymes associated with granular haemocytes of marine mussel *Mytilus edulis*. *Histochem J* 1990;**22**:595–603.
9. Cajaraville MP, Pal SG. Morphofunctional study of the haemocytes of the bivalve mollusc *Mytilus galloprovincialis* with emphasis on the endolysosomal compartment. *Cell Struct Funct* 1995;**20**:355–67.
10. Carballal MJ, López MC, Azevedo C, Villalba A. Hemolymph cell types of the mussel *Mytilus galloprovincialis*. *Dis Aquat Org* 1997;**29**:127–35.
11. Tripp MR. Phagocytosis by hemocytes of the hard clam, *Mercenaria mercenaria*. *J Invertebr Pathol* 1992;**59**:222–7.
12. Ford SE, Ashton-Alcox KA, Kanaley SA. Comparative cytometric and microscopic analyses of oyster hemocytes. *J Invertebr Pathol* 1994;**64**:114–22.
13. Lopez C, Carballal MJ, Azevedo C, Villalba A. Morphological characterisation of the haemocytes of the clam, *Ruditapes decussatus* (Mollusca: Bivalvia). *J Invertebr Phatol* 1997;**69**:51–7.
14. Cima F, Matozzo V, Marin MG, Ballarin L. Haemocytes of the clam *Tapes philippinarum* (Adams & Reeve, 1850): morphofunctional characterisation. *Fish Shellfish Immunol* 2000;**10**:677–93.
15. Matozzo V, Rova G, Marin MG. Haemocytes of the cockle *Cerastoderma glaucum*: morphological characterisation and involvement in immune responses. *Fish Shellfish Immunol* 2007;**23**:732–46.

16. Pampanin DM, Marin MG, Ballarin L. Morphological and cytoenzymatic characterization of haemocytes of the venus clam *Chamelea gallina*. *Dis Aquat Org* 2002;**49**:227–34.

17. Chang SJ, Tseng SM, Chou HY. Morphological characterization via light and electron microscopy of the hemocytes of two cultured bivalves: a comparison study between the hard clam (*Meretrix lusoria*) and Pacific oyster (*Crassostrea gigas*). *Zool Stud* 2005;**44**:144–53.

18. Hong HK, Kang HS, Le TC, Choi KS. Comparative study on the hemocytes of subtropical oysters *Saccostrea kegaki* (Torigoe & Inaba, 1981), *Ostrea circumpicta* (Pilsbry, 1904), and *Hyotissa hyotis* (Linnaeus, 1758) in Jeju Island, Korea: morphology and functional aspects. *Fish Shellfish Immunol* 2013;**35**:2020–5.

19. Ottaviani E, Franchini A, Barbieri D, Kletsas D. Comparative and morphofunctional studies on *Mytilus galloprovincialis* hemocytes: presence of two aging-related hemocyte stages. *Ital J Zool* 1998;**65**:349–54.

20. Jauzein C, Donaghy L, Volety AK. Flow cytometric characterization of hemocytes of the sunray venus clam *Macrocallista nimbosa* and influence of salinity variation. *Fish Shellfish Immunol* 2013;**35**:716–24.

21. Rebelo MD, Figueiredo ED, Mariante RM, Nóbrega A, de Barros CM, Allodi S. New insights from the oyster *Crassostrea rhizophorae* on bivalve circulating hemocytes. *PLoS One* 2013; **8**(2):e57384.

22. Voltzow J. Gastropoda: Prosobranchia. In: Harrison FW, Kohn AJ, editors. *Microscopic anatomy of invertebrates*. New York: Wiley-Liss Inc.; 1994. p. 111–252.

23. Martin GG, Oakes CT, Tousignant HR, Crabtree H, Yamakawa R. Structure and function of haemocytes in two marine gastropods, *Megathura crenulata* and *Aplysia californica*. *J Mollus Stud* 2007;**73**:355–65.

24. Accorsi A, Bucci L, de Eguileor M, Ottaviani E, Malagoli D. Comparative analysis of circulating hemocytes of the freshwater snail *Pomacea canaliculata*. *Fish Shellfish Immunol* 2013;**34**:1260–8.

25. Travers MA, Mirella da Silva P, Le Goïc N, Marie D, Donval A, Huchette S, et al. Morphologic, cytometric and functional characterisation of abalone (*Haliotis tuberculata*) haemocytes. *Fish Shellfish Immunol* 2008;**24**:400–11.

26. Matricon-Gondran M, Letocart M. Internal defenses of the snail *Biomphalaria glabrata* I. Characterization of haemocytes and fixed phagocytes. *J Invertebr Pathol* 1999;**74**:224–34.

27. Sminia T. Hematopoiesis in the freshwater snail *Lymnaea stagnalis* studied by electron microscopy and autoradiography. *Cell Tissue Res* 1974;**150**:443–54.

28. Sahaphong S, Linthong V, Wanichanon C, Riengrojpitak S, Kangwanrangsan N, Viyanant V, et al. Morphofunctional study of the hemocytes of *Haliotis asinina*. *J Shellfish Res* 2001;**20**: 711–6.

29. Pengsakul T, Suleiman YA, Cheng Z. Morphological and structural characterization of haemocytes of *Oncomelania hupensis* (Gastropoda: Pomatiopsidae). *Ital J Zool* 2013;**80**:494–502.

30. Di GL, Zhang ZX, Ke CH, Guo JR, Xue M, Ni JB, et al. Morphological characterization of the haemocytes of the ivory snail, *Babylonia areolata* (Neogastropoda: Buccinidae). *J Mar Biol Assoc UK* 2011;**91**:1489–97.

31. Ottaviani E. Haemocytes of the freshwater snail *Viviparus ater* (Gastropoda, Prosobranchia). *J Mollus Stud* 1989;**55**:379–82.

32. Ottaviani E, Franchini A. Ultrastructural study of haemocytes of the freshwater snail *Planorbarius corneus* (L.) (Gastropoda, Pulmonata). *Acta Zool* 1988;**69**:157–62.

33. Phillips DJH. The chemistries and environmental fates of trace metals and organochlorines in aquatic ecosystem. *Mar Pollut Bull* 1995;**31**:193–200.

34. Gagné F, Auclair J, Fortier M, Bruneau A, Fournier M, Turcotte P, et al. Bioavailability and immunotoxicity of silver nanoparticles to the freshwater mussel *Elliptio complanata*. *J Toxicol Environ Health A* 2013;**76**:767–77.

35. Canesi L, Ciacci C, Fabbri R, Marcomini A, Pojana G, Gallo G. Bivalve molluscs as a unique target group for nanoparticle toxicity. *Mar Environ Res* 2012;**76**:16–21.

36. Mydlarz LD, Jones LE, Harvell CD. Innate immunity environmental drivers and disease ecology of marine and freshwater invertebrates. *Ann Rev Ecol Evol Syst* 2006;**37**:251–88.

37. Hoek RM, Smit AB, Frings H, Vink JM, de Jong-Brink M, Geraerts WP. A new Ig-superfamily member, molluscan defence molecule (MDM) from *Lymnaea stagnalis*, is down-regulated during parasitosis. *Eur J Immunol* 1996;**26**:939–44.

38. Gust M, Fortier M, Garric J, Fournier M, Gagné F. Effects of short-term exposure to environmentally relevant concentrations of different pharmaceutical mixtures on the immune response of the pond snail *Lymnaea stagnalis*. *Sci Total Environ* 2013;**445 and 446**:210–8.

39. Kruse M, Steffen R, Batel R, Müller IM, Müller WE. Differential expression of allograft inflammatory factor 1 and of glutathione peroxidase during auto- and allograft response in marine sponges. *J Cell Sci* 1999;**112**:4305–13.

40. De Zoysa M, Nikapitiya C, Kim Y, Oh C, Kang DH, Whang I, et al. Allograft inflammatory factor-1 in disk abalone (*Haliotis discus discus*): molecular cloning, transcriptional regulation against immune challenge and tissue injury. *Fish Shellfish Immunol* 2010;**29**:319–26.

41. Matozzo V, Marin MG, Cima F, Ballarin L. First evidence of cell division in circulating haemocytes from the Manila clam *Tapes philippinarum*. *Cell Biol Int* 2008;**32**:865–8.

42. Jemaà M, Morin N, Cavelier P, Cau J, Strub JM, Delsert C. Adult somatic progenitor cells and hematopoiesis in oysters. *J Exp Biol* 2014;**217**:3067–77.

43. Binelli A, Cogni D, Parolini M, Riva C, Provini A. Cytotoxic and genotoxic effects of in vitro exposure to triclosan and trimethoprim on zebra mussel (*Dreissena polymorpha*) hemocytes. *Comp Biochem Physiol C* 2009;**150**:50–6.

44. Gust M, Gélinas M, Fortier M, Fournier M, Gagné F. *In vitro* immunotoxicity of environmentally representative antibiotics to the freshwater mussel *Elliptio complanata*. *Environ Pollut* 2012;**169**:50–8.

45. Matozzo V, Rova S, Marin MG. The nonsteroidal anti-inflammatory drug, ibuprofen, affects the immune parameters in the clam *Ruditapes philippinarum*. *Mar Environ Res* 2012;**79**:116–21.

46. Aguirre-Martínez GV, Buratti S, Fabbri E, DelValls AT, Martín-Díaz ML. Using lysosomal membrane stability of haemocytes in *Ruditapes philippinarum* as a biomarker of cellular stress to assess contamination by caffeine, ibuprofen, carbamazepine and novobiocin. *J Environ Sci* 2013;**25**:1408–18.

47. Parolini M, Binelli A, Provini A. Chronic effects induced by ibuprofen on the freshwater bivalve *Dreissena polymorpha*. *Ecotox Environ Safe* 2011;**74**:1586–94.

48. Parolini M, Binelli A, Provini A. Assessment of the potential cyto-genotoxicity of the nonsteroidal anti-inflammatory drug (NSAID) diclofenac on the zebra mussel (*Dreissena polymorpha*). *Water Air Soil Pollut* 2011;**217**:589–601.

49. Parolini M, Binelli A, Cogni D, Provini A. Multi-biomarker approach for the evaluation of the cyto-genotoxicity of paracetamol on the zebra mussel (*Dreissena polymorpha*). *Chemosphere* 2010;**79**:489–98.

50. Parolini M, Binelli A. Sub-lethal effects induced by a mixture of three non-steroidal anti-inflammatory drugs (NSAIDs) on the freshwater bivalve *Dreissena polymorpha*. *Ecotoxicology* 2012;**21**:379–92.

51. Luna-Acosta A, Renault T, Thomas-Guyon H, Faury N, Saulnier D, Budzinski H, et al. Detection of early effects of a single herbicide (diuron) and a mix of herbicides and pharmaceuticals (diuron, isoproturon, ibuprofen) on immunological parameters of Pacific oyster (*Crassostrea gigas*) spat. *Chemosphere* 2012;**87**:1335–40.
52. Canty MN, Hutchinson TH, Brown RJ, Jones MB, Jha AN. Linking genotoxic responses with cytotoxic and behavioural or physiological consequences: differential sensitivity of echinoderms (*Asterias rubens*) and marine molluscs (*Mytilus edulis*). *Aquat Toxicol* 2009;**94**:68–76.
53. Canesi L, Lorusso LC, Ciacci C, Betti M, Regoli F, Poiana G, et al. Effects of blood lipid lowering pharmaceuticals (bezafibrate and gemfibrozil) on immune and digestive gland functions of the bivalve mollusc, *Mytilus galloprovincialis*. *Chemosphere* 2007;**69**:994–1002.
54. Parolini M, Quinn B, Binelli A, Provini A. Cytotoxicity assessment of four pharmaceutical compounds on the zebra mussel (*Dreissena polymorpha*) haemocytes, gill and digestive gland primary cell cultures. *Chemosphere* 2011;**84**:91–100.
55. Franzellitti S, Fabbri E. Cyclic-AMP mediated regulation of ABCB mRNA expression in mussel haemocytes. *PLoS One* 2013;**8**(4):e61634.
56. Munari M, Marin MG, Matozzo V. Effects of the antidepressant fluoxetine on the immune parameters and acetylcholinesterase activity of the clam *Venerupis philippinarum*. *Mar Environ Res* 2014;**94**:32–7.
57. Gagné F, Blaise C, Fournier M, Hansen PD. Effects of selected pharmaceutical products on phagocytic activity in *Elliptio complanata* mussels. *Comp Biochem Physiol C* 2006;**143**:179–86.
58. Martin-Diaz L, Franzellitti S, Buratti S, Valbonesi P, Capuzzo A, Fabbri E. Effects of environmental concentrations of the antiepileptic drug carbamazepine on biomarkers and cAMP-mediated cell signaling in the mussel *Mytilus galloprovincialis*. *Aquat Toxicol* 2009;**94**:177–85.
59. Minguez L, Halm-Lemeille MP, Costil K, Bureau R, Lebel JM, Serpentini A. Assessment of cytotoxic and immunomodulatory properties of four antidepressants on primary cultures of abalone hemocytes (*Haliotis tuberculata*). *Aquat Toxicol* 2014;**153**:3–11.
60. Gaume B, Bourgougnon N, Auzoux-Bordenave S, Roig B, Le Bot B, Bedoux G. In vitro effects of triclosan and methyl-triclosan on the marine gastropod *Haliotis tuberculata*. *Comp Biochem Physiol C* 2012;**156**:87–94.
61. Matozzo V, Costa Devoti A, Marin MG. Immunotoxic effects of triclosan in the clam *Ruditapes philippinarum*. *Ecotoxicology* 2012;**21**:66–74.
62. Binelli A, Cogni D, Parolini M, Riva C, Provini A. In vivo experiments for the evaluation of genotoxic and cytotoxic effects of triclosan in zebra mussel hemocytes. *Aquat Toxicol* 2009;**91**:238–44.
63. Gust M, Fortier M, Garric J, Fournier M, Gagné F. Immunotoxicity of surface waters contaminated by municipal effluents to the snail *Lymnaea stagnalis*. *Aquat Toxicol* 2012;**126**:393–403.
64. Canesi L, Frenzilli G, Balbi T, Bernardeschi M, Ciacci C, Corsolini S, et al. Interactive effects of n-TiO$_2$ and 2,3,7,8-TCDD on the marine bivalve *Mytilus galloprovincialis*. *Aquat Toxicol* 2014;**153**:53–65.
65. Marisa I, Marin MG, Caicci F, Franceschinis E, Martucci A, Matozzo V. In vitro exposure of haemocytes of the clam *Ruditapes philippinarum* to titanium dioxide (TiO2) nanoparticles: nanoparticle characterisation, effects on phagocytic activity and internalisation of nanoparticles into haemocytes. *Mar Environ Res* 2015;**103**:11–7.
66. Barmo C, Ciacci C, Canonico B, Fabbri R, Cortese K, Balbi T, et al. In vivo effects of n-TiO$_2$ on digestive gland and immune function of the marine bivalve *Mytilus galloprovincialis*. *Aquat Toxicol* 2013;**132 and 133**:9–18.

67. Chalew TEA, Galloway JF, Graczyk TK. Pilot study on effects of nanoparticle exposure on *Crassostrea virginica* hemocyte phagocytosis. *Mar Pollut Bull* 2012;**64**:2251–3.
68. Ciacci C, Canonico B, Bilaničová D, Fabbri R, Cortese K, Gallo G, et al. Immunomodulation by different types of n-oxides in the hemocytes of the marine bivalve *Mytilus galloprovincialis*. *PLoS One* 2012;**7**(5):e36937.
69. Couleau N, Techer D, Pagnout C, Jomini S, Faocaud L, Laval-Gilly P, et al. Hemocyte responses of *Dreissena polymorpha* following a short-term *in vivo* exposure to titanium dioxide nanoparticles: preliminary investigations. *Sci Total Environ* 2012;**438**:490–7.
70. Katsumiti A, Gilliland D, Arostegui I, Cajaraville MP. Cytotoxicity and cellular mechanisms involved in the toxicity of CdS quantum dots in hemocytes and gill cells of the mussel *Mytilus galloprovincialis*. *Aquat Toxicol* 2014;**153**:39–52.
71. Rocha TL, Gomes T, Cardoso C, Letendre J, Pinheiro JP, Sousa VS, et al. Immunocytotoxicity, cytogenotoxicity and genotoxicity of cadmium-based quantum dots in the marine mussel *Mytilus galloprovincialis*. *Mar Environ Res* 2014;**101**:29–37.
72. Gagnè F, Auclair J, Turcotte P, Fournier M, Gagnon C, Sauvè S, et al. Ecotoxicity of CdTe quantum dots to freshwater mussel: impacts on immune system, oxidative stress and genotoxicity. *Aquat Toxicol* 2008;**86**:333–40.
73. Munari M, Sturve J, Frenzilli G, Sanders MB, Christian P, Nigro M, et al. Genotoxic effects of Ag_2S and CdS nanoparticles in blue mussel (*Mytilus edulis*) haemocytes. *Chem Ecol* 2014;**30**:719–25.
74. Gomes T, Araújo O, Pereira R, Almeida AC, Cravo A, Bebianno MJ. Genotoxicity of copper oxide and silver nanoparticles in the mussel *Mytilus galloprovincialis*. *Mar Environ Res* 2013;**84**:51–9.
75. Roh JY, Sim SJ, Yi J, Park K, Chung KH, Ryu DY, et al. Ecotoxicity of silver nanoparticles on the soil nematode *Caenorhabditis elegans* using functional ecotoxicogenomics. *Environ Sci Technol* 2009;**43**:3933–40.
76. Hannam ML, Bamber SD, Sundt RC, Galloway TS. Immune modulation in the blue mussel *Mytilus edulis* exposed to North Sea produced water. *Environ Pollut* 2009;**157**:1939–44.
77. Donaghy L, Lambert C, Choi K-S, Soudant P. Hemocytes of the carpet shell clam (*Ruditapes decussatus*) and the Manila clam (*Ruditapes philippinarum*): current knowledge and future prospects. *Aquaculture* 2009;**297**:10–24.
78. Matozzo V, Giacomazzo M, Finos L, Marin MG, Bargelloni L, Milan M. Can ecological history influence immunomarker responses and antioxidant enzyme activities in bivalves that have been experimentally exposed to contaminants? A new subject for discussion in "eco-immunology" studies. *Fish Shellfish Immunol* 2013;**35**:126–35.
79. Brousseau-Fournier C, Alix G, Beaudry A, Gauthier-Clerc S, Duchemin M, Fortier M, et al. Role of confounding factors in assessing immune competence of bivalves (*Mya arenaria, Mytilus edulis*) exposed to pollutants. *J Xenobiotics* 2013;**3**(s1):e2. 3–5.
80. Matozzo V, Marin MG. First evidence of gender-related differences in immune parameters of the clam *Ruditapes philippinarum* (Mollusca, Bivalvia). *Mar Biol* 2010;**157**:1181–9.
81. Fraser M, Rault P, Roumier P-H, Fortier M, André C, Brousseau P, et al. Decrease in phagocytosis capacity of hemocyte during spawning in *Mytilus edulis*: a pilot study. *J Xenobiotics* 2013;**3**(1S):e12. 31–3.
82. Fraser M, Rault P, Fortier M, Brousseau P, Fournier M, Surette C, et al. Immune response of blue mussels (*Mytilus edulis*) in spawning period following exposure to metals. *J Xenobiotics* 2014;**4**(4895):65–7.
83. Alix G, Beaudry A, Brousseau-Fournier C, Fortier M, Auffret M, Fournier M, et al. Increase sensitivity to metals of hemocytes obtained from *Mya arenaria* collected at different distances from the shore. *J Xenobiotics* 2013;**3**(1S):e11;29–30.

84. Beaudry A, Brousseau-Fournier C, Alix G, Fortier M, Auffret M, Brousseau P, et al. Influence of tidal stress on the immunocompetence of hemocytes in soft-shell clam (*Mya arenaria*). *J Xenobiotics* 2013;**3**(1S):e13;34–5.

85. Gagné F, Blaise C, Pellerin J, Fournier M, Gagnon C, Sherry J, et al. Impacts of pollution in feral *Mya arenaria* populations: the effects of clam bed distance from the shore. *Sci Total Environ* 2009;**407**:5844–54.

86. Matozzo V, Binelli A, Parolini M, Previato M, Masiero L, Finos L, et al. Biomarker responses in the clam *Ruditapes philippinarum* and contamination levels in sediments from seaward and landward sites in the Lagoon of Venice. *Ecol Indic* 2012;**19**:191–205.

87. Brousseau P, Pillet S, Frouin H, Auffret M, Gagné F, Fournier M. Linking immunotoxicity and ecotoxicological effects at higher biological levels. In: Amiard-Triquet C, Amiard J-C, Rainbow PS, editors. *Ecological biomarkers: indicators of ecotoxicological effects*. Boca Raton: CRC Press; 2012. p. 131–54.

88. Blaise C, Gagné F, Pellerin J. Bivalve population status and biomarker responses in *Mya arenaria* clams (Saguenay Fjord, Quebec, Canada). *Fresenius Environ Bull* 2003;**12**:956–60.

89. Gagné F, Blaise C, Pellerin J, Fournier M, Durand MJ, Talbot A. Relationships between intertidal clam population and health status of the soft-shell clam *Mya arenaria* in the St. Lawrence Estuary and Saguenay Fjord (Québec, Canada). *Environ Int* 2008;**34**:30–42.

Chapter 4

New Aspects of Earthworm Innate Immunity: Novel Molecules and Old Proteins With Unexpected Functions

Péter Engelmann
University of Pécs, Pécs, Hungary

Yuya Hayashi
Aarhus University, Aarhus, Denmark; Karlsruhe Institute of Technology (KIT), Karlsruhe, Germany

Kornélia Bodó, László Molnár
University of Pécs, Pécs, Hungary

ESSENTIALS OF EARTHWORM IMMUNITY: A CONCISE INTRODUCTION

Earthworms as a Research Model in Life Sciences

Invertebrates are the major components of marine, freshwater, and terrestrial communities. Some invertebrates such as earthworms (Annelida, Clitellata, Oligochaeta) are frequently referred to as ecosystem engineers for their pivotal role in maintaining ecosystem wellness. Indeed, the mystery of earthworms' key role in soil formation was what excited Charles Darwin most in his late scientific career.[1] Earthworms are found worldwide, their life cycles are short, and they have a wide temperature and moisture tolerance range,[2] which has made them a popular research model in environmental biology. They are also sensitive to environmental contamination,[3-5] and together these factors are favored by researchers and regulators in ecotoxicology. To this end, the two closely related species *Eisenia andrei* and *Eisenia fetida* have been recommended by the Organisation for Economic Co-operation and Development since 1984 for toxicity testing of chemicals in soil environments.[6] Earthworms are, however, less evident research subjects in other life science areas. For instance, several

Lessons in Immunity: From Single-Cell Organisms to Mammals
http://dx.doi.org/10.1016/B978-0-12-803252-7.00004-7
53

studies have attempted to dissect the immune components of earthworms, but the precise molecular data are relatively limited compared to other "classical" invertebrate model organisms such as the *Drosophila* fruit fly or the nematode *Caenorhabditis elegans*.[7,8] In this chapter, we focus on this facet of earthworms, and by reviewing the state of the art, we aim to present the knowledge gap as well as future perspectives in earthworm innate immunity.

Historical Foundation of Earthworm Immunity Research

Historically, earthworm immunity was established upon the morphological observations and descriptions of the cellular elements harbored in the coelomic cavity (so-called coelomocytes) by Cuénot, Rosa, and Liebmann.[9]

Earthworm immune mechanisms were further evidenced in connection with transplantation experiments. As one of the pioneers in invertebrate immunology, Edwin L. Cooper observed graft rejections when body wall tissues were exchanged as allograft or xenograft in earthworms.[10,11] Interestingly, in the course of graft rejection, mononuclear cells invaded the grafting area indicating the direct involvement of immune cells in this process.[12]

In contrast to other invertebrate models (cnidarians and ascidians) that provided precise data about the molecular recognition involved during tissue rejection,[13,14] the molecular basis of the self/nonself recognition of grafted tissues in earthworms is largely unexplored.

Following the established roots, several research groups have been organized in different locations (France, Germany, Czech Republic).[15–17]

Major Constituents of Earthworm Immune Response

Earthworm immune components consist of cellular and humoral elements (antimicrobial and pattern recognition molecules)[7,8,18–20] located in the coelomic cavity (Fig. 4.1). Previously, we have characterized the coelomocyte subpopulations (hyaline amoebocytes, granular amoebocytes, and eleocytes) using cytochemical, immunological (applying specific monoclonal antibodies, mAbs), and functional approaches.[21–25] With respect to the functions, hyaline and granular amoebocytes are capable of phagocytosis[26] and encapsulation although granular amoebocytes engulf less foreign particles than hyaline cells do[27] (Fig. 4.2A). Eleocytes show no phagocytic activities,[28] but they undertake metabolic functions as well as the production of bioactive molecules.[29,30] In addition, cellular cytotoxic effects of coelomocytes have been demonstrated in xenogeneic and allogeneic cultures.[31,32]

In parallel to those cellular studies, the humoral counterpart—molecular components of coelomic fluid—have been examined extensively. For example, it is now known that earthworm coelomic fluid possesses a wide range of biological functions in addition to antimicrobial activities,[20] including mitogenic, antioxidative, proteolytic, hemolytic, cytotoxic, and nutritive activities.[8,33,34]

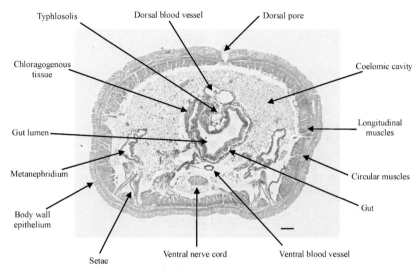

FIGURE 4.1 Cross section of an *Eisenia andrei* earthworm. Main organs and tissues are marked. Hematoxylin-eosin staining. Note that the coelomic cavity is filled with coelomocytes. Scale bar: 100 μm.

In the following sections, we provide a quick snapshot of the novel findings that have drastically advanced our understanding of cellular and humoral immune functions in earthworms.

"STARS AND STRIPES" OR PATTERN RECOGNITION IN EARTHWORMS

Coelomic Cytolytic Factor: The Unique Earthworm Pattern Recognition Receptors

Innate immune response is the first line of active defense against infections. Germ line-encoded receptors are the key elements to initiate the immune response by recognizing conserved molecular motifs from both exogenous and endogenous sources. Pattern recognition receptors (PRRs) can be subdivided into various classes[35]: Toll-like receptors (TLRs), peptidoglycan recognition receptors (PGRPs), nucleotide-binding leucine-rich repeat containing receptors (NLRs), retinoic acid-inducible gene I (RIG-I)-like receptors (RLRs), C-type lectins, and scavenger receptors (SRs).

Until recently, only one unique type of PRR was known from *Eisenia* earthworms, and it has been designated as coelomic cytolytic factor 1 (CCF1).[36] Interestingly, this 42 kDa protein contains lipopolysaccharide, peptidoglycan, and β-1,3-glucan/N,N'-diacetylchitobiose-binding domains. Basically, this means CCF is able to bind a wide range of microbes, including gram-positive and

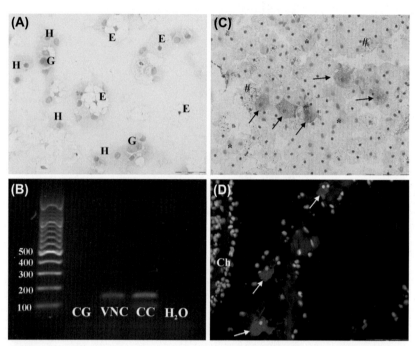

FIGURE 4.2   Elements of earthworm immunity: coelomocytes, pattern recognition receptors, and humoral factors. (A) Free-floating coelomocyte subtypes harbored in the coelomic cavity: hyaline amoebocytes (H), granular amoebocytes (G), and eleocytes (E). Hematoxylin-eosin staining, scale bar: 50 μm. (B) Toll-like receptor expression is demonstrated (targeting the Toll/interleukin-1 receptor domain) in the neural tissues and coelomocytes of *Eisenia* earthworms by semiquantitative RT-PCR. (To avoid any contamination, sequential isolation steps were performed: first, coelomocytes were isolated. Next the chloragogenous tissue was removed, and then the gut was detached. At last the nerve cord was removed. Between the steps careful washings with a *Lumbricus*-balanced salt solution buffer were performed.) *CG*, cerebral ganglion; *VNC*, ventral nerve cord; *CC*, coelomocytes. (C) Lysenin expression is restricted mainly to eleocytes (*arrows*) among free-floating coelomocytes, while some eleocytes are negative (*number signs*). Hyaline amoebocytes are consistently negative (*asterisks*). Immunocytochemical staining is performed by lysenin specific a-EFCC5 monoclonal antibody. Hematoxylin counterstaining, scale bar: 100 μm. (D) Sessile chloragocytes (Ch) are negative for lysenin demonstrated by immunofluorescence staining on the earthworm cross section. Only free-floating coelomocytes (*arrows*) were labeled with the polyclonal antilysenin antibody. DAPI counterstaining, scale bar: 200 μm.

gram-negative bacteria and yeast.[36] Homologues of CCF have been described for other earthworm species such as *Lumbricus terrestris*, *Lumbricus rubellus*, and *Dendrobaena veneta* with certain differences in the domain structures compared to *Eisenia* sp. that could be explained by the different ecology of this species.[37] It has been postulated that CCF initiates the prophenoloxidase cascade; however, this effector mechanism seems to be not so efficient in earthworms compared to other invertebrates (eg, arthropods).[38,39]

Variations on a Theme: Not Just Coelomic Cytolytic Factor Anymore

In contrast to other invertebrate models, TLRs were described relatively belatedly in annelids.[40] The first evidence of the presence of TLRs in annelids was derived during the genome analysis of *Capitella* polychaeta and *Helobdella* hirudean species.[41] In addition, neural regeneration experiments revealed the expression of TLR (and NLR) in leeches.[42] Finally, diverse coding sequences of TLRs were cloned from the coelomocytes of *E. andrei*.[43] Protein prediction analysis has presumed that this earthworm TLR contains seven extracellular leucine-rich repeats. Bacterial challenge modulated the level of TLR transcripts; however, it was only significant in the case of the *Bacillus subtilis* treatment.[43] Besides this information, the exact ligand specificity of these TLRs is not yet known.

Meanwhile, genome amplification experiments of *D. veneta* revealed several homologous sequences that proved the conservation of TLRs among various earthworm species.[44]

Toll-like Receptors Expression in Nonimmune Tissues

It is known that the expression of TLRs (and other PRRs) is not restricted to the hematopoietic tissues, but it is present in the central nervous system (CNS) as well.[45] Similar trends can be observed in invertebrates, as we mentioned earlier (TLR molecules are present in leech CNS).[42] In fact, several different organs express TLRs in earthworms,[43] but whether these molecules are located in extracellular and/or intracellular membranes remains unanswered. Our initial results correspond to the TLR expression in the coelomocytes of *E. andrei* (Fig. 4.2B). Additionally, we confirmed Toll/interleukin-1 receptor (TIR) transcript expression in the peripheral nerve cord but not in the cerebral ganglion. This result complements those findings in leech that also demonstrated PRR expression in nonimmune tissues.[46]

Another interesting question relates to the task of TLRs. The function of this ectopic TLR is still a matter to be investigated. This book is dedicated entirely to the evolution of immunity; yet we should not forget that Toll was initially described as a dorsoventral body plan determining factor involved in fruit fly development.[47] Until now, very limited information has been available for the evolutionary conservation of Toll in this developmental process.[48]

LYSENIN: A MULTITASKING PROTEIN IN *EISENIA* EARTHWORMS

Cellular Expression of Lysenin

Earthworm coelomic fluid is rich in bioactive molecules; however, its exact nature and full spectrum is still only partly understood. One major constituent of the coelomic fluid is a sphingomyelin (and phosphocholine)-binding protein family[49] consisting of lysenin, lysenin-related proteins, and fetidin. They are known to have cytotoxic, hemolytic, and smooth muscle contraction activities.[51] Initially, lysenin was described as a smooth muscle contraction protein from coelomic fluid. Following studies revealed that lysenin mediates (temperature-dependent) hemolysis, and it strongly targets erythrocytes of sheep rather than those of humans or rats. Its cytotoxicity was reported for insect hemocytes, vertebrate fibroblasts, and tumor cells but not against *Lumbricus* coelomocytes or molluskan hemocytes.[50] An interesting remark is, however, that the presence of sphingomyelin is limited to vertebrate taxa, and all those sphingomyelin-targeted activities of lysenin demand further explanations in an ecophysiological context in earthworms. An in situ hybridization study showed that its expression was restricted to the central chloragocytes (chloragocytes located in the typhlosolis, as opposed to peripheral chloragocytes facing to the coelomic cavity).[51] In contrast, our immunohistochemical analysis (applying in-house-raised a-lysenin mAb designated as a-EFCC5) revealed that subgroups of free-floating coelomocytes (in particular the eleocytes) were lysenin-expressing cells (Fig. 4.2C).[52] Central chloragocytes located in the typhlosolis were consistently negative in our experiments when we applied our mAb or the commercially available a-lysenin polyclonal antibody (Fig. 4.2D). To resolve this discrepancy, one could hypothesize that the expression of lysenin mRNA in the central chloragocytes exists only during their maturation, and the mature, free-floating chloragocytes (eleocytes) undertake its transcription. Indeed, this is an option to consider, however, there is no experimental evidence to prove this idea. Moreover, the exact origin of eleocytes was debated.[9] Some literature claims that eleocytes are free-floating chloragocytes derived from the sessile chloragogenous tissue[53]; yet this hypothesis needs to be supported by robust experimental observations.[54]

Antimicrobial Induction of Lysenin

In parallel to lysenin, another bioactive protein harbored in the coelomic fluid was described and named fetidin.[55] Although it was thought to be a new molecule, it turned out that this molecule shared strong molecular homology with lysenin. Now it is considered that in earthworms, lysenin belongs to a multiprotein family with at least four members sharing molecular homology.[56] Little is known about lysenin's antimicrobial activity, but the bacterial challenge of the coelomocytes seems to trigger the expression of lysenin. Interestingly, gram-positive bacteria exposure evoked increased lysenin expression in coelomocytes, while exposure to gram-negative bacteria attenuated the level of lysenin expression.[53] In support of our observation of the latter, a mass spectrometry-based proteomic study revealed that the expression of lysenin was also suppressed in vivo upon *Escherichia coli* challenge.[57] Furthermore, when different culture (soil) conditions were applied to earthworms, there was a fluctuation in the transcriptional profile of lysenin suggesting that lysenin is a stress-induced factor.[4]

Inhibitors and Possible Regulators of Lysenin-Mediated Cell Lysis

Screening of natural products has uncovered candidates for possible inhibitors of lysenin oligomerization and lysenin-evoked cell lysis.[58] Among 1580 samples a plant- and a microorganism-derived compound retain the potential inhibition of lysenin's action. Interestingly enough, it is not known what type of inhibitory molecules exist in the earthworms themselves to rescue self-structures from unintended pore formation by lysenin. Indeed, the lack of sphingomyelin in the membranes would explain this issue. Yet, earthworms are equipped with inhibitors of pore-forming molecules (eg, eiseniapore) in general.[59] Amoebapores and perforin are among the functional homologues of lysenin. Perforin is a well-known lytic protein secreted by NK-cells and cytotoxic T-lymphocytes.[60] Indeed, effector immune cells should be rescued from self-damage after releasing the cytotoxic content of their cytoplasmic granules. Now, it is known that lysosomal proteases are anchored to the membrane of the effector immune cells, and these proteases, namely cathepsins, are able to diminish the self-destruction effect of the secreted perforin.[60] Cathepsins are a conserved group of proteases described in many species. Cathepsin B is the most typical member of this extensive molecular family involved in this process; however, other cathepsins also participate in the immune response (eg, intracellular antigen processing). Cathepsin L from the leech *Theromyzon tessulatum* is involved in the phagocytic response,[61] and homologues with a similar role probably exist in other annelids including earthworms. However, whether any of the postulated cathepsins have a regulatory role in the inhibition of the lysenin-mediated cytotoxic process is only a hypothesis that should be experimentally proven.

LYSENIN MEETS NANOPARTICLES: UNEXPECTED RISE OF A NEW FUNCTION

Lysenin and the Concept of the Biomolecular Corona

It was a great surprise when the multitasking protein lysenin revealed yet another role in immunity toward nanoparticles. This relatively new finding was first uncovered by a simple experiment in which nanosized particles of silver were incubated with secretory proteins from *E. fetida*.[62] The study sought a unique interaction of earthworm proteins with nanoparticles, for we knew that an array of different types of biomolecules (mainly proteins) binds to a nanoparticle spontaneously forming a biomolecule–nanoparticle complex or a "biomolecular corona." The theory and experimental evidence of biomolecular coronas around nanoparticles have been an active area of bionanoscience research and are well documented elsewhere.[63] Although those observations were limited to mammalian proteins (mostly human plasma/serum proteins and fetal bovine serum (FBS) proteins), the universal tendency seems to be preferential binding of lipoproteins and immunological proteins such as opsonins (immunoglobulins and complement proteins), coagulation proteins, and acute-phase proteins.[64]

Much less known, however, is how proteins from invertebrate organisms behave when they meet nanoparticles. The proteomes that nanoparticles encounter can differ in many aspects from the spatiotemporal profile of the animal's physiology to species differences in the protein repertoire. To examine the latter in this context using earthworms, we focused on the immune-competent fluid in which immunocytes reside and circulate: the coelomic fluid in comparison to FBS.[62]

The High Affinity of Lysenin for Silver Nanoparticles

Two methods were examined for the harvesting of coelomic fluid proteins, and we concluded that secreted proteins from a primary culture of *E. fetida* coelomocytes were favored for our experimental purposes and reproducibility rather than the conventional method of needle-aspiration of the coelomic fluid.[62] In both cases, lysenin was one of the two major constituents of the coelomic fluid proteins, as anticipated from the relative abundance of lysenin-producing eleocytes among the coelomocyte subpopulations.[52] More striking is the selective enrichment of lysenin at silver nanoparticles following incubation of the nanoparticles in the secretory proteins from the coelomocytes.[62] The strong binding of lysenin was surprisingly explicit since it was only the family of lysenin and a few minor proteins that were "fished" by silver nanoparticles leaving the other major proteins behind. In general, abundant proteins are frequently found in the nanoparticle's coronas as they have higher chances to encounter the nanoparticle surface than minor proteins do. The classical theory of the Vroman effect[65] can be readily applied here, by which sequential replacement of bound proteins occurs according to the relative abundance and the affinity for the surface. To test the high affinity of lysenin, we incubated the nanoparticles in a biased mixture of secretory coelomic proteins (low abundance) and FBS (high abundance) and observed a gradual accumulation of lysenin over time, likely displacing the early arriving proteins such as serum albumin.[62] The implication is that lysenin is not adsorbing to silver nanoparticles purely by its relative abundance but rather by a specific parameter, which makes it favorable to adsorb. Currently, we do not know the mechanism behind this selective binding, as lysenin's crystal structure (RCSB Protein Data Bank ID: 3ZXD)[49] does not provide any clues on particular sites of potential silver-specific association (eg, via cysteine-rich pockets). We do, however, speculate that the unique hydropathicity profile of lysenin (eg, alternate hydrophilic/hydrophobic residue sequence[49]) may allow the local enrichment of the protein at silver nanoparticles.

The Unexpected Role of Lysenin in the Accumulation of Nanoparticles

As mentioned earlier, earthworms have acquired an ability to opsonize microbial particles by means of the extracellular receptor protein CCF, of which two motifs encompass a versatile pattern recognition repertoire.[7] The production of melanin downstream of the CCF-triggered prophenoloxidase cascade has been considered responsible for the subsequent phagocytosis of the opsonized particles.[7] Surprisingly, upon incubation of synthetic particles in the coelomic fluid, CCF was also deposited onto the particle surface in a manner that was recognizable by CCF-specific monoclonal antibodies (ie, CCF was adsorbed without a significant loss of its native conformation).[66] This adhesion capability of CCF was an early (and to our knowledge, only) example of pattern recognition-independent opsonization of nonbiological particles. Using secretory proteins from coelomocytes (which were comparable to needle-aspirated coelomic fluid proteins), we preformed coronas of the coelomic proteins (or recombinant lysenin) on silver nanoparticles and showed that coelomocytes accumulated those nanoparticles significantly more than when the coronas were preformed of FBS.[62] Notably, when recombinant lysenin was used in place of the coelomic proteins, the accumulation was even greater in eleocytes in comparison to amoebocyte populations (capable of phagocytosis).[62] In our previous transmission electron microscopic study, similar-sized silver nanoparticles were clearly visible in the intracellular compartments of amoebocytic cells but not in eleocytes, suggesting the importance of phagocytic activities over receptor-mediated endocytosis.[67] Although the precise mechanism remains unclear, it seems likely that lysenin is involved in opsonization-induced cellular interactions of silver nanoparticles and that the related mechanism may not be the same between amoebocytes and eleocytes (Fig. 4.3). The local enrichment of lysenin

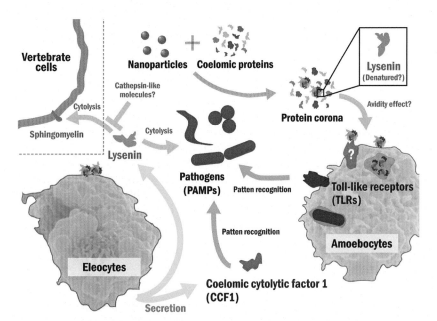

FIGURE 4.3 **A schematic illustrating the novel and known pattern recognition strategies involved in earthworm immunity toward environmental pathogens and foreign materials (nanoparticles).** Headings with question marks represent the mechanisms that are less understood in the course of immune response in earthworms.

at silver nanoparticles would certainly facilitate the presentation of repetitive motifs (or avidity effect[68]) that may possibly be detected by known or unidentified pattern recognition machinery of the coelomocytes. Interestingly, our latest study revealed a negative feedback cycle of *lysenin* expression and time-lagged induction of the *TLR* in the coelomocytes exposed to a low-cytotoxic concentration of silver nanoparticles.[69] As yet, we do not know whether there is a biological link between the two phenomena or if the contrasting regulation of the two genes is simply an independent response. Given that lysenin is a pore-forming protein that works in an oligomerization state,[67] it may be interesting to study whether it could act as a "find-me/eat-me" signal to guide scavenger cells for immediate phagocytic clearance. Lysenin is an old molecule into which many researchers have long dug in search of novel medicine, but its original role in earthworm immunity is much less understood. This unexpected finding of lysenin's role toward nanoparticles begins to illuminate its unexplored facet in immunity.

CONCLUSIONS AND PERSPECTIVES

Undoubtedly, these new discoveries have given a tremendous boost to earthworm immunity research. Although rapidly emerging, the available molecular data are as yet scarce. For instance, the aforementioned novel findings related to Toll would certainly advance the research of earthworm immunity to discover Toll ligands and mediators of intracellular signaling following Toll receptor/ligand engagements. Moreover, TLRs are just one characteristic group of PRRs, and we should keep in mind that the other PRRs (eg, PGRPs, NLRs, RLRs, and SRs) are also conserved in the course of evolution. They can be considered as potential but undiscovered candidates involved in earthworm immunity against extracellular and intracellular pathogens. Last, the unexpected observation of lysenin's strong interaction with silver nanoparticles and subsequent cellular association has driven us to rethink its original role in earthworm immunity. The emergence of new earthworm PRRs would also offer intriguing insights into how nanoparticles are detected via ligand–receptor interactions. The unique and conserved recognition strategies reviewed here have certainly opened up new research avenues and potentially harbor an intriguing clue for better elucidating the vertebrate immune response toward various antigens.

ACKNOWLEDGMENTS

We gratefully acknowledge the financial support of the Medical Faculty Research Foundation, University of Pécs (PTE-ÁOK-KA 34039/10-06 and 2013/09), the János Bolyai Research Scholarship of the Hungarian Academy of Sciences, and the Danish Council for Independent Research. The present scientific contribution is dedicated to the 650th anniversary of the foundation of the University of Pécs, Hungary. We also thank the helpful comments of the anonymous reviewer to improve our work.

REFERENCES

1. Darwin CR. In: Murray J, editor. *The formation of vegetable mould, through the action of worms.* 1883. London.
2. Dominguez J. State-of-the-art and new perspectives on vermicomposting research. In: Edwards CA, editor. *Earthworm ecology.* Boca Raton: CRC Press; 2004. p. 401–24.
3. Spurgeon DJ, Hopkin SP. Tolerance to zinc in populations of the earthworms *Lumbricus rubellus* from uncontaminated and metal-contaminated ecosystems. *Arch Environ Contam Toxicol* 1999;**37**:332–7.
4. Brulle F, Mitta G, Cocquerelle C, Vieau D, Lemière S, Leprêtre A, et al. Cloning and real-time PCR testing of 14 potential biomarkers in *Eisenia fetida* following cadmium exposure. *Environ Sci Technol* 2006;**40**:2844–50.
5. Ricketts HJ, Morgan AJ, Spurgeon DJ, Kille P. Measurement of annetocin gene expression: a new reproductive biomarker in earthworm ecotoxicology. *Ecotoxicol Environ Saf* 2004;**57**: 4–10.
6. OECD. *OECD guideline for testing chemicals. Section 2: effects on biotic systems. Method, 207. Earthworm, acute toxicity tests.* Paris (France). 1984.
7. Bilej M, Procházková P, Silerová M, Josková R. Earthworm immunity. *Adv Exp Med Biol* 2010;**708**:66–79.
8. Cooper EL, Kauschke E, Cossarizza A. Digging for innate immunity since Darwin and Metchnikoff. *Bioessays* 2002;**24**:319–33.
9. Liebmann E. The coelomocytes of Lumbricidae. *J Morphol* 1942;**71**:221–49.
10. Cooper EL. Transplantation immunity in annelids-I. Rejection of xenografts exchanged between *Lumbricus terrestris* and *Eisenia foetida*. *Transplantation* 1968;**6**:322–37.
11. Cooper EL. Chronic allograft rejection in *Lumbricus terrestris*. *J Exp Zool* 1969;**171**:69–73.
12. Cooper EL, Roch P. Earthworm leukocyte interactions during early stages of graft rejection. *J Exp Zool* 1984;**232**:67–72.
13. Voskoboynik A, Newman AM, Corey DM, Sahoo D, Pushkarev D, Neff NF, et al. Identification of a colonial chordate histocompatibility gene. *Science* 2013;**341**:384–7.
14. Rosengarten RD, Nicotra ML. Model systems of invertebrate allorecognition. *Curr Biol* 2011;**21**:82–92.
15. Roch P, Valembois P. Evidence for concanavalin A-receptors and their redistribution on lumbricid leukocytes. *Dev Comp Immunol* 1978;**2**:51–63.
16. Mohrig W, Kauschke E, Ehlers M. Rosette formation of the coelomocytes of the earthworm *Lumbricus terrestris* L. with sheep erythrocytes. *Dev Comp Immunol* 1984;**8**:471–6.
17. Tucková L, Rejnek J, Síma P, Ondrejová R. Lytic activities in coelomic fluid of *Eisenia foetida* and *Lumbricus terrestris*. *Dev Comp Immunol* 1986;**10**:181–9.
18. Jarosz J, Gliński Z. Earthworm immune responses. *Folia Biol (Krakow)* 1997;**45**:1–9.
19. Cooper EL. Earthworm immunity. *Prog Mol Subcell Biol* 1996;**15**:10–45.
20. Bilej M, De Baetselier P, Beschin A. Antimicrobial defense of the earthworm. *Folia Microbiol (Praha)* 2000;**45**:283–300.
21. Engelmann P, Molnár L, Pálinkás L, Cooper EL, Németh P. Earthworm leukocyte populations specifically harbor lysosomal enzymes that may respond to bacterial challenge. *Cell Tissue Res* 2004;**316**:391–401.
22. Engelmann P, Pálinkás L, Cooper EL, Németh P. Monoclonal antibodies identify four distinct annelid leukocyte markers. *Dev Comp Immunol* 2005;**29**:599–614.
23. Opper B, Németh P, Engelmann P. Calcium is required for coelomocyte activation in earthworms. *Mol Immunol* 2010;**47**:2047–56.

24. Engelmann P, Cooper EL, Opper B, Németh P. Earthworm innate immune system. In: Karaca A, editor. *Biology of earthworms*. Berlin Heidelberg: Springer Verlag; 2011. p. 229–45.
25. Engelmann P, Cooper EL, Németh P. Anticipating innate immunity without a Toll. *Mol Immunol* 2005;**42**:931–42.
26. Fuller-Espie SL. Using flow cytometry to measure phagocytic uptake in earthworms. *J Microbiol Biol Educ* 2010;**11**:144–51.
27. Cooper EL, Stein EA. Oligochaeta. In: Ratcliffe NA, Rowley AF, editors. *Invertebrate blood cells*. San Diego: Academic Press; 1981. p. 75–140.
28. Stein E, Avtalion RR, Cooper EL. The coelomocytes of the earthworm *Lumbricus terrestris*: morphology and phagocytic properties. *J Morphol* 1977;**153**:467–77.
29. Valembois P, Roch P, Lasségues M, Cassand P. Antibacterial activity of the haemolytic system from the earthworm *Eisenia fetida andrei*. *J Invertebr Pathol* 1982;**40**:21–7.
30. Çotuk A, Dales RP. Lysozyme activity in the coelomic fluid and coelomocytes of the earthworm *Eisenia foetida* Sav., in relation to bacterial infection. *Comp Biochem Physiol* 1984;**78A**: 469–74.
31. Cossarizza A, Cooper EL, Suzuki MM, Salvioli S, Capri M, Gri G, et al. Earthworm leukocytes that are not phagocytic and cross-react with several human epitopes can kill human tumor cell lines. *Exp Cell Res* 1996;**224**:174–82.
32. Suzuki MM, Cooper EL. Allogeneic killing by earthworm effector cells. *Nat Immun* 1995;**14**:11–9.
33. Hrzenjak T, Hrzenjak M, Kasuba V, Efenberger-Marinculić P, Levanat S. A new source of biologically active compounds–earthworm tissue (*Eisenia foetida, Lumbricus rubellus*). *Comp Biochem Physiol* 1992;**102A**:441–7.
34. Kauschke E, Mohrig W, Cooper EL. Coelomic fluid proteins as basic components of innate immunity in earthworms. *Eur J Soil Biol* 2007;**43**:110–5.
35. Bryant CE, Monie TP. Mice, men and the relatives: cross-species studies underpin innate immunity. *Open Biol* 2012;**2**:120015.
36. Beschin A, Bilej M, Hanssens F, Raymakers J, Van Dyck E, Drevets H, et al. Identification and cloning of a glucan- and LPS-binding protein from *Eisenia fetida* earthworms involved in the activation of prophenoloxidase cascade. *J Biol Chem* 1998;**273**:24948–54.
37. Silerová M, Procházková P, Josková R, Josens G, Beschin A, De Baetselier P, et al. Comparative study of the CCF-like pattern recognition protein in different Lumbricid species. *Dev Comp Immunol* 2006;**30**:765–71.
38. Procházková P, Silerová M, Stijlemans B, Dieu M, Halada P, Josková R, et al. Evidence for proteins involved in prophenoloxidase cascade *Eisenia fetida* earthworms. *J Comp Physiol B* 2006;**176**:581–7.
39. Beschin A, Bilej M, Brys L, Torreele E, Lucas R, Magez S, et al. Convergent evolution of cytokines. *Nature* 1999;**400**:627–8.
40. Cooper EL, Kvell K, Engelmann P, Nemeth P. Still waiting for the toll? *Immunol Lett* 2006;**104**:18–28.
41. Davidson CR, Best NM, Francis JW, Cooper EL, Wood TC. Toll-like receptor genes (TLRs) from *Capitella capitata* and *Helobdella robusta* (Annelida). *Dev Comp Immunol* 2008;**32**: 608–12.
42. Cuvillier-Hot V, Boidin-Wichlacz C, Slomianny C, Salzet M, Tasiemski A. Characterization and immune function of two intracellular sensors, HmTLR1 and HmNLR, in the injured CNS of an invertebrate. *Dev Comp Immunol* 2011;**35**:214–26.
43. Škanta F, Roubalová R, Dvořák J, Procházková P, Bilej M. Molecular cloning and expression of TLR in the *Eisenia andrei* earthworm. *Dev Comp Immunol* 2013;**41**:694–702.

44. Fjøsne TF, Stenseth EB, Myromslien F, Rudi K. Gene expression of TLR homologues identified by genome-wide screening of the earthworm *Dendrobaena veneta*. *Innate Immun* 2015;**21**:161–6.
45. Kielian T. Overview of toll-like receptors in the CNS. *Curr Top Microbiol Immunol* 2009;**336**:1–14.
46. Schikorski D, Cuvillier-Hot V, Boidin-Wichlacz C, Slomianny C, Salzet M, Tasiemski A. Deciphering the immune function and regulation by a TLR of the cytokine EMAPII in the lesioned central nervous system using a leech model. *J Immunol* 2009;**183**:7119–28.
47. Anderson KV, Bokla L, Nüsslein-Volhard C. Establishment of dorsal-ventral polarity in the Drosophila embryo: the induction of polarity by the Toll gene product. *Cell* 1985;**42**:791–8.
48. Imler JL, Zheng L. Biology of Toll receptors: lessons from insects and mammals. *J Leukoc Biol* 2004;**75**:18–26.
49. De Colibus L, Sonnen Andreas FP, Morris Keith J, Siebert CA, Abrusci P, Plitzko J, et al. Structures of lysenin reveal a shared evolutionary origin for pore-forming proteins and its mode of sphingomyelin recognition. *Structure* 2012;**20**:1498–507.
50. Kobayashi H, Ohta N, Umeda M. Biology of lysenin, a protein in the coelomic fluid of the earthworm *Eisenia foetida*. *Int Rev Cytol* 2004;**236**:45–99.
51. Ohta N, Shioda S, Sekizawa Y, Nakai Y, Kobayashi H. Sites of expression of mRNA for lysenin, a protein isolated from the coelomic fluid of the earthworm *Eisenia foetida*. *Cell Tissue Res* 2000;**302**:263–70.
52. Opper B, Bognár A, Heidt D, Németh P, Engelmann P. Revising lysenin expression of earthworm coelomocytes. *Dev Comp Immunol* 2013;**39**:214–8.
53. Jamieson BGM. Chloragocytes. In: Jamieson BGM, editor. *The ultrastructure of the oligochaete*. New York: Academic Press; 1981. p. 96–118.
54. Homa J, Bzowska M, Klimek M, Plytycz B. Flow cytometric quantification of proliferating coelomocytes non-invasively retrieved from the earthworm, *Dendrobaena veneta*. *Dev Comp Immunol* 2008;**32**:9–14.
55. Lassegues M, Milochau A, Doignon F, Du Pasquier L, Valembois P. Sequence and expression of an *Eisenia fetida*-derived cDNA clone that encodes the 40-kDa fetidin antibacterial protein. *Eur J Biochem* 1997;**246**:756–62.
56. Bruhn H, Winkelmann J, Andersen C, Andrä J, Leippe M. Dissection of the mechanisms of cytolytic and antibacterial activity of lysenin, a defence protein of the annelid *Eisenia fetida*. *Dev Comp Immunol* 2006;**30**:597–606.
57. Wang X, Chang L, Sun Z, Zhang Y. Comparative proteomic analysis of differentially expressed proteins in the earthworm *Eisenia fetida* during *Escherichia coli* O157:H7 stress. *J Proteome Res* 2010;**9**:6547–60.
58. Sukumwang N, Umezawa K. Earthworm-derived pore-forming toxin lysenin and screening of its inhibitors. *Toxins* 2013;**5**:1392–401.
59. Lange S, Kauschke E, Mohrig W, Cooper EL. Biochemical characteristics of Eiseniapore, a pore-forming protein in the coelomic fluid of earthworms. *Eur J Biochem* 1999;**262**:547–56.
60. Balaji KN, Schaschke N, Machleidt W, Catalfamo M, Henkart PA. Surface cathepsin B protects cytotoxic lymphocytes from self-destruction after degranulation. *J Exp Med* 2002;**196**:493–503.
61. Lefebvre C, Vandenbulcke F, Bocquet B, Tasiemski A, Desmons A, Verstraete M, et al. Cathepsin L and cystatin B gene expression discriminates immune coelomic cells in the leech *Theromyzon tessulatum*. *Dev Comp Immunol* 2008;**32**:795–807.
62. Hayashi Y, Miclaus T, Scavenius C, Kwiatkowska K, Sobota A, Engelmann P, et al. Species differences take shape at nanoparticles: protein corona made of the native repertoire assists cellular interaction. *Environ Sci Technol* 2013;**47**:14367–75.

63. Monopoli MP, Aberg C, Salvati A, Dawson KA. Biomolecular coronas provide the biological identity of nanosized materials. *Nat Nano* 2012;**7**:779–86.
64. Tenzer S, Docter D, Kuharev J, Musyanovych A, Fetz V, Hecht R, et al. Rapid formation of plasma protein corona critically affects nanoparticle pathophysiology. *Nat Nano* 2013; **8**:772–81.
65. Vroman L, Adams A, Fischer G, Munoz P. Interaction of high molecular weight kininogen, factor XII, and fibrinogen in plasma at interfaces. *Blood* 1980;**55**:156–9.
66. Bilej M, Brys L, Beschin A, Lucas R, Vercauteren E, Hanušová R, et al. Identification of a cyto-lytic protein in the coelomic fluid of *Eisenia foetida* earthworms. *Immunol Lett* 1995;**45**:123–8.
67. Hayashi Y, Engelmann P, Foldbjerg R, Szabó M, Somogyi I, Pollák E, et al. Earthworms and humans in vitro: characterizing evolutionarily conserved stress and immune responses to silver nanoparticles. *Environ Sci Technol* 2012;**46**:4166–73.
68. Shemetov AA, Nabiev I, Sukhanova A. Molecular interaction of proteins and peptides with nanoparticles. *ACS Nano* 2012;**6**:4585–602.
69. Hayashi Y, Miclaus T, Engelmann P, Autrup H, Sutherland DS, Scott-Fordsmand JS. Nanosil-ver pathophysiology in earthworms: transcriptional profiling of secretory proteins and the implication for the protein corona. *Nanotoxicology* 2015:1–9 (Epub ahead of print).

Chapter 5

Neuroprotection and Immunity in the Medicinal Leech *Hirudo medicinalis*: What About Microglia?

Jacopo Vizioli, Francesco Drago, Christophe Lefebvre
University of Lille – Science and Technology, Villeneuve D'Ascq, France

THE MEDICINAL LEECH CENTRAL NERVOUS SYSTEM

Hirudo medicinalis, and all other leeches, belong to the phylum Annelida and are members of the Lophotrochozoa, which also includes mollusks, brachiopods, flatworms, and nemerteans. The medicinal leech, *H. medicinalis*, was studied initially in the field of neuroscience because of the particular structure of its central nervous system (CNS).[1] The leech CNS is a tubular nerve cord composed of 1 head ganglion, 21 body ganglia, and 7 merged tail ganglia. All these ganglia are connected by a beam of fibers termed the connectives consisting of two large lateral bundles of nerve fibers and the medial Faivre's nerve. The neuronal cell bodies are located within the ganglia and extend their own axons into the connectives. In addition to the neurons, a few giant glial cells surround the axons in the connectives and six-packet glial cells sheathe the neuronal cell bodies in each ganglion. Another type of small resident immune cell, the microglia, is found in each connective and ganglion. The leech nerve cells were studied notably for their electrophysiological properties. Because the nerve cord accessibility allows for the chemical destruction of single cells, specific neurons were discriminated functionally and mapped in each ganglion, leading to the description of three groups of sensory neurons—named touch (T), pressure (P), and nociceptive (N) cells—and one type of motor neuron (M).[2] In vivo electrophysiological measures of single-altered neurons were correlated to locomotive behavior. The leech CNS undergoes synapse regeneration as a natural and functional mechanism leading to the restoration of locomotion. In this context, some authors showed that individual neurons develop new synaptic connections with a high degree of specificity following a lesion.[3,4]

Lessons in Immunity: From Single-Cell Organisms to Mammals
http://dx.doi.org/10.1016/B978-0-12-803252-7.00005-9

This ability to regenerate was also verified by valuable in vitro experiments from leech ganglia isolated and maintained in culture.[5–7] The nerve repair processes were progressively investigated by taking into account the importance of glial cell types. The individual destruction of giant glial cells showed no alteration in the mechanism of synaptic reconnection suggesting that these cells are not essential in this process.[8,9] In contrast, the involvement of the microglia is very important, as described below.

MICROGLIA AS BRAIN IMMUNE CELLS

Microglial cells are brain-resident macrophages involved in neurogenesis, neuronal growth, and immune-related functions. These CNS-resident immune cells were first named "microglia" by del Rio-Hortega who studied them in the medicinal leech using the silver carbonate method.[10] In mammals, they are described generally as the first effectors in the case of inflammation, trauma, or other neuronal pathologies,[11] but microglia should be mostly considered as multitasking cells involved in a large panel of functions under physiological and pathological states (eg, phagocytosis, vessel patterning, synaptic refinement, or immunosurveillance).[12] The origin of microglia is linked to yolk-derived macrophages that, through blood circulation, migrate and colonize the brain.[13] Subsequently, the resident microglia help neurogenesis and axonal growth and release neurotrophic factors necessary for brain development. In the adult brain, two populations of macrophage/microglia exist, commonly described as resident and infiltrating cells. Resident microglia constitute a pool of macrophages tightly associated with neurons and act as sentinel cells in homeostasis and brain protection. In the case of nerve tissue injury, microglia are activated: the resident cells develop a ramified shape, transform into a retracted form devoid of filopodia, and start migrating toward the affected area, becoming "reactive microglia." When disease or injury occurs (trauma, infectious, or autoimmune diseases), blood-derived monocytes and bone marrow-derived cells infiltrate the brain, pass through the blood–brain barrier, and migrate to the affected area. The resident and infiltrating macrophages/microglia are similar morphologically and are not easily distinguishable, but the expression of specific surface molecules permits differentiation between them.[14,15] The end result is a large panel of microglia/macrophages that exhibit both neuroprotective and neurotoxic effects. The discrimination of functional features between these two cell types—usually classified in specific "microglial phenotype"—is essential for elucidating neuroimmune responses involving activated cells. This is why alternative models, such as the medicinal leech, which present negligible infiltration of blood immune cells, are advantageous in developing new insights into the CNS-resident immune cell response. Microglia-like cells have been reported occasionally in some invertebrate species. Indeed, the presence of a subset of glial cells sharing structural and functional similarities with vertebrate microglia was identified in mollusks and insects, but their characterization remains poorly explored.[16] These cells are now studied principally in vertebrates such as the mouse and zebra fish.[17] The second one, in particular, is a promising model for structural and functional studies on microglia because of the possibility to couple genetic approaches with neuroimaging techniques.[18] The leech remains the only invertebrate model for the study of microglia functions due to the structure of its CNS.[17] The comparison between leech and mouse/zebra fish models would help the understanding of evolutionary-conserved processes regulating microglia functions in brain immunity.

In *H. medicinalis*, resident microglia are the "immune triggers" for axonal regeneration since a very low number of blood cells infiltrates the CNS upon injury.[19] Within 24 h following damage to the connectives, resident microglial cells migrate to the lesion. When microglial accumulation is inhibited, a significant reduction in axonal sprouting of damaged neurons occurs, which illustrates the importance of microglia in the natural repair of injured axons.[20] As previously mentioned, the giant glial cells are not involved in the initiation of nerve repair.[8,9] The neuroimmune response in leeches is supported by microglia as well as by neurons. Taking into account the nerve repair process, we may suggest a particular neuroprotective phenotype for leech microglia.

IMMUNE RESPONSE AGAINST PATHOGENS

Differential display proteomic analyses showed that the leech CNS is an immunocompetent organ able to respond to bacterial challenges by modulating the profile of several proteins, including cytoskeletal and metabolic proteins, foldases, kinases, and neurohemerythrin.[21] The modulation of these molecules might reflect a cytoskeletal reorganization linked to cell migration, vesicular trafficking, and/or phagocytosis. Some of the regulated proteins, such as neurohemerythrin and gliarin, are expressed specifically in glial and microglial cells suggesting that, as in the vertebrates, these cells are involved in leech CNS immune responses.[22]

The immune competency of the leech nervous system and its role in producing antimicrobial peptides (AMPs) upon bacterial challenges have been demonstrated.[23] Two AMPs called neuromacin and *Hm*lumbricin (*Hm* for *Hirudo medicinalis*) were purified and identified from the nerve cord of immune-challenged leeches. Neuromacin is active only against gram-positive bacteria. *Hm*lumbricin, because of the similarity to its earthworm counterpart, is predicted to be active against fungi, gram-positive bacteria, and gram-negative bacteria. Both AMPs were observed in the injured area of connectives a few hours after axotomy while only neuromacin was detected in microglia surrounding neuron bodies. *Hm*lumbricin and neuromacin genes were not modulated by the axotomy itself, but they were rapidly upregulated upon an immune challenge. Both genes were induced by gram-positive bacteria stimulation, and the *Hm*lumbricin expression was also upregulated by CNS exposure to zymosan. These results indicate that the leech CNS is able to mount a pathogen-specific response that discriminates among different microbial components.[21]

Interestingly, the addition of native *Hm*lumbricin and neuromacin promoted the wound healing of an injured nervous system, and this effect is inhibited by the addition of specific antibodies. While it is doubtful that these AMPs contribute to axonal outgrowth directly, their presence in the injured area might improve the cleansing events associated with a lesion and thus enhance the nerve repair process in *H. medicinalis*.

Analysis of the leech genome revealed the presence of key molecules involved in pathogen recognition, which is necessary to establish a specific neuroimmune response toward microbial components.[24–26] Two members of the MyD88 family (*Hm*MyD88 and *Hm*SARM), adaptors of Toll-like receptors (TLRs), were characterized.[27] Lipopolysaccharide (LPS) may induce a redistribution of *Hm*MyD88 at the surface of neurons demonstrating for the first time the response of neurons to LPS exposure through a MyD88-dependent signaling pathway. Thus leech neurons and microglia express pattern recognition receptors regulating the differential production of AMPs, such as neuromacin and *Hm*lumbricin, as well as the release of the cytokine *Hm* endothelial monocyte-activating polypeptide II (*Hm*EMAPII).[23,24,28] These results indicate that a neuroimmune response is specifically triggered in leeches upon a septic challenge or CNS injury.[25,26,29]

The antimicrobial response triggered by pathogens is also associated with a cell-mediated immune response. In mammals, microglial cells have an important phagocytic role in the CNS, removing damaged neurons, cell debris, and apoptotic cells.[30] Similarly, in leeches, microglia gathered at the lesion to clear the cellular debris associated to tissue damage.[31] In vitro, leech microglia can phagocytize fluorescein isothiocyanate-labeled bacteria (*Aeromonas hydrophila*).[29] Bacteria were detectable inside the cells within 10 min of incubation and the phagocytosis process continued for at least 6 h. These data suggest a rapid clearing mechanism by resident microglia that in a short time phagocytizes the debris issued from the lesion and cleans the area.

MICROGLIA RECRUITMENT

The previous data show that leech microglial cells have properties similar to their mammalian counterparts through their mobility, phagocytic activity, and morphological changes during the activation processes.

Following an experimental lesion, a massive accumulation of microglial cells can be observed at the injury site (Fig. 5.1A). Microglia start moving within a few minutes postaxotomy. Their accumulation can be observed at the lesion site within 2 h and continues up to 24 h. As indicated earlier, this mechanism is essential for synapse reconstitution, axonal sprouting, and functional recovery in leeches.[18] This mobility postinjury was functionally investigated in order to specify the molecular mechanisms mediating their time-course accumulation. Several chemotactic signals coming from neurons or glial cells were identified.

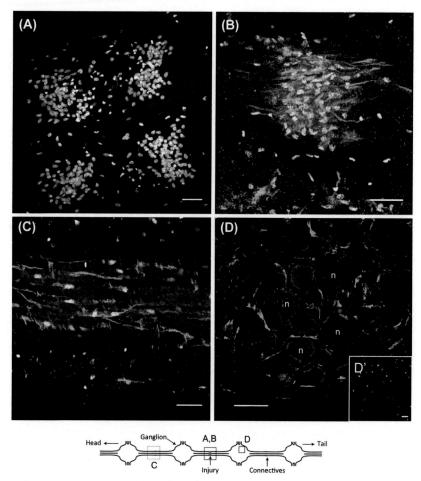

FIGURE 5.1 Confocal microscopy imaging showing the activated microglia from *Hirudo medicinalis* nerve cords cultured at different time points. (A) Nuclear staining of connective microglial cells accumulated at the lesion site in the leech CNS (24h postaxotomy). (B–D) Immunohistochemistry on whole-mounted leech CNS carried out with anti-*Hm*Iba1 antibodies. (B) Accumulation of *Hm*Iba1-positive cells at the lesion site (6h postaxotomy). (C) Immunostaining of resident microglia in a nonlesioned connective segment (24-h-cultured nerve cord). (D) *Hm*Iba1-positive microglial cells surrounding neuron bodies (n) of a ganglion (3-day-cultured nerve cord). (D′) *Hm*Iba1 immunostaining of a freshly dissected ganglion (T0h). Cell nuclei in A, B, C, and D′ were counterstained with Hoechst 33342. Scale bars correspond to 20 μm. In the bottom, a schematic representation of leech CNS organization indicating (boxes) the connective sites and the ganglion area illustrated in figures (A)–(D).

ATP is considered a general microglial activator exerting a "go" signal for migration. Its extracellular release by nerve cells is regulated through innexin/pannexin channels.[32] Its recognition by microglia might require purinergic receptors since a specific antagonist was observed to attenuate the migration.[33]

Nitric oxide (NO) is responsible for recruiting leech microglia within the first minutes following a lesion.[34,35] In addition, NO activates the accumulation of microglia at low concentrations far from the lesion site and stops their migration at high concentrations at the injury site.[34] These data suggest that NO contributes to microglial cell movement by regulating their directionality, and NO has been identified as the first diffusible molecule for the microglial movement toward the lesion.

Furthermore, the balance of NO and ATP-release, contributing to the microglia accumulation at the injury site, might be regulated by endocannabinoids, namely, N-arachidonylethanolamide and 2-arachidonoyl glycerol.[36] Arachidonic acid is also involved in this regulatory process. Indeed, injury releases arachidonic acid that blocks the ATP-release through the inhibition of innexin/pannexin channels. Consequently, arachidonic acid acts as an endogenous regulator spreading out a stop signal to microglia at lesions.[37] In addition, the involvement of ATP and NO correlates the microglial recruitment with the initiation of axonal sprouting.[20]

Other immune effectors homologous to vertebrate molecules (called *Hm*E-MAPII, *Hm*IL-16, and *Hm*C1q) playing an important role in the microglia recruitment were identified in the leech CNS.

EMAPII is a marker of microglial cell reactivity[38] and is highly produced by activated microglia in neurodegenerative pathologies.[39] The first chemotactic function of EMAPII on microglia has been described in the leech CNS.[28] *Hm*E-MAPII production in leeches is associated with TLR-dependent pathways.[24,28]

Interleukin-16 (IL-16) was initially identified in mammals as a lymphocyte chemoattractant factor,[40,41] and it is produced by lymphocytes and microglia as a proinflammatory cytokine.[42] Human IL-16 attracts CD4+ lymphocytes under pathological conditions.[43] In the brain, it would regulate inflammatory processes after axonal damage.[44,45] Its leech homolog, *Hm*IL-16, is produced in neurons following a lesion, is released at the axonal ends, and serves to chemoattract microglia.[46] Studies using neutralizing antibodies on leech microglia accumulation suggest the involvement of receptors homologous to CXCR3 and CD4 that are used for mammalian EMAPII and IL-16, respectively.[28,46]

C1q is considered as an inflammatory mediator in mammals and seems to be a key molecule in neurodegenerative pathologies.[47,48] As shown in the leech CNS for *Hm*C1q,[49] its mammalian form is known to drive microglial activation after neuronal and/or microglial production.[50] Two different receptors, called *Hm*C1qBP and *Hm*CalR (calreticulin), were characterized in *H. medicinalis* and would be expressed by distinct microglial subpopulations.[51,52] In mammals, these C1q-interacting receptors have not been demonstrated in nerve cells but only in peripheral dendritic cells.[53]

In *H. medicinalis*, ex vivo experiments can be performed on cultured segments of isolated nerve cords, and microglial cells are still able to accumulate following the experimental lesion of the tissue. This ex vivo approach using nuclear dyes allows us to observe the recruitment of microglia under different conditions. In vitro chemotactic assays were developed as well using primary cultures of leech microglia. Both approaches showed that leech microglia can be partially chemoattracted by the human forms of EMAPII, IL-16, and C1q.[28,46,49]

As explained earlier, cells gather at an experimental lesion under specific chemoattractant signals, suggesting the existence of several microglia subpopulations that differ in migration chronology and activation patterns. This differential reactivity indicates that specific microglial cells may have different functions in the context of axonal repair in early (minutes/hours) as well as late (days) events.

As suggested in mammals, resident microglia must be considered as a mosaic of different reactive subsets responsive to several neurochemical signals.[54] Since a high conservation of recognition mechanisms for chemotactic signals was observed between leeches and mammals, the *H. medicinalis* microglia represent an interesting model to decipher the molecular signaling in microglia recruitment.

NEUROINFLAMMATORY MARKERS

Similarly to vertebrates, the microglia of *H. medicinalis* are activated upon bacterial challenges or CNS injury. The processes associated with a CNS lesion involve the reactivity of several hundreds of microglial cells. In the first hours following the injury, the activation process is linked to (1) a morphological modification of cells that undergo a change from a stellate to a spindled shape, (2) a migration along connective fibers toward the injured area, and (3) their accumulation in the axotomy zone (Fig. 5.1A). For 20 years, gliarin was the only general glial marker described in the leech CNS.[55,56] This molecule, belonging to the intermediate filament protein superfamily, highlighted the different morphologies of microglial cells according to their location and the lesion status of the nerve cord.[29] A novel microglial marker, *Hm*Iba1, was characterized in *Hirudo*.[57] This protein is significantly similar to the vertebrate ionized calcium-binding adaptor molecule 1 (Iba1), also known as Aif-1 (allograft inflammatory factor 1). Iba1 is a largely used microglial marker in mammalian models because of its specific expression in activated cells. The expression of Iba1 in mammals is linked to different pathologies such as cancer, autoimmune diseases, or brain injuries, but its function remains poorly understood.[58] Similarly to its vertebrate counterpart, *Hm*Iba1 is specifically expressed in leech microglia upon an experimental lesion (Fig. 5.1). *Hm*Iba1 is the first marker for activated microglia described to date in invertebrates, and its modulation upon inflammatory conditions looks similar to that which occurs in rodent models.[57] Interestingly, this protein is only present in some of the hundreds of cells gathered at the lesion site a few hours postaxotomy (Fig. 5.1B). Other microglial cells accumulate at the lesion despite their lack of *Hm*Iba1 signals. This result supports the hypothesis of different microglial populations migrating to the challenged area and displaying different functions and/or activation states.

Indeed, *Hm*Iba1 immunostaining is not specifically associated to migrating cells but only indicates their activation state. Fig. 5.1C shows some *Hm*Iba1-positive cells in a nonlesioned connective 24 h after lesion of the neighboring connective. A similar result was observed for resident microglia in ganglia (Fig. 5.1D) that indicates that microglia that are not directly involved in migration and accumulation events are nonetheless in an activated state. In naïve conditions, these cells in both connectives (data not shown) and ganglia (Fig. 5.1D') show a weak expression level of *Hm*Iba1.

Similarly to vertebrate Iba1, the leech gene is induced by ATP.[57] Because of the similarities of leech and mammalian microglia described earlier, novel activation markers associated to neuroinflammatory events in the leech have been identified. Preliminary studies from leech CNS suggest the presence of some additional proteins (CD11b, CD45, progranulin), generally expressed in vertebrate macrophages and microglia upon inflammatory conditions.[26,59] These results suggest a conservation of basic mechanisms controlling cell activation and inflammation during postaxotomy events in leech microglia compared to mammalian models.

TOWARD NERVE REPAIR: MICROGLIA/NEURONS CROSSTALK INTO THE SPOTLIGHT

Upon an experimental lesion, leech microglia promote wound repair and axonal sprouting. The molecular crosstalk between microglia and neurons in this neuroprotection is largely unknown. In the CNS, intercellular communication is mediated by (1) synapses, (2) the secretion of soluble molecules, or (3) the release of extracellular vesicles (EVs) containing various effectors. The third mechanism seems to be important in the leech: a massive presence of EV-related structures interacting with the neuron surface was observed during the coculture of leech microglia and neurons.[60] When neurons were cultured alone, many fewer EVs were detected, suggesting that EVs mainly derive from microglial cells.

Under physiological conditions and various disease states, cells secrete two types of EVs. The first type, the exosomes (50–100 nm in diameter), are generated inside multivesicular bodies (MVBs) and are released upon MVB fusion with the plasma membrane. The second type of EVs, the ectosomes, also called shed vesicles/particles (100 nm–1 μm in diameter), bud from the plasma membrane. The protein composition of EVs varies depending on the cellular origin and plays a role in the phenotypic response or programmed cell death events. Moreover, the EVs contain (1) mRNAs that can be translated to proteins by cells receiving the vesicles and (2) miRNAs that regulate posttranscriptional processes in target cells. The EVs, released from many cell types, are being studied as potential markers of physiological and pathological conditions. Their relevance in neurogenesis, as well as in pathogenesis of several CNS disorders, has only begun to be explored, according to their production by neurons and glial cells.[61,62] The EVs are involved in neurite outgrowth after axonal damage as well as during axonal regeneration.[63] Moreover, the ability of EVs to cross the blood–brain barrier and their potential to be manipulated genetically have created a great interest in EVs as natural vectors for the delivery of therapeutic agents (RNAs and/or proteins).[64,65] Proteomic studies are currently being undertaken to investigate the content of leech-activated microglia EVs associated to general (ATP) or specific (C1q, EMAPII, and IL-16) stimulation.[66] The characterization of EV contents (proteins and RNAs) and their correlation with neurite outgrowth constitute an interesting approach to bringing new insights into the microglial role leading to neuroprotection and highlight their functions in the leech as well as in vertebrate models.

CONCLUSIONS

The medicinal leech represents an intriguing model to study different phenomena in neurobiology from immune response to nerve repair. Its CNS constitutes a relatively simple system easily accessible in vivo and very useful for ex vivo studies. It has multiple roles, including as an immune competent organ able to mount an effective humoral and cell-mediated immune response against pathogens. The *H. medicinalis* CNS is particularly interesting because of its ability to repair itself naturally following injury. In this context, microglial cells play a pivotal role, being at the interface between immunity and axonal repair. These resident cells exhibit multiple functions. Their study will bring new insights into the comprehension of neuroimmune and neuroinflammatory mechanisms controlling nerve repair in several animal models.

REFERENCES

1. Coggeshall RE, Fawcett DW. The fine structure of the central nervous system of the leech, *Hirudo Medicinalis*. *J Neurophysiol* 1964;**27**:229–89.
2. Nicholls JG, Baylor DA. Specific modalities and receptive fields of sensory neurons in CNS of the leech. *J Neurophysiol* 1968;**31**:740–56.
3. Baylor DA, Nicholls JG. Patterns of regeneration between individual nerve cells in the central nervous system of the leech. *Nature* 1971;**232**:268–70.
4. Jansen JK, Nicholls JG. Regeneration and changes in synaptic connections between individual nerve cells in the central nervous system of the leech. *Proc Natl Acad Sci USA* 1972;**69**: 636–9.
5. Wallace BG, Adal MN, Nicholls JG. Regeneration of synaptic connections by sensory neurons in leech ganglia maintained in culture. *Proc R Soc Lond B Biol Sci* 1977;**199**:567–85.
6. Muller KJ, Scott SA. Correct axonal regeneration after target cell removal in the central nervous system of the leech. *Science* 1979;**206**:87–9.
7. Muller KJ, Scott SA. Removal of the synaptic target permits terminal sprouting of a mature intact axon. *Nature* 1980;**283**:89–90.
8. Elliot EJ, Muller KJ. Synapses between neurons regenerate accurately after destruction of ensheathing glial cells in the leech. *Science* 1982;**215**:1260–2.
9. Elliott EJ, Muller KJ. Sprouting and regeneration of sensory axons after destruction of ensheathing glial cells in the leech central nervous system. *J Neurosci* 1983;**3**:1994–2006.

10. Del Rio-Hortega P. Cytology and cellular pathology of the nervous system. In: Penfield W, editor. *Microglia*. New York (NY): P.B. Hoebaer; 1932. p. 483–534.

11. Kettenmann H, Hanisch UK, Noda M, Verkhratsky A. Physiology of microglia. *Physiol Rev* 2011;**91**:461–553.

12. Casano AM, Peri F. Microglia: multitasking specialists of the brain. *Dev Cell* 2015;**32**:469–77.

13. Swinnen N, Smolders S, Avila A, et al. Complex invasion pattern of the cerebral cortex bymicroglial cells during development of the mouse embryo. *Glia* 2013;**61**:150–63.

14. Prinz M, Priller J, Sisodia SS, Ransohoff RM. Heterogeneity of CNS myeloid cells and their roles in neurodegeneration. *Nat Neurosci* 2011;**14**:1227–35.

15. Butovsky O, Jedrychowski MP, Moore CS, et al. Identification of a unique TGF-beta-dependent molecular and functional signature in microglia. *Nat Neurosci* 2014;**17**:131–43.

16. Sonetti D, Ottaviani E, Bianchi F, et al. Microglia in invertebrate ganglia. *Proc Natl Acad Sci USA* 1994;**91**:9180–4.

17. Sieger D, Peri F. Animal models for studying microglia: the first, the popular, and the new. *Glia* 2013;**61**:3–9.

18. Eyo UB, Dailey ME. Microglia: key elements in neural development, plasticity, and pathology. *J Neuroimmune Pharmacol* 2013;**8**:494–509.

19. Boidin-Wichlacz C, Vergote D, Slomianny C, Jouy N, Salzet M, Tasiemski A. Morphological and functional characterization of leech circulating blood cells: role in immunity and neural repair. *Cell Mol Life Sci* 2012;**69**:1717–31.

20. Ngu EM, Sahley CL, Muller KJ. Reduced axon sprouting after treatment that diminishes microglia accumulation at lesions in the leech CNS. *J Comp Neurol* 2007;**503**:101–9.

21. Vergote D, Macagno ER, Salzet M, Sautiere PE. Proteome modifications of the medicinal leech nervous system under bacterial challenge. *Proteomics* 2006;**6**:4817–25.

22. Vergote D, Sautiere PE, Vandenbulcke F, et al. Up-regulation of neurohemerythrin expression in the central nervous system of the medicinal leech, *Hirudo medicinalis*, following septic injury. *J Biol Chem* 2004;**279**:43828–37.

23. Schikorski D, Cuvillier-Hot V, Leippe M, et al. Microbial challenge promotes the regenerative process of the injured central nervous system of the medicinal leech by inducing the synthesis of antimicrobial peptides in neurons and microglia. *J Immunol* 2008;**181**:1083–95.

24. Cuvillier-Hot V, Boidin-Wichlacz C, Slomianny C, Salzet M, Tasiemski A. Characterization and immune function of two intracellular sensors, *Hm*TLR1 and *Hm*NLR, in the injured CNS of an invertebrate. *Dev Comp Immunol* 2011;**35**:214–26.

25. Tasiemski A, Salzet M. Leech immunity: from brain to peripheral responses. *Adv Exp Med Biol* 2010;**708**:80–104.

26. Macagno ER, Gaasterland T, Edsall L, et al. Construction of a medicinal leech transcriptome database and its application to the identification of leech homologs of neural and innate immune genes. *BMC Genomics* 2010;**11**:407.

27. Rodet F, Tasiemski A, Boidin-Wichlacz C, et al. *Hm*-MyD88 and *Hm*-SARM: two key regulators of the neuroimmune system and neural repair in the medicinal leech. *Sci Rep* 2015;**5**:9624.

28. Schikorski D, Cuvillier-Hot V, Boidin-Wichlacz C, Slomianny C, Salzet M, Tasiemski A. Deciphering the immune function and regulation by a TLR of the cytokine EMAPII in the lesioned central nervous system using a leech model. *J Immunol* 2009;**183**:7119–28.

29. Le Marrec-Croq F, Drago F, Vizioli J, Sautiere PE, Lefebvre C. The leech nervous system: a valuable model to study the microglia involvement in regenerative processes. *Clin Dev Immunol* 2013;**2013**:274019.

30. Fu R, Shen Q, Xu P, Luo JJ, Tang Y. Phagocytosis of microglia in the central nervous system diseases. *Mol Neurobiol* 2014;**49**:1422–34.

31. Morgese VJ, Elliott EJ, Muller KJ. Microglial movement to sites of nerve lesion in the leech CNS. *Brain Res* 1983;**272**:166–70.
32. Samuels SE, Lipitz JB, Dahl G, Muller KJ. Neuroglial ATP release through innexin channels controls microglial cell movement to a nerve injury. *J Gen Physiol* 2010;**136**:425–42.
33. Duan Y, Sahley CL, Muller KJ. ATP and NO dually control migration of microglia to nerve lesions. *Dev Neurobiol* 2009;**69**:60–72.
34. Chen A, Kumar SM, Sahley CL, Muller KJ. Nitric oxide influences injury-induced microglial migration and accumulation in the leech CNS. *J Neurosci* 2000;**20**:1036–43.
35. Kumar SM, Porterfield DM, Muller KJ, Smith PJ, Sahley CL. Nerve injury induces a rapid efflux of nitric oxide (NO) detected with a novel NO microsensor. *J Neurosci* 2001;**21**:215–20.
36. Arafah K, Croix D, Vizioli J, Desmons A, Fournier I, Salzet M. Involvement of nitric oxide through endocannabinoids release in microglia activation during the course of CNS regeneration in the medicinal leech. *Glia* 2013;**61**:636–49.
37. Samuels SE, Lipitz JB, Wang J, Dahl G, Muller KJ. Arachidonic acid closes innexin/pannexin channels and thereby inhibits microglia cell movement to a nerve injury. *Dev Neurobiol* 2013;**73**:621–31.
38. Schluesener HJ, Seid K, Meyermann R. Effects of autoantigen and dexamethasone treatment on expression of endothelial-monocyte activating polypeptide II and allograft-inflammatory factor-1 by activated macrophages and microglial cells in lesions of experimental autoimmune encephalomyelitis, neuritis and uveitis. *Acta Neuropathol* 1999;**97**:119–26.
39. Mueller CA, Schluesener HJ, Conrad S, Meyermann R, Schwab JM. Spinal cord injury induces lesional expression of the proinflammatory and antiangiogenic cytokine EMAP II. *J Neurotrauma* 2003;**20**:1007–15.
40. Center DM, Cruikshank W. Modulation of lymphocyte migration by human lymphokines. I. Identification and characterization of chemoattractant activity for lymphocytes from mitogen-stimulated mononuclear cells. *J Immunol* 1982;**128**:2563–8.
41. Cruikshank W, Center DM. Modulation of lymphocyte migration by human lymphokines. II. Purification of a lymphotactic factor (LCF). *J Immunol* 1982;**128**:2569–74.
42. Center DM, Kornfeld H, Ryan TC, Cruikshank WW. Interleukin 16: implications for CD4 functions and HIV-1 progression. *Immunol Today* 2000;**21**:273–80.
43. Schluesener HJ, Seid K, Kretzschmar J, Meyermann R. Leukocyte chemotactic factor, a natural ligand to CD4, is expressed by lymphocytes and microglial cells of the MS plaque. *J Neurosci Res* 1996;**44**:606–11.
44. Mittelbronn M, Dietz K, Schluesener HJ, Meyermann R. Local distribution of microglia in the normal adult human central nervous system differs by up to one order of magnitude. *Acta Neuropathol* 2001;**101**:249–55.
45. Skundric DS, Cai J, Cruikshank WW, Gveric D. Production of IL-16 correlates with CD4$^+$ Th1 inflammation and phosphorylation of axonal cytoskeleton in multiple sclerosis lesions. *J Neuroinflammation* 2006;**3**:13.
46. Croq F, Vizioli J, Tuzova M, et al. A homologous form of human interleukin 16 is implicated in microglia recruitment following nervous system injury in leech *Hirudo medicinalis*. *Glia* 2010;**58**:1649–62.
47. Bergamaschini L, Donarini C, Gobbo G, Parnetti L, Gallai V. Activation of complement and contact system in Alzheimer's disease. *Mech Ageing Dev* 2001;**122**:1971–83.
48. Kishore U, Gaboriaud C, Waters P, et al. C1q and tumor necrosis factor superfamily: modularity and versatility. *Trends Immunol* 2004;**25**:551–61.
49. Tahtouh M, Croq F, Vizioli J, et al. Evidence for a novel chemotactic C1q domain-containing factor in the leech nerve cord. *Mol Immunol* 2009;**46**:523–31.

50. Farber K, Cheung G, Mitchell D, et al. C1q, the recognition subcomponent of the classical pathway of complement, drives microglial activation. *J Neurosci Res* 2009;**87**:644–52.
51. Tahtouh M, Garcon-Bocquet A, Croq F, et al. Interaction of *Hm*C1q with leech microglial cells: involvement of C1qBP-related molecule in the induction of cell chemotaxis. *J Neuroinflammation* 2012;**9**:37.
52. Le Marrec-Croq F, Bocquet-Garcon A, Vizioli J, et al. Calreticulin contributes to C1q-dependent recruitment of microglia in the leech *Hirudo medicinalis* following a CNS injury. *Med Sci Monit* 2014;**20**:644–53.
53. Vegh Z, Kew RR, Gruber BL, Ghebrehiwet B. Chemotaxis of human monocyte-derived dendritic cells to complement component C1q is mediated by the receptors gC1qR and cC1qR. *Mol Immunol* 2006;**43**:1402–7.
54. Pannell M, Szulzewsky F, Matyash V, Wolf SA, Kettenmann H. The subpopulation of microglia sensitive to neurotransmitters/neurohormones is modulated by stimulation with LPS, interferon-gamma, and IL-4. *Glia* 2014;**62**:667–79.
55. Xu Y, Bolton B, Zipser B, Jellies J, Johansen KM, Johansen J. Gliarin and macrolin, two novel intermediate filament proteins specifically expressed in sets and subsets of glial cells in leech central nervous system. *J Neurobiol* 1999;**40**:244–53.
56. Luthi TE, Brodbeck DL, Jeno P. Identification of a 70kD protein with sequence homology to squid neurofilament protein in glial cells of the leech CNS. *J Neurobiol* 1994;**25**:70–82.
57. Drago F, Sautiere PE, Le Marrec-Croq F, et al. Microglia of medicinal leech (*Hirudo medicinalis*) express a specific activation marker homologous to vertebrate ionized calcium-binding adapter molecule 1 (Iba1/alias aif-1). *Dev Neurobiol* 2014;**74**:987–1001.
58. Zhao YY, Yan DJ, Chen ZW. Role of AIF-1 in the regulation of inflammatory activation and diverse disease processes. *Cell Immunol* 2013;**284**:75–83.
59. Vizioli J, Accorsi A, Croq F, et al. Neuroinflammation and microglia activation studies: a novel strategy using an invertebrate model, the medicinal leech. *Glia* 2011;**59–S1**:S153.
60. Le Marrec-Croq F, Van Camp C, Drago F, et al. Extracellular vesicles (EVs) from leech microglia: a tool for understanding the dialog with damaged neurons. *Glia* 2015;**63–S1**:E212–3.
61. Bahrini I, Song JH, Diez D, Hanayama R. Neuronal exosomes facilitate synaptic pruning by up-regulating complement factors in microglia. *Sci Rep* 2015;**5**:7989.
62. Gupta A, Pulliam L. Exosomes as mediators of neuroinflammation. *J Neuroinflammation* 2014;**11**:68.
63. Lopez-Verrilli MA, Picou F, Court FA. Schwann cell-derived exosomes enhance axonal regeneration in the peripheral nervous system. *Glia* 2013;**61**:1795–806.
64. El Andaloussi S, Mager I, Breakefield XO, Wood MJ. Extracellular vesicles: biology and emerging therapeutic opportunities. *Nat Rev Drug Discov* 2013;**12**:347–57.
65. Hu G, Drescher KM, Chen XM. Exosomal miRNAs: Biological properties and therapeutic potential. *Front Genet* 2012;**3**:56.
66. Drago F, Arab T, Van Camp C, et al. Differentially activated microglia release Extracellular Vesicles (EVs) showing specific contents and functions in a model of nerve repair. *Glia* 2015;**63–S1**:E321–2.

Chapter 6

Specificity of Innate Immunity in Bivalves: A Lesson From Bacteria

Laura Canesi, Carla Pruzzo
University of Genova, Genova, Italy

INNATE IMMUNITY IN BIVALVES: DIVERSITY AND COMPLEXITY

Bivalves (Mollusca, Lophotrochozoa) are an important ecological group, widespread in freshwater, estuarine, and marine ecosystems, with many edible species. Like all other invertebrate groups, bivalves lack adaptive immunity; however, they are endowed with an effective and complex innate immune system (humoral and cellular defenses) similar to that of vertebrates.[1] The lack of acquired immunity and the capacity to form antibodies (specific response) does not mean a lack of specificity: invertebrates have evolved genetic mechanisms capable of producing thousands of different proteins from a small number of genes. This diversity allows them to recognize and eliminate a wide range of different pathogens.[2]

Bivalve hemocytes are responsible for cell-mediated immunity through the combined action of the phagocytic process with humoral defense factors such as agglutinins (eg, lectins), lysosomal enzymes (eg, acid phosphatase, lysozyme), toxicoxygen intermediates, and various antimicrobial peptides (AMPs).[3] The morphology, ultrastructure, and functions of bivalve hemocytes were reviewed by Hine.[4] Granular hemocytes (basophilic and acidophilic granulocytes) form a distinct group, whereas agranular hemocytes are heterogeneous in appearance and ultrastructure (blast-like cells, basophilic macrophage-like cells, hyalinocytes). Not all types occur in each bivalve species; scallops lack granulocytes, and the hyalinocyte is a poorly defined cell type in several groups. Moreover, due to functional heterogeneity, the functions of each hemocyte type cannot be reliably extrapolated between species. In the last decade, the application of flow cytometry analysis and molecular characterization of different immune-related molecules have greatly improved our knowledge of the functional characterization of hemocytes, underlying both common and distinct features of the immune system in different bivalve species.[1,5–8]

Lessons in Immunity: From Single-Cell Organisms to Mammals
http://dx.doi.org/10.1016/B978-0-12-803252-7.00006-0

In bivalves, innate immunity promotes generalized protection against not only pathogenic organisms (eg, protozoa, bacteria, viruses) but also environmental stressors (eg, the presence of contaminants, algal toxins, air exposure, mechanical stress, high temperatures, changes in salinity).[9] To afford protection in this fluctuating environment, bivalve immunity displays a wide variety of sensitive receptors, selective effectors, and synergistic genetic regulatory networks. Moreover, as filter feeders, bivalves can accumulate large numbers of microorganisms from the aquatic environment; this may result in a concentration of potential pathogens, mainly bacteria, that can either establish a commensal relationship with the host without causing diseases or proliferate and invade soft tissues, resulting in high mortality. For edible species (such as oysters, mussels, and clams), understanding the relationship between the immune system and bacteria has two main implications: (1) to ensure a better protection in the intensive breeding of economically important species, and (2) to control the potential accumulation of human pathogens of concern for public health. In this chapter, available data underlying the specificity of the bivalve immune response to bacterial challenges will be summarized.

BIVALVES AND MARINE BACTERIA

A rich and diverse microbiota is present in the aquatic environment, and bivalves can ingest many different kinds of bacteria, including some that can be pathogenic to the bivalve host.[10] Bacterial pathogens can affect larvae cultured in hatchery and adults cultured in the natural environment; generally, they are the most virulent during the larval stages. Larval pathogens include members of the *Vibrio, Pseudomonas, Alteromonas, Moraxella,* and *Aeromonas* genera.[11] Vibrios are also involved in diseases of juvenile and adult bivalves together with, but to a lower extent, bacteria belonging to other genera.[11–13]

Vibrios are gram-negative marine bacteria widely distributed in estuarine and coastal waters and sediments. The genus comprises human pathogens (*Vibrio cholerae, Vibrio vulnificus, Vibrio parahaemolyticus*) and species pathogenic for aquatic animals[9] (eg, *Vibrio splendidus, Vibrio aestuarianus*). Vibrios tend to be most common in warmer waters (above 17°C) and depending on the species, they tolerate a wide range of salinities.[10] A common trait is the presence of multiple lifestyles: a planktonic, free-swimming state and an adhering form on biotic and abiotic surfaces. Vibrios represent a high proportion of bacteria isolated from healthy and diseased bivalves, with 100-fold higher concentration than in the surrounding water. For some of the bivalve-associated vibrios, the precise role as commensal, opportunistic, or pathogenic organisms remains to be defined.

Vibrio species associated with bivalve larvae diseases include *Vibrio anguillarum, Vibrio alginolyticus, Vibrio tubiashii, V. splendidus, Vibrio pectenicida,* and *Vibrio neptunius.*[9–11] The pathogen source has been reported to be from brood stock, seawater, and algal food.[14] Larval vibriosis is an aggressive and rapidly progressing infection that affects different species and is best documented in oysters. Disease outbreaks are characterized by bacterial swarming around the velum, loss of larval motility, extensive soft tissue necrosis, and rapid mortality (up to 90% within 24 h of initial exposure to the most pathogenic strains). Oyster larvae cannot repair damage to the mantle during the early stages of infection; this capacity increases with the increasing size of the juveniles.[11] The higher susceptibility of developing larvae to bacterial infection may be due to an immature immune system and an investment of energy in a fast metabolic development for settlement. Metamorphosis was identified as a crucial stage when larvae increased the expression of immune-related genes and responded to environmental signals[15]; however, information on ontogeny of the immune response in different species is still scarce.

Vibriosis has also been described in juvenile and adult oysters, clams, and mussels.[11,12] Vibrios are associated with the syndrome known as brown ring disease (BRD) in adult clams[12,16] and summer mortality in juvenile oysters.[13,17–19] BRD affects both reared and wild clams (*Ruditapes philippinarum* and *Ruditapes decussatus*); it is caused by *Vibrio tapetis* that was shown to be capable of reproducing the disease in healthy animals.[11,20] Interestingly, secreted proteins contribute to the virulence of this species.[20] An alteration of the calcification process of the inner surface of the valves and the presence of a brown deposit of conchiolin between the shell edge and the pallial line are typical of the disease.[11] The geographical origin of the clams and environmental factors (ie, temperature and salinity) seem to play a role in sensitivity to infections.[10,11] Resistance to BRD in different clam species and stocks may be also related to the capacity of shell repair as well as to the phagocytic activity of the hemocytes.[21,22] Information on virulence factors of *V. tapetis* is scant; recently, several protein fractions from extracellular products were shown to display biological activity toward clam hemocytes.[20]

The physiological and/or genetic status of the oysters, and multiple stressors such as elevated temperature, low dissolved oxygen, and limited energy resources after spawning were associated with summer mortality events.[13] In addition, one or more infectious agents, such as herpes virus, OsHV1[19], and different *Vibrio* species (eg, *V. aestuarianus*, *V. splendidus* clade, *Vibrio harveyi*) have been implicated as etiological agents.[17,18] High temperatures might be important stressors by affecting the host physiology and susceptibility to infection and supporting the proliferation, spread, and virulence of thermodependent *Vibrio* spp.[23]

The so-called *V. splendidus* clade constitutes a complex of phenotypically and genetically related species,[24] with several members causing significant losses in the aquaculture industry worldwide. Studies with the *V. splendidus* LGP32 strain (recently assigned to the species *V. tasmaniensis*, belonging to the same clade[25]) indicated that its virulence is linked to the outer membrane protein OmpU.[26] Other virulence factors are the metalloprotease Vsm[27] and an invasive serine protease Vsp specifically secreted through outer membrane vesicle production.[28] A recent 2-year sampling campaign in the northern Adriatic Sea (Italy)[29] showed that genes encoding OmpU protein and zinc metalloprotease are present in strains belonging to different species of the clade. Nasfi et al.[26] suggested that diverse clones of the *V. splendidus* clade can replace each other during different mortality outbreaks, probably favored by a massive lateral transfer of virulence factors thus underlying the epidemiological risk of an emergence of new virulent strains.

The species *V. aestuarianus* is ubiquitous in different geographic areas. It was associated with oyster summer mortalities, and its pathogenic potential was shown in experimental oyster challenges.[30,31] Isolates show variable virulence likely linked to the varying toxicity of the bacterial extracellular products. Those produced by *V. aestuarianus* 01/032, a strain isolated during a mortality outbreak in an experimental hatchery, caused morphological changes and immunosuppression in *Crassostrea gigas* hemocytes in vitro.[32] These effects were ascribed to the capacity of the strain to produce a Vam metalloprotease that affects hemocyte morphology and impairs phagocytic function. N-acetyl glucosamine binding protein and/or mannose sensitive hemagglutinin (MSHA) adhesins are present in a large proportion of *V. aestuarianus* isolates[29]; both ligands are involved in interactions with environmental surfaces (eg, chitin), which might contribute to their persistence in the environment.[9] Moreover, these adhesins may play a role in mediating surface interactions between bacteria and bivalve hemocytes, thus affecting the immune response (see section: Immune Recognition).

IMMUNE RECOGNITION

Immune recognition is the first step of the immune response, allowing the discrimination of self/not-self substances. Pattern recognition receptors (PRRs) on the hemocyte membrane and in hemolymph serum play a crucial role in activating the immune system to eliminate pathogens. PRRs selectively recognize a large family of conserved foreign molecules called pathogen-associated molecular patterns (PAMPs), such as lipopolysaccharides, lipoproteins, peptidoglycans, lipoteichoic acids, viral dsRNA, unmethylated bacterial DNA, zymosans, and heat shock proteins. Several groups of distinct PRRs have been identified in bivalves, including lectins, peptidoglycan recognition proteins, gram-negative binding proteins, Toll-like receptors (TLRs), scavenger receptors, rig-like receptors, and NOD-like receptors.[1,8,33] The most studied PRRs show a high versatility and flexibility; however, some degree of specificity could be identified.

Calcium-dependent (C-type) lectins are a superfamily of proteins that can bind PAMPs through the recognition of carbohydrates, thus promoting their agglutination/immobilization and triggering successive immune functions, such as opsonization and phagocytosis. Multiple lectin-related transcripts have been identified in different bivalve species that are upregulated by immune challenges, showing a broad specificity toward microorganisms but a remarkable carbohydrate-binding specificity.[34]

TLRs are involved in the molecular recognition of pathogens as well as in cell adhesion, signal transduction, and cell growth.[35] The search for components of the Toll signaling pathway has recently led to their discovery in many bivalve models: transcriptome analysis using next generation sequencing (NGS) technologies led to the identification of a vast repertoire of putative TLRs encoding sequences for *Mytilus edulis*,[33] *R. philippinarum*,[36] and *Crassostrea virginica*.[37] TLRs and components of the Toll-activated pathways were upregulated in the hemocytes of marine bivalves following a single in vivo injection with different bacteria and PAMPs, with the majority of the challenges involving Vibrios as predominant marine bacteria.[38]

The complement system pathway relies on several interacting proteins to recognize and then eliminate foreign microorganisms, with a pivotal role in the initiation of defense mechanisms, including agglutination, adhesion, opsonization, and cell lysis. Once activated, the complement system promotes target proteolytic reactions that operate following classical, lectin, or alternative pathways. C1q, a subcomponent of the complement C1 complex, is considered to be a versatile PRP, binding directly to a broad range of PAMPs of bacteria, viruses, and parasites as well as enhancing pathogen phagocytosis.[39] Some C1q proteins with specific ligand recognition properties have been also described and characterized in bivalves: similar expression changes were observed in the hemocytes challenged with both gram-positive and gram-negative bacteria.[40,41]

IMMUNE SIGNALING

Upon the successful recognition of foreign compounds, activated PRRs trigger different intracellular signaling pathways that are required for the immune response. This may lead to the rapid activation of phagocytosis, reactive oxygen species (ROS) production, release of preexisting enzymes, or antimicrobial molecules as well as to changes in the transcription of immune or stress response genes at the nuclear level.[42] Among immune signaling pathways, the mitogen-activated protein kinase (MAPK), nuclear factor kB (NF-kB), the complement component, and the Toll pathways have been investigated in bivalves. For a discussion of the NF-kB, complement, and Toll pathways, see Refs 1,8.

Studies on the components of kinase-mediated transduction pathways first revealed specificities in the bivalve immune response to different bacteria. In *Mytilus galloprovincialis* hemocytes, exposure to different bacterial species and strains, heterologous cytokines and natural hormones, and organic environmental chemicals underlined the role of conserved cytosolic kinases (such as MAPKs and protein kinase C-PKC) and kinase-activated transcription factors (such as signal transducers and activators of transcription (STATs), c-AMP responsive element (CREB)) in the immune response.[42] In particular, in vitro studies showed rapid phosphorylation/dephosphorylation of these signaling components in response to different stimuli, with specific time courses and resulting in the activation of different functional immune parameters. Challenges with different bacteria (*Escherichia coli* and *V. cholerae*) resulted in differential activation/inactivation of cytosolic kinases as well as of the transcription factors STAT1 and CREB.[42] In particular, different strains of *E. coli* and *V. cholerae* (*E. coli* MG155, a wild-type strain carrying type 1 fimbriae, and its unfimbriated derivative, AAEC072 Δfim; *V. cholerae* O1 El Tor biotype strain N16961, carrying MSHA, and its ΔMSHA mutant) induced distinct patterns of phosphorylation of MAPKs, in particular of the stress-activated p38 and JNKs as well as PKC isoforms that were related to differences in bactericidal activity.[43] The lower antibacterial activity of hemocytes toward the mutant *E. coli* strain and wild-type *V. cholerae* compared with wild-type *E. coli* was associated with a reduced capacity of activating MAPKs. Moreover, the ΔMSHA *V. cholerae* strain that was the most resistant to the hemocyte bactericidal activity induced downregulation of cell signaling, strong lysosomal damage, and reduced hydrolytic enzyme release.[44] These results underlined how not only different bacteria but also different bacterial strains can elicit specific responses in terms of the activation of cytosolic components of kinase-mediated signaling: these effects were ascribed to specific surface interactions between hemocytes and bacteria. Interestingly, the differential effects on immune signaling and the resulting immune response observed in vitro well correlated with the capacity of mussels to clear different *E. coli* and *V. cholerae* strains from their hemolymph in vivo.[45,46]

Differential responses were also observed in *Mytilus* hemocytes challenged with two different bivalve pathogens, *V. splendidus* LGP32 and *V. anguillarum* (ATCC 19264). Functional responses were first observed in vivo after a challenge with heat-killed bacteria.[47] The underlying mechanisms were investigated in vitro, with live bacteria, revealing the differential activation of immune signaling by the two vibrio species.[48] *Vibrio splendidus* LGP32 rapidly induced significant changes in hemocyte adhesion, lysosomal membrane stability, lysozyme release, extracellular ROS, and NO production. These responses were associated with rapid and persistent activation of p38 MAPK and PKC isoforms. On the other hand, *V. anguillarum* showed a reduced capacity to stimulate functional immune responses, in line with a reduced activation of p-38 MAPK and PKC with respect to *V. splendidus*.

Overall, these studies underlined the specificity of kinase-mediated signaling activated by bacterial challenges in mussel hemocytes; however, the identification of these signaling components, evaluation of protein expression, and their activation state (phosphorylation) were based on the utilization of heterologous antibodies and on the use of specific pharmacological inhibitors of their mammalian counterparts. Homologues to MAPK pathway constituents were first sequenced in oyster[49] and manila clam.[50] More recently, NGS analyses on *R. philippinarum*[51] and *C. virginica*[52] have helped to finally identify a functionally conservative set of regulated transcripts associated with MAPK pathways. Recent advancements in transcriptomics and data mining pipelines have also enabled the discovery of JAK/STAT homologues in *M. edulis*.[33]

IMMUNE EFFECTORS

Defense responses involve phagocytosis of foreign materials and the ROS production and release of hydrolytic enzymes, lectins, and antimicrobial peptides by the hemocytes.[3] Bivalve hemolymph serum contains a wide range of different secreted components that participate in agglutination, opsonization, degradation, and encapsulation of microorganisms as well as in clotting and wound healing.[3,9] An overview of the most recent accomplishments in the fields of AMPs, lysozymes, cytokines and acute phase processes that depend on perforins, immune cell activation, and antioxidant enzymes is given by Bassim et al.[8] Additionally, proteins involved in metal homeostasis, such as ferritin and metallothionein, were identified in bivalves following exposure to pathogens or PAMPs and are thought to be part of the elicited antimicrobial processes.[51]

Induction of many cellular and serum functional immune parameters by different stimuli, including in vitro and in vivo challenges with live and heat-killed bacteria and PAMPs, has been evaluated in a large number of studies on different bivalve species. Although quantitative differences could be observed in different experimental conditions, no clear evidence of specificity emerged from these studies, and therefore data are not reported in this chapter. An exception to this is represented by AMPs, small cationic peptides with a remarkable structural diversity, engaged in the destruction of bacteria inside phagocytes, before being released into hemolymph to participate in systemic responses.[1] In *Mytilus*, different AMPs (including defensins, mytilins, and myticins) share antibacterial and antifungal properties; on the other hand, mytimycin was identified as the first strictly antifungal protein from mollusks.[52]

SPECIFICITY OF THE IMMUNE RESPONSE TO PATHOGENIC VIBRIOS: ROLE OF SURFACE INTERACTIONS AND SERUM-SOLUBLE COMPONENTS

The specificity of the bivalve immune response has been investigated mainly in bivalve species susceptible to infection by certain *Vibrio* spp. and strains. However, a limited number of studies focused on the mechanisms underlying differential responses of bivalves to different pathogenic vibrios, in particular with those strains associated with oyster summer mortalities as described in the section Bivalves and Marine Bacteria. The first work describing specific mechanisms involved in the interactions between bivalve hemocytes and bacteria was that of Duperthuy et al.,[26] with oysters and the oyster pathogen *V. splendidus* LGP32. In *C. gigas*, LGP32 uses the OmpU protein to attach and invade the hemocytes through Cg-EcSOD (extracellular superoxide dismutase), the major plasma protein that acts as an opsonin mediating recognition and promoting phagocytosis. In this process, Cg-EcSOD is recognized through its RGD (Arg-Gly-Asp) sequence by hemocyte β-integrins, leading to subversion of the cell actin cytoskeleton, inducing the expression of trafficking genes, and resulting in actin and clathrin polymerization. Capable of intracellular survival, LGP32 was shown to escape from host cellular defenses by avoiding acidic vacuole formation and by limiting ROS production.

A different situation was observed in *M. galloprovincialis* that is resistant to LGP32 infection.[53] LGP32 was rapidly phagocytized by the hemocytes, where it induced lysosomal damage; when internalized, it remained viable and culturable within intracellular vacuoles apparently escaping lysosomal degradation through disregulation of phosphatidylinositol 3 kinase signaling, leading to impairment of the endolysosomal system. However, interactions with hemolymph soluble factors were not crucial in determining the effects of this strain on mussel hemocytes. Actually, in mussels, the major plasma protein is the "extrapallial fluid major protein" (EP protein) that shares no sequence homology with CgEcSOD.[54] The effects of LGP32 in mussels were confirmed in vivo, following injection with bacteria, where no bactericidal activity toward *V. splendidus* was observed at different times postinjection; this strain was actually able to grow within mussel hemolymph, leading to stressful conditions in the hemocytes. However, this effect was transient, and hemocytes showed the capacity to recover at longer times postinjection. Overall, these data indicated that the mechanisms involved in promoting LGP32 adhesion and invasion in oyster and mussel hemocytes may be profoundly different, resulting in different effects. Moreover, these data underlined the role of species-specific interactions of soluble hemolymph proteins with different *vibrio* strains.

Previous studies showed that, in mussels, soluble hemolymph components can play a key role in mediating the interactions between bacteria and hemocytes. In *M. galloprovincialis*, serum soluble factors specifically bind mannose-sensitive bacterial ligands (ie, type 1 fimbriae of *E. coli* and MSHA pilus of *V. cholerae*), thus promoting efficient adhesion to and killing by hemocytes.[43–46] Preliminary data indicated that a thermolabile protein fraction with an MW >10kD may be involved in this process.[55] The possible interactions between mussel hemocytes, soluble opsonins, and MSHA carrying bacteria are depicted in Fig. 6.1.

As mentioned above, MSHA adhesins are also present in a large proportion of environmental isolates of *V. aestuarianus*.[29] *V. aestuarianus* pathogenicity to *C. gigas* has been demonstrated by experimental challenges[32]; on the other hand, *V. aestuarianus* isolates were only moderately pathogenic to *M. galloprovincialis*.[18,56] The different sensitivity to infection of the two bivalve species may partly depend on their different capability to kill invading pathogens through the action of soluble hemolymph components.[3,44]

The role of mannose-sensitive interactions in *V. aestuarianus* 01/032 sensitivity to killing by *M. galloprovincialis* and *C. gigas* hemolymph was recently investigated.[57] Although 01/032 bacteria adhered to hemocytes of both bivalves, they were sensitive to the bactericidal activity of whole hemolymph from mussel but not from oyster; in addition, adhesion to mussel (but not

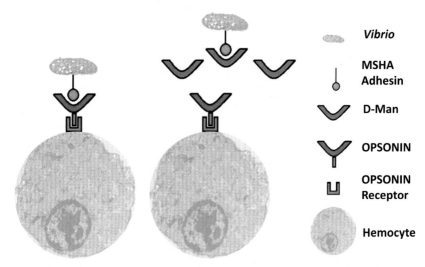

FIGURE 6.1   Schematic representation of the interactions between *Mytilus* hemocytes, soluble hemolymph components, and bacteria carrying the D-mannose-sensitive mannose sensitive hemagglutinin (MSHA) adhesin.

oyster) hemocytes was affected by D-mannose. The mussel hemolymph protein responsible for promoting mannose-sensitive interactions of *V. aestuarianus* 01/032 with the hemocytes, thus serving as an opsonin, was identified as the extrapallial protein precursor (EP) of *M. edulis*.[57] EP, the major plasma protein in *Mytilus*, is an acidic glycoprotein with a high histidine content that can bind Ca^{2+} and heavy metals.[54] Recently, by an MS-based approach, a complex and anomalous N-glycan structure was determined in *M. edulis* EP. Such unique structure and calcium and heavy metal binding properties suggest a possible role for this protein in multiple biological functions, including shell formation, metal ion transportation, and detoxification.[58] Interestingly, EP also shows a conserved domain homologous to MgC1q6, a complement component identified in *M. galloprovincialis*.[41] These data ascribe to mussel EP the additional role of mediating specific immune interactions against bacteria carrying D-mannose-sensitive ligands.

CONCLUSIONS

Increasing knowledge of bivalve immunity is revealing a complex innate immune system able to recognize and eliminate a wide range of invading microorganisms in a fluctuating environment. Studies with different bacterial species and strains will help in understanding the mechanisms underlying the specificity of bivalve immune response, thus contributing to developing innovative solutions and tools for the prevention, control, and mitigation of bivalve disease in farmed species.

REFERENCES

1. Song L, Wang L, Qiu L, Zhang H. Bivalve immunity. *Adv Exp Med Biol* 2010;**708**:44–65.
2. Ghosh J, Lun CM, Majeske AJ, Sacchi S, Schrankel CS, Smith LC. Invertebrate immune diversity. *Dev Comp Immunol* 2011;**35**:959–74.
3. Canesi L, Gallo G, Gavioli M, Pruzzo C. Bacteria-hemocyte interactions and phagocytosis in marine bivalves. *Microsc Res Tech* 2002;**57**:469–76.
4. Hine PM. The inter-relationships of bivalve haemocytes. *Fish Shellfish Immunol* 1999;**9**: 367–85.
5. Allam B, Ashton-Alcox KA, Ford SE. Flow cytometric comparison of haemocytes from three species of bivalve molluscs. *Fish Shellfish Immunol* 2002;**13**:141–58.
6. Parisi MG, Li H, Jouvet LB, Dyrynda EA, Parrinello N, Cammarata M, et al. Differential involvement of mussel hemocyte sub-populations in the clearance of bacteria. *Fish Shellfish Immunol* 2008;**25**:834–40.
7. Hong HK, Kang HS, Le TC, Choi KS. Comparative study on the hemocytes of subtropical oysters *Saccostrea kegaki* (Torigoe & Inaba, 1981), *Ostrea circumpicta* (Pilsbry, 1904), and *Hyotissahyotis* (Linnaeus, 1758) in Jeju Island, Korea: morphology and functional aspects. *Fish Shellfish Immunol* 2013;**35**:2020–5.
8. Bassim S, Tanguy A, Genard B, Moraga D, Tremblay R. Identification of *Mytilus edulis* genetic regulators during early development. *Gene* 2014;**551**:65–78.
9. Ellis RP, Parry H, Spicer JI, Hutchinson TH, Pipe RK, Widdicombe S. Immunological function in marine invertebrates: responses to environmental perturbation. *Fish Shellfish Immunol* 2011;**3**:1209–22.
10. Pruzzo C, Huq A, Colwell RR, Donelli G. Pathogenic Vibrio species in marine and estuarine environment. In: Colwell R, Belkin S, editors. *Oceans and health: pathogens in the marine environment*. New York: Kluwer Academic/Plenum Publishers; 2005. p. 217–52.
11. Beaz-Hidalgo R, Balboa S, Romalde JL, Figueras MJ. Diversity and pathogenicity of *Vibrio* species in cultured bivalve molluscs. *Environ Microbiol Rep* 2010;**2**:34–43.
12. Paillard C, Le Roux F, Borrego JJ. Bacterial disease in marine bivalves, a review of recent studies: trends and evolution. *Aquat Living Resour* 2004;**17**:477–98.
13. Wendling CC, Batista FM, Wegner KM. Persistence, seasonal dynamics and pathogenic potential of Vibrio communities from Pacific oyster hemolymph. *PLoS One* 2014;**9**:e94256.
14. Elston RA, Frelier P, Cheney D. Extrapallial abscesses associated with chronic bacterial infections in the intensively cultured juvenile Pacific oyster *Crassostrea gigas*. *Dis Aquat Org* 1999;**37**:115–20.
15. Balseiro P, Moreira R, Chamorro R, Figueras A, Novoa B. Immune responses during the larval stages of *Mytilus galloprovincialis*: metamorphosis alters immunocompetence, body shape and behavior. *Fish Shellfish Immunol* 2013;**35**:438–47.
16. Richard G, Le Bris C, Guérard F, Lambert C, Paillard C. Immune responses of phenoloxidase and superoxide dismutase in the manila clam *Venerupis philippinarum* challenged with *Vibrio tapetis* - Part II: combined effect of temperature and two *V. tapetis* strains. *Fish Shellfish Immunol* 2015;**44**:79–87.
17. Lacoste A, Jalabert F, Malham S, Cueff A, Gelebart F, Cordevant C, et al. A *Vibrio splendidus* strain is associated with summer mortality of juvenile oysters *Crassostrea gigas* in the Bay of Morlaix (North Brittany, France). *Dis Aquat Organ* 2001;**46**:139–45.
18. Garnier M, Labreuche Y, Garcia C, Robert M, Nicolas JL. Evidence for the involvement of pathogenic bacteria in summer mortalities of the Pacific oyster *Crassostrea gigas*. *Microb Ecol* 2007;**53**:187–96.

19. Schikorski D, Faury N, Pépin JF, Saulnier D, Tourbiez D, Renault T. Experimental ostreid herpesvirus 1 infection of the Pacific oyster *Crassostrea gigas*: kinetics of virus DNA detection by q-PCR in seawater and in oyster samples. *Virus Res* 2011;**155**:28–34.
20. Madec S, Pichereau V, Jacq A, Paillard M, Boisset C, Guerard G, et al. Characterization of the secretomes of two vibrios pathogenic to mollusks. *PLoS One* 2014;**9**:e113097.
21. Jeffroy F, Brulle F, Paillard C. Differential expression of genes involved in immunity and biomineralization during Brown Ring Disease development and shell repair in the Manila clam, *Ruditapes philippinarum*. *J Invertebr Pathol* 2013;**113**:129–36.
22. Allam B, Ford SE. Effects of the pathogenic *Vibrio tapetis* on defence factors of susceptible and non-susceptible bivalve species: I. Haemocyte changes following in vitro challenge. *Fish Shellfish Immunol* 2006;**20**:374–83.
23. Vezzulli L, Brettar I, Pezzati E, Reid PC, Colwell RR, et al. Long-term effects of ocean warming on the prokaryotic community: evidence from the vibrios. *ISME J* 2012;**6**:21–30.
24. Nasfi H, Travers MA, de Lorgeril J, Habib C, Sannie T, Sorieul L, et al. European epidemiological survey of *Vibrio splendidus* clade shows unexplored diversity and massive exchange of virulence factors. *World J Microbiol Biotechnol* 2015;**31**:461–75.
25. Sawabe T, Ogura Y, Matsumura Y, Feng G, Amin AR, Mino S, et al. Updating the Vibrio clades defined by multilocus sequence 512 phylogeny: proposal of eight new clades, and the description of *Vibrio tritonius* sp.nov.513. *Front Microbiol* 2013;**4**:414.
26. Duperthuy M, Schmitt P, Garzón E, Caro A, Rosa RD, Le Roux F, et al. Use of OmpU porins for attachment and invasion of *Crassostrea gigas* immune cells by the oyster pathogen *Vibrio splendidus*. *Proc Natl Acad Sci USA* 2011;**108**:2993–8.
27. Le Roux F, Binesse J, Saulnier D, Mazel D. Construction of a *Vibrio splendidus* mutant lacking the metalloprotease gene vsm by use of a novel counter selectable suicide vector. *Appl Environ Microbiol* 2007;**73**:777–84.
28. Vanhove AS, Duperthuy M, Charriere GM, Le Roux F, Goudenege D, Gourbal B, et al. Outer membrane vesicles are vehicles for the delivery of *Vibrio tasmaniensis* virulence factors to oyster immune cells. *Environ Microbiol* 2015;**17**:1152–65.
29. Vezzulli L, Pezzati E, Stauder M, Stagnaro L, Venier P, Pruzzo C. Aquatic ecology of the oyster pathogens *Vibrio splendidus* and *Vibrio aestuarianus*. *Environ Microbiol* 2015;**17**(4):1065–80.
30. Labreuche Y, Soudant P, Gonçalves M, Lambert C, Nicolas JL. Effects of extracellular products from the pathogenic *Vibrio aestuarianus* strain 01/32 on lethality and cellular immune responses of the oyster *Crassostrea gigas*. *Dev Comp Immunol* 2006;**30**:367–79.
31. Garnier M, Labreuche Y, Nicolas JL. Molecular and phenotypic characterization of *Vibrio aestuarianus* subsp. francensis subsp nov., a pathogen of the oyster *Crassostrea gigas*. *Syst Appl Microbiol* 2008;**31**:358–65.
32. Labreuche Y, Le Roux F, Henry J, Zatylny C, Huvet A, Lambert C, et al. *Vibrio aestuarianus* zinc metalloprotease causes lethality in the Pacific oyster *Crassostreagigas* and impairs the host cellular immune defenses. *Fish Shellfish Immunol* 2010;**29**:753–8.
33. Philipp EE, Kraemer L, Melzner F, Poustka AJ, Thieme S, Findeisen U, et al. Massively parallel RNA sequencing identifies a complex immune gene repertoire in the lophotrochozoan *Mytilus edulis*. *PLoS One* 2012;**7**:e33091.
34. Huang M, Song X, Zhao J, Mu C, Wang L, Zhang H, et al. A C-type lectin (AiCTL-3) from bay scallop *Argopecten irradians* with mannose/galactose binding ability to bind various bacteria. *Gene* 2013;**531**:31–8.
35. Cooper EL, Kvell K, Engelmann P, Nemeth P. Still waiting for the toll? *Immunol Lett* 2006;**104**:18–28.

36. Moreira R, Balseiro P, Romero A, Dios S, Posada D, Novoa B, et al. Gene expression analysis of clams *Ruditapes philippinarum* and *Ruditapes decussatus* following bacterial infection yields molecular insights into pathogen resistance and immunity. *Dev Comp Immunol* 2012;**36**:140–9.
37. Zhang L, Li L, Zhang G. A *Crassostrea gigas* Toll-like receptor and comparative analysis of TLR pathway in invertebrates. *Fish Shellfish Immunol* 2011;**30**:653–60.
38. Toubiana M, Rosani U, Giambelluca S, Cammarata M, Gerdol M, Pallavicini A, et al. Toll signal transduction pathway in bivalves: complete cds of intermediate elements and related gene transcription levels in hemocytes of immune stimulated *Mytilus galloprovincialis*. *Dev Comp Immunol* 2014;**45**:300–12.
39. Nayak A, Pednekar L, Reid KB, Kishore U. Complement and non-complement activating functions of C1q: a prototypical innate immune molecule. *Innate Immun* 2012;**18**:350–63.
40. Gestal C, Pallavicini A, Venier P, Novoa B, Figueras A. MgC1q, a novel C1q-domain-containing protein involved in the immune response of *Mytilus galloprovincialis*. *Dev Comp Immunol* 2010;**34**:926–34.
41. Gerdol M, Venier P, Pallavicini A. The genome of the Pacific oyster *Crassostrea gigas* brings new insights on the massive expansion of the C1q gene family in Bivalvia. *Dev Comp Immunol* 2015;**49**:59–71.
42. Canesi L, Betti M, Ciacci C, Lorusso LC, Pruzzo C, Gallo G. Cell signaling in the immune response of mussel hemocytes. *Invertebr Surviv J* 2006;**3**:40–9.
43. Canesi L, Betti M, Ciacci C, Lorusso LC, Gallo G, Pruzzo C. Interactions between *Mytilus* haemocytes and different strains of *Escherichia coli* and *Vibrio cholerae* O1 El Tor: role of kinase-mediated signalling. *Cell Microbiol* 2005;**7**:667–74.
44. Pruzzo C, Gallo G, Canesi L. Persistence of vibrios in marine bivalves: the role of interactions with haemolymph components. *Environ Microbiol* 2005;**7**:761–72.
45. Canesi L, Pruzzo C, Tarsi R, Gallo G. Surface interactions between *Escherichia coli* and hemocytes of the Mediterranean mussel *Mytilus galloprovincialis* Lam. leading to efficient bacterial clearance. *Appl Environ Microbiol* 2001;**67**:464–8.
46. Zampini M, Canesi L, Betti M, Ciacci C, Tarsi R, Gallo G, et al. Role for mannose-sensitive hemagglutinin in promoting interactions between *Vibrio cholerae* El Tor and mussel hemolymph. *Appl Environ Microbiol* 2003;**69**:5711–5.
47. Ciacci C, Citterio B, Betti M, Canonico B, Roch P, Canesi L. Functional differential immune responses of *Mytilus galloprovincialis* to bacterial challenge. *Comp Biochem Physiol B Biochem Mol Biol* 2009;**153**:365–71.
48. Ciacci C, Betti M, Canonico B, Citterio B, Roch P, Canesi L. Specificity of anti-Vibrio immune response through p38 MAPK and PKC activation in the hemocytes of the mussel *Mytilus galloprovincialis*. *J Invertebr Pathol* 2010;**105**:49–55.
49. Tanguy A, Boutet I, Laroche J, Moraga D. Molecular identification and expression study of differentially regulated genes in the Pacific oyster *Crassostrea gigas* in response to pesticide exposure. *FEBS J* 2004;**272**:390–403.
50. Kang Y-S, Kim Y-M, Park K-I, Cho SK, Choi K-S, Cho M. Analysis of EST and lectin expressions in hemocytes of manila clams (*Ruditapes philippinarum*) (bivalvia: Mollusca) infected with *Perkinsus olseni*. *Dev Comp Immunol* 2006;**30**:1119–31.
51. Perrigault M, Allam B. Differential immune response in the hard clam (*Mercenaria Mercenaria*) against bacteria and the protistan pathogen QPX (quahog parasite unknown). *Fish Shellfish Immunol* 2012;**32**:1124–34.
52. Sonthi M, Cantet F, Toubiana M, Trapani MR, Parisi MG, Cammarata M, et al. Gene expression specificity of the mussel antifungal mytimycin (MytM). *Fish Shellfish Immunol* 2012;**32**:45–50.

53. Balbi T, Fabbri R, Cortese K, Smerilli A, Ciacci C, Grande C, et al. Interactions between *Mytilus galloprovincialis* hemocytes and the bivalve pathogens *Vibrio aestuarianus* 01/032 and *Vibrio splendidus* LGP32. *Fish Shellfish Immunol* 2013;**35**:1906–15.

54. Itoh N, Xue QG, Schey KL, Li Y, Cooper RK, La Peyre JF. Characterization of the major plasma protein of the eastern oyster, *Crassostrea virginica*, and a proposed role in host defense. *Comp Biochem Physiol B Biochem Mol Biol* 2011;**158**:9–22.

55. Canesi L, Pezzati E, Stauder M, Grande C, Bavestrello M, Papetti A, et al. *Vibrio cholerae* interactions with *Mytilus galloprovincialis* hemocytes mediated by serum components. *Front Microbiol* 2013;**4**:371.

56. Romero A, Costa M, Forn-Cuni G, Balseiro P, Chamorro R, Dios S, et al. Occurrence, seasonality and infectivity of Vibrio strains in natural populations of mussels *Mytilus galloprovincialis*. *Dis Aquat Organ* 2014;**108**:149–63.

57. Pezzati E, Canesi L, Damonte G, Salis A, Marsano F, Grande C, et al. Susceptibility of *Vibrio aestuarianus* 01/032 to the antibacterial activity of *Mytilus* hemolymph: identification of a serum opsonin involved in mannose-sensitive interactions. *Environ Microbiol* February 5, 2015. http://dx.doi.org/10.1111/1462-2920.12750.

58. Zhou H, Hanneman AJ, Chasteen ND, Reinhold VN. Anomalous N-Glycan structures with an internal fucose branched to GlcA and GlcN residues isolated from a mollusk shell-forming fluid. *J Proteome Res* 2013;**12**:4547–55.

Chapter 7

Immune-Related Signaling in Mussel and Bivalves

Paola Venier, Stefania Domeneghetti, Nidhi Sharma
University of Padova, Padova, Italy

Alberto Pallavicini, Marco Gerdol
University of Trieste, Trieste, Italy

List of Abbreviations

AIF-1 Allograft inflammatory factor-1
AMPs Antimicrobial peptides
Apaf-1 Apoptotic protease-activating factor 1
ATGs Autophagy-related genes
BAX Bcl2-associated X protein
Bcl-2 B-cell lymphoma 2 protein
Dff-A DNA fragmentation factor 45
ds Double stranded
FADD Fas (TNFRSF6)-associated via death domain
IAPs Apoptosis inhibitors
IFN, IFNs Interferon, Interferons
IL-1β Interleukin-1β
IL-17 Interleukin 17
IRF IFN regulatory factor
ISGs IFN-stimulated genes
JAK-STAT Janus-activated kinase–signal transducer and activator of transcription
MAPKs Mitogen-activated protein kinases
MIF Macrophage migration inhibitory factor
miRNA microRNA
NGF Nerve growth factor
NLRs NOD-like receptors
OsHV-1 Ostreid herpesvirus type 1
PAMPs Pathogen-associated molecular patterns
PDRG p53 and DNA-damage regulated protein
PGRPs Peptidoglycan recognition proteins
RLRs RIG-like receptors
RNAi RNA interference

Lessons in Immunity: From Single-Cell Organisms to Mammals
http://dx.doi.org/10.1016/B978-0-12-803252-7.00007-2

siRNA Small inhibitory RNA
SOCS Suppressor of cytokine signaling proteins
ss Single stranded
STING Stimulator of interferon genes
TLRs Toll-like receptors
TNF Tumor necrosis factor

PREMISE

Animal immune systems allow efficient functional reactions against infective agents, parasites, or excessive amounts of opportunistic microbes; however, at the same time, symbiotic bacteria and viruses in the latency phase maintain successful ecological niches in their hosts.[1,2] Any imbalance in the complex relationships between hosts and their microorganism associations, including the occurrence of novel host–pathogen interactions, can lead to the emergence of diseases and mortality outbreaks.[3,4,5]

Current advances in the life sciences and the still mounting wave of molecular data for a variety of nonmodel organisms demonstrate the fundamental role of immunity in animal life.[6,7] In regard to marine bivalve mollusks, the available sequence data now include several transcriptomes, which have been recently reviewed[8,9]: the genomes of *Crassostrea gigas*,[10] *Pinctada fucata*,[11] *Mytilus galloprovincialis*,[12] and the upcoming genome of *Crassostrea virginica*.[13] These resources not only offer the opportunity to speed up the identification of protein domains and genes involved in fundamental cell processes[14,15] but also bring new clarity to understanding the genetic population structure[16] and to developing marker-assisted selection programs.[12,17]

MULTIPLE LAYERS OF BIOLOGICAL SIGNALING

Host–microorganism interactions are fundamental drivers of animal life and evolution.[18,19] The terms "interspecies" and "interkingdom signaling" have been used to indicate the signaling role of molecules derived from bacteria toward similar or dissimilar bacterial strains, single-cell, and multicellular eukaryotes.[20] Peptidoglycan provides a paradigmatic example of structural and signaling molecules. It composes the cell wall of most bacteria in the form of an extracellular polymer, more abundant in gram-positive than in gram-negative bacteria, and it is actively replaced at each generation. Peptidoglycan fragments called muropeptides can (1) indicate growth-promoting conditions to nongrowing bacteria, (2) mediate diverse processes including the selective recognition of symbiotic luminescent bacteria, and (3) allow the sensing of a "nonself" cell in the host via Toll-like receptors (TLRs), peptidoglycan recognition proteins (PGRPs), and cytosolic NOD-like receptors (NLRs), ultimately shaping the host immunity through the modulated expression of antimicrobial peptides (AMPs) and other effector proteins.[20]

In multicellular eukaryotes, mainly humans, there is increasing evidence of bidirectional signaling between the immune and the neuroendocrine system in both physiological and pathological conditions. Actually, nerve growth factor (NGF, a signaling molecule also produced by macrophages and mast cells) and known proinflammatory cytokines, such as tumor necrosis factor (TNF) and interleukin-1β (IL-1β), can act as pain mediators by activating and sensitizing sensory neurons called nociceptors (enhancing the expression and release of neuropeptides, among other cellular changes).[21] Other lines of evidence suggest direct and indirect influences of chemokines, secreted proteins able to attract and activate immune cells, on the nociceptor excitability.[21] The specific interaction of bacterial products such as the α-hemolysin toxin and formylated peptides on neuronal membrane proteins allows the peripheral network of nociceptors to integrate the sensing of local infections and inflammatory reactions.[22,23] Data obtained on mammalian cells suggest that nociceptors would represent the very first line of defense against infective agents and that released neuropeptides could modulate the activity of innate and adaptive immune cells in multiple ways, leading for instance to cell priming or immune tolerance.[21,24] As a whole, the signals provided to various target cells by hormones, neurotransmitters and neuropeptides, and several cytokines produced by different cell types give shape to ordinary and atypical immune responses and to related systemic phenotypes.

In *Mytilus* spp., the identification of transcript sequences encoding for receptors of neurotransmitters, such as glutamate, or similar to neuropeptide Y, a sympathetic peptide possibly contributing to neurogenic inflammation,[24] stimulates new studies on the cross talk between sensory and immune systems. In addition to insulin-related peptides and cysteine-knot protein hormones, the inspection of genome and transcriptome data sets has revealed several dozen putative genes for neuropeptide precursors in the limpet *Lottia gigantea*,[25] in the oysters *P. fucata* and *C. gigas*,[26] and in the land snail *Theba pisana*.[27] In general, neuropeptides encompass chemically diverse messengers instrumental to complex physiological events: whether the putative mollusk neuropeptides act in a similar fashion to the arthropod and mammalian homologues and to what extent they can influence invertebrate immunity are questions that remain to be solved with appropriate studies.

A recent survey aiming to identify bivalve cytokines by systematic screening of their functional motifs in genomic and transcriptome data sets demonstrated the presence and remarkable evolutionary conservation of interleukin 17 (IL-17) and proximate signaling components in *M. galloprovincialis*.[28] Such proinflammatory cytokines have been traced in oysters,[29,30] abalone,[31] and other invertebrates. The existence of six putative/ predicted IL-17s in *M. galloprovincialis* and 10 putative/predicted IL-17s in *C. gigas* suggests the possibility of different ligand–receptor combinations with pleiotropic effects on the target cells, as reported in mammals.

Indeed, various expression patterns were detected for ligands and receptors in hemocytes and gills of mussels immunostimulated with heat-killed bacteria (*Micrococcus lysodeyticus, Vibrio splendidus, Vibrio anguillarum*).[28] Moreover, the general overexpression of IL-17s and downstream signaling components in *C. gigas* spat actively infected by Ostreid herpesvirus type 1 (OsHV-1) confirm the importance of this molecular pathway in the antiviral bivalve response.[28]

Previously, transcript sequences for the macrophage migration inhibitory factor (MIF) with predicted tautomerase and oxidoreductase activities were identified in *M. galloprovincialis*.[32,33] Mussel MIF, constitutively expressed in hemocytes and mantle, was closely related to that of *P. fucata* and *Haliotis diversicolor* but not to that of *Chlamys farreri* and *Biomphalaria glabrata*.[34–37] In addition to a better understanding of the regulatory role of MIF in the mussel immune system, it would be worth investigating if mussel MIF can attenuate the antinociceptive action of morphine and opioids.[38]

Mussels and a number of other mollusk species possess homologues of the allograft inflammatory factor-1 (AIF-1), a calcium-binding cytokine participating in the inflammatory response and activation of immune cells.[10,32,39–45] CgAIF-1 displays constitutive transcription in the main oyster tissues, particularly in hemocytes. It is inducible by various pathogen-associated molecular patterns (PAMPs) and it is able to enhance both granulocyte-mediated phagocytosis and transcript levels of oyster MIF, IL-17, and TNF.[43] The upregulation of OeAIF in hemocytes and the mantle of flat oysters with heavy bonamiosis is consistent with the maintenance of the inflammatory status in response to the parasitic protist.[45]

In addition, a transcript for a TNF orthologue was upregulated in the hemocytes of the highly parasitized flat oysters.[45] TNFs represent an important family of pleiotropic cytokines. Protein coding sequences, with a typical TNF domain and a short N-terminal hydrophobic stretch for membrane anchoring, have been involved in cell proliferation, immune regulation, inflammation, cell death, and apoptosis. Human TNFα is mainly secreted by macrophages. After ligand–receptor binding, specific protein–protein interactions relating to interconnected signaling pathways drive the cell to its fate (apoptotic death or cell survival with expression of proinflammatory or immunomodulatory genes). Numerous TNF superfamily genes have been identified in various bivalve spp., such as *Mytilus edulis, Mytilus californianus*, and *C. gigas*, where tandem gene duplication events probably generated 23 distinct TNF superfamily genes.[10,46,47] Although early approaches of EST Sanger sequencing only allowed the identification of TNF-interacting molecules in *M. gall provicialis*,[32] deep sequencing technologies coupled with protein domain analysis were more exhaustive and revealed at least three TNF superfamily transcript sequences.[8] Overall, the number of TNF genes identified in *C. gigas* and other mollusks, and their differential transcription under biotic or abiotic challenges and during development, support the hypothesis of taxon-specific expansion and functional diversification of these genes.[10,14,46,47]

The existence of invertebrate cytokines has been a lively debated issue since no structural homologues could be identified for a very long time, albeit the evolutionary conservation of intracellular signaling pathways, which would hypothetically trigger their expression. Despite the substantial lack of sequence similarity with their vertebrate counterparts, current data demonstrate the presence of such gene-encoded signaling factors in mollusks while the bioinformatics analysis is already expanding to neurohormones and neuropeptides. The elucidation of the gene structure, functional properties, and involvement of these regulatory proteins in mussel immunity certainly require genuine research work.

In regard to interferons (IFNs), these cytokines are typically produced by virus-infected cells. They interfere with viral replication and counteract other nonself elements such as bacteria, parasites, and tumor cells by sustaining the activation of immune cells and modulating different aspects of the innate and adaptive immunity. Following receptor binding, members of the Janus-activated kinase–signal transducer and activator of the transcription family (JAK-STAT) mediate the expression of many IFN-stimulated genes (ISGs) including those involved in signal transduction (mitogen- and stress-activated protein kinases, among others) as well as genes encoding for antimicrobial and antiviral proteins (eg, guanylate-binding proteins including small immunity-related GTPases, or IRGs, and Mx proteins). Among human IFNs, the IFNα secreted by macrophages has a clear antiviral activity, whereas IFNβ is proapoptotic and can antagonize some of the proinflammatory effects of IFNγ. Although transcript sequences for IFN-inducible proteins and IFN regulatory factors (IRFs) have been identified in mussel[8,32] and oyster,[10,47,48] respectively, the search for mollusk IFNs did not give significant results. Indeed, the evolutionary history of IFNγ can be traced back to the onset of the gnathostome lineage as no IFN-like sequences can be detected in agnathans nor in basal deuterostomes[49]: any protostome molecule functionally homologous to vertebrate IFNs, if present, might be structurally divergent. Despite only indirect data suggesting an IFN-like response in *M. galloprovincialis*,[50] the identification and functional analysis of an IFN-like protein[51] and of downstream signaling elements[52] in *C. gigas* currently stimulate the scientific debate.

IMMUNE SIGNALING AND RELATED CELL PROCESSES

Recent papers offer an updated view of key molecules and main events shaping the immune responses in bivalve spp.[8,9,47,53,54] Inside the cells, interconnected signaling pathways translate the signals referring to normal functioning and alarm/stress situations in concerted waves of gene expression and, therefore, condition-dependent transcriptomes, proteomes, and metabolomes. According to what we know about model organisms, the role of some signal transduction pathways in the animal immune responses is well recognized. However, numerous signaling intermediates and the complexity of protein–protein interactions within redundant pathways of response make an overall mechanistic picture impossible, in particular for invertebrate species, which testify their own evolutionary solutions for life.

Marine bivalves bear endosymbiotic bacteria and live surrounded by microbes and viruses, which fluctuate with the season and habitat features. Recent studies have revealed that the Toll/NF-kB signaling, an ancient defense pathway whose key elements can be found in most protostomes, is present and well developed in *Mytilus* spp.[55–58] While the presence of TLRs and intracellular signaling components is not surprising by itself, the multiplicity of the TLR genes, observed in mussel and confirmed in the oyster genome,[47] can be interpreted as a strategy to better cope with a challenging habitat. In the Mediterranean mussel, the analysis of constitutive and inducible gene expression levels indicated the activation of the Toll/NF-kB pathway against gram-negative and gram-positive bacteria as well as fungi.[57,58] At the present time, it is not known if this pathway can be uniformly activated in different cell types, if endosome-specific TLRs exist in mussels, and how TLRs operate during multiple defensive events.[59] Although transcript sequences for intermediate elements homologous to the insect IMD pathway are detectable in mussel, transcripts for molecules with a role homologous to the insect Spätzle and to the IMD/RIP adaptor could not be identified by comparative sequence analysis,[8] possibly because of the large evolutionary divergence between Ecdysozoa and Lophotrochozoa.

The MAPK signaling, generally activated in response to stimuli related to cell growth, differentiation, and survival processes, can also be activated downstream of TLRs. Moreover, one recent study performed in mussel and oysters supports the functional connection between the IL-17 and MAPK signaling pathways.[28] The MAPK signaling elements identified in *Mytilus* and other bivalve spp. are detailed elsewhere.[8]

Mytilus transcript sequences encoding proteins like cytosolic RIG-like receptors (RLRs), JAK 2, STAT, the suppressor of cytokine signaling SOCS, the helicase DDX41, and the stimulator of interferon genes STING support the presence of multiple antiviral signaling pathways, which ensures the expression of proinflammatory cytokines and antiviral effector genes.[8,55]

In the complexity of cell processes, the overall balance of molecular events mediated by interconnected signal transduction pathways more or less involved in the immune responses (eg, MAPK, P13K/AKT, etc.) can eventually drive the apoptotic death of infected cells or the fight against pathogens and parasites able to counteract and elude the host defense mechanisms.[59–62]

Cell death is essential to the immune host response, and it can occur in different modes, which are most often genetically regulated.[63] Apoptosis eliminates atypical, damaged, and infected cells without inflammation, and it can be stimulated in mollusks by reactive oxygen intermediates during phagocytosis or by other stress signals.[64] A regulatory network for cell apoptosis has been supposed to exist in a common metazoan ancestor, with a mixture of evolutionary events believed to have given origin to lineage-specific apoptotic pathways, such as the complex machinery described in mollusks.[55,65,66] The various apoptosis-related transcripts identified in *Mytilus* spp. (ie, sequences for TNF receptor like, Fas (TNFRSF6) associated via death domain FADD, initiator and effector cysteine peptidases or caspases, apoptosis inhibitors or IAPs, p53, p53 and DNA damage regulated protein or PDRG, Bcl-2, Bcl2-associated X protein or BAX, Bax inhibitor-1, apoptotic protease-activating factor 1 or Apaf-1, DNA fragmentation factor 45 or Dff-A, and other proteins) indicate the existence of both the extrinsic and intrinsic mechanisms.[55,66,67]

Autophagy is a common response to external or intracellular stress signals such as those resulting from starvation, growth factor deprivation, and infections. This kind of self-degradation facilitates the selective clearance of senescent cells and organelles and does not necessarily imply cell death. A main hallmark of this process is the formation of autophagosomes from the fusion of cytoplasmic contents with lysosomes. From yeast to mammals, interconnected signaling pathways lead to an induced or modulated expression of many autophagy-related genes (ATGs). Besides its role in the turnover of cellular organelles, proteins, and membranes, the autophagic machinery can be activated in the context of innate immunity and, more specifically, by the sensing of exogenous nucleic acids (including viral RNAs) or bacterial components by endosomal TLRs and cytosolic receptors such as STING and NLRs.[68] When autophagy leads to the elimination of intracellular pathogens, this process is usually named xenophagy. In mussels, the extent of lysosomal damage has been used for a long time as a measure of the cell condition in relation to the exposure to chemical pollutants, and it has been proposed that increased autophagic removal of oxidatively damaged components should be considered as an additional mechanism of defense against oxidative stress.[69] During xenophagy, the transcription of genes involved in basic cell functioning and redox homeostasis could reinforce the host defense by supporting pathogen clearance and by regulating innate immune responses. Several ATGs have been identified so far in the *C. gigas* genome (beclin, P13K, Akt, mTOR, ATG1 or ULK1, ATG8 or LC3, among others) and experimental data suggest that autophagy plays a protective role against *Vibrio aestuarianus* and OsHV-1 infections.[15,52] Transcripts sequences for 10 ATGs, Beclin 1, and the target of rapamycin or mTOR have been identified in *M. edulis*,[55] and the study of ATGs is in progress in *M. galloprovincialis*. Recent findings confirmed the role of autophagy in the host defense against microbial infections but also pointed out the need to understand how viral pathogens can evade this process.[70]

HOW SMALL RNAs CAN INFLUENCE THE IMMUNE HOST RESPONSE

In eukaryotes, genes transcribed into mRNA might not be translated owing to RNA interference (RNAi) by small inhibitory RNA (siRNA) or by microRNA (miRNA). Although these two types of single stranded (ss) RNAs have different origins, they both result from the cleavage of double stranded (ds) precursors and act, combined with proteins, in the so-called RISC complex.[71]

Following binding to complementary mRNA regions, siRNAs (21–25 nt) induce the nucleolytic degradation of a single targeted mRNA molecule, whereas the imperfect binding of a given miRNA (21–22 nt) to many target mRNAs inhibits their translation. While more than 1000 human miRNAs act as extensive negative regulators of the expression of protein-coding genes, particularly during development, siRNAs enter a cellular RNAi pathway essentially aimed at removing exogenous nucleic acids, including infectious viral sequences, and aberrant endogenous transcripts such as those from transposons and pre-miRNAs.[71]

On one hand, miRNAs can target immune-related and stress-related genes, thus repressing protein translation and influencing the cell response. On the other hand, miRNA and siRNA could be exploited to improve our knowledge of the function and regulation of many key players in cell functioning and to seek new strategies for the bivalve farming industry.[52,72] Despite the still very limited knowledge of such important cellular regulators in mollusks, a pioneer study identified a total of 199 oyster miRNAs (71 known and 128 new) in the hemocytes of *C. gigas* subjected to bacterial challenges and heat stress,[73] and the discovery of novel miRNAs in other marine bivalves is in progress.[74]

Another emerging type of noncoding RNAs, present but still to be explored in bivalve transcriptomes, is represented by endogenous long noncoding RNAs (lncRNAs, >200 nt), which encompass not only antisense, intronic, and intergenic transcripts but also transcribed pseudogenes and retrotransposons. It is expected to influence gene expression via chromatin remodeling, transcriptional, and posttranscriptional regulation.[75]

PERSPECTIVES

Fig. 7.1 depicts in essence the variety of molecules (and related processes) acting outside and inside of a hypothetical mussel cell, with more emphasis to gene-encoded products, which have already been identified. While offering functional hints, it should recall the joined evolution of a host organism with its associated microorganisms, as holobiome, and the need to accurately disentangle the complex gene–environment interactions occurring in the early onset of infectious and parasitic bivalve diseases in marketed bivalves.

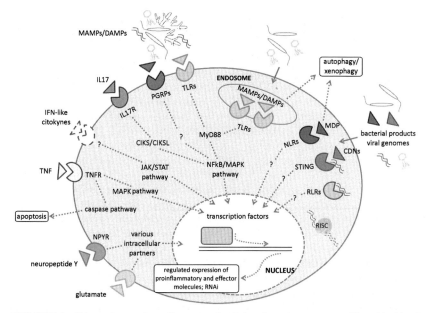

FIGURE 7.1 Schematic overview of immune-related signaling components outside and inside of a theoretical mussel cell. *MAMPs*, microorganisms associated molecular patterns; *DAMPs*, damage associated molecular patterns; *MDP*, muramyl dipeptide; *CDNs*, cyclic di-nucleotides; *NPYR*, neuropeptide Y receptor. For other acronyms see the List of Abbreviations.

ACKNOWLEDGMENTS

We are grateful to Marco Scocchi for the critical reading. SD and NS are supported by PRAT2012 (CPDA 128951) and by the Young Researcher Mobility Program India/Nepal of the University of Padova, respectively.

REFERENCES

1. Sonnenburg ED, Sonnenburg JL. Gut microbes take their vitamins. *Cell Host Microbe* 2014;**15**:5–6.
2. Aranda AM, Epstein AL. Herpes simplex virus type 1 latency and reactivation: an update. *Med Sci (Paris)* 2015;**31**:506–14.
3. Segarra A, Pépin JF, Arzul I, Morga B, Faury N, Renault T. Detection and description of a particular Ostreid herpesvirus 1 genotype associated with massive mortality outbreaks of Pacific oysters, *Crassostrea gigas*, in France in 2008. *Virus Res* 2010;**153**:92–9.
4. Di Prisco G, Cavaliere V, Annoscia D, Varricchio P, Caprio E, Nazzi F, et al. Neonicotinoid clothianidin adversely affects insect immunity and promotes replication of a viral pathogen in honey bees. *Proc Natl Acad Sci USA* 2013;**110**:18466–71.
5. Staley M, Bonneaud C. Immune responses of wild birds to emerging infectious diseases. *Parasite Immunol* 2015;**37**:242–54.
6. Flajnik MF, Kasahara M. Origin and evolution of the adaptive immune system: genetic events and selective pressures. *Nat Rev Genet* 2010;**11**:47–59.

7. Loker ES. Macroevolutionary immunology: a role for immunity in the diversification of animal life. *Front Immunol* 2012;**3**:25.

8. Gerdol M, Venier P. An updated molecular basis for mussel immunity. *Fish Shellfish Immunol* 2015;**46**:17–38. http://dx.doi.org/10.1016/j.fsi.2015.02.013.

9. Gómez-Chiarri M, Guo X, Tanguy A, He Y, Proestou D. The use of -omic tools in the study of disease processes in marine bivalve mollusks. *J Invertebr Pathol* 2015;**131**:137–154. http://dx.doi.org/10.1016/j.jip.2015.05.007. [Epub ahead of print].

10. Zhang G, Fang X, Guo X, Li L, Luo R, Xu F, et al. The oyster genome reveals stress adaptation and complexity of shell formation. *Nature* 2012;**490**:49–54.

11. Takeuchi T, Kawashima T, Koyanagi R, Gyoja F, Tanaka M, Ikuta T, et al. Draft genome of the pearl oyster *Pinctada fucata*: a platform for understanding bivalve biology. *DNA Res* 2012;**19**:117–30.

12. Nguyen TTT, Hayes BJ, Ingram BA. Genetic parameters and response to selection in blue mussel (*Mytilus galloprovincialis*) using a SNP-based pedigree. *Aquaculture* 2014;**420–421**:295–301.

13. Gómez-Chiarri M, Warren WC, Guo X, Proestou D. Developing tools for the study of molluscan immunity: the sequencing of the genome of the eastern oyster, *Crassostrea virginica*. *Fish Shellfish Immunol* 2015;**46**:2–4.

14. Gao D, Qiu L, Gao Q, Hou Z, Wang L, Song L. Repertoire and evolution of TNF superfamily in *Crassostrea gigas*: implications for expansion and diversification of this superfamily in Mollusca. *Dev Comp Immunol* 2015;**51**:251–60.

15. Moreau P, Moreau K, Segarra A, Tourbiez D, Travers MA, Rubinsztein DC, et al. Autophagy plays an important role in protecting Pacific oysters from OsHV-1 and *Vibrio aestuarianus* infections. *Autophagy* 2015;**11**:516–26.

16. Huang X, Wu S, Guan Y, Li Y, He M. Identification of sixteen single-nucleotide polymorphism markers in the pearl oyster, *Pinctada fucata*, for population genetic structure analysis. *J Genet* 2014;**93**:e1–4.

17. Li Y, He M. Genetic mapping and QTL analysis of growth-related traits in *Pinctada fucata* using restriction-site associated DNA sequencing. *PLoS One* 2014;**9**:e111707.

18. Rosenberg E, Koren O, Reshef L, Efrony R, Zilber-Rosenberg I. The role of microorganisms in coral health, disease and evolution. *Nat Rev Microbiol* 2007;**5**:355–62.

19. Bosch TC, Grasis JA, Lachnit T. Microbial ecology in *Hydra*: why viruses matter. *J Microbiol* 2015;**53**:193–200.

20. Dworkin J. The medium is the message: interspecies and interkingdom signaling by peptidoglycan and related bacterial glycans. *Annu Rev Microbiol* 2014;**68**:137–54.

21. McMahon SB, Russa FL, Bennett DL. Crosstalk between the nociceptive and immune systems in host defence and disease. *Nat Rev Neurosci* 2015;**16**:389–402.

22. Chiu IM, Heesters BA, Ghasemlou N, Von Hehn CA, Zhao F, Tran J, et al. Bacteria activate sensory neurons that modulate pain and inflammation. *Nature* 2013;**501**:52–7.

23. Steinberg BE, Tracey KJ, Slutsky AS. Bacteria and the neural code. *N Engl J Med* 2014;**371**:2131–3.

24. Augustyniak D, Nowak J, Lundy FT. Direct and indirect antimicrobial activities of neuropeptides and their therapeutic potential. *Curr Protein Pept Sci* 2012;**13**:723–38.

25. Veenstra JA. Neurohormones and neuropeptides encoded by the genome of *Lottia gigantea*, with reference to other mollusks and insects. *Gen Comp Endocrinol* 2010;**167**:86–103.

26. Stewart MJ, Favrel P, Rotgans BA, Wang T, Zhao M, Sohail M, et al. Neuropeptides encoded by the genomes of the Akoya pearl oyster *Pinctada fucata* and Pacific oyster *Crassostrea gigas*: a bioinformatic and peptidomic survey. *BMC Genomics* 2014;**15**:840.

27. Adamson KJ, Wang T, Zhao M, Bell F, Kuballa AV, Storey KB, et al. Molecular insights into land snail neuropeptides through transcriptome and comparative gene analysis. *BMC Genomics* 2015;**16**:308.
28. Rosani U, Varotto L, Gerdol M, Pallavicini A, Venier P. IL-17 signaling components in bivalves: comparative sequence analysis and involvement in the immune responses. *Dev Comp Immunol* 2015;**52**:255–68.
29. Wu SZ, Huang XD, Li Q, He MX. Interleukin-17 in pearl oyster (*Pinctada fucata*): molecular cloning and functional characterization. *Fish Shellfish Immunol* 2013;**34**:1050–6.
30. Li J, Zhang Y, Zhang Y, Xiang Z, Tong Y, Qu F, et al. Genomic characterization and expression analysis of five novel IL-17 genes in the Pacific oyster, *Crassostrea gigas*. *Fish Shellfish Immunol* 2014;**40**:455–65.
31. Valenzuela-Muñoz V, Gallardo-Escárate C. Molecular cloning and expression of IRAK-4, IL-17 and I-κB genes in *Haliotis rufescens* challenged with *Vibrio anguillarum*. *Fish Shellfish Immunol* 2014;**36**:503–9.
32. Venier P, Varotto L, Rosani U, Millino C, Celegato B, Bernante F, et al. Insights into the innate immunity of the Mediterranean mussel *Mytilus galloprovincialis*. *BMC Genomics* 2011;**12**:69.
33. Parisi MG, Toubiana M, Mangano V, Parrinello N, Cammarata M, Roch P. MIF from mussel: coding sequence, phylogeny, polymorphism, 3D model and regulation of expression. *Dev Comp Immunol* 2012;**36**:688–96.
34. Wang B, Zhang Z, Wang Y, Zou Z, Wang G, Wang S, et al. Molecular cloning and characterization of macrophage migration inhibitory factor from small abalone *Haliotis diversicolor* supertexta. *Fish Shellfish Immunol* 2009;**27**:57–64.
35. Baeza Garcia A, Pierce RJ, Gourbal B, Werkmeister E, Colinet D, Reichhart JM, et al. Involvement of the cytokine MIF in the snail host immune response to the parasite *Schistosoma mansoni*. *PLoS Pathog* 2010;**6**(9):e1001115.
36. Li F, Huang S, Wang L, Yang J, Zhang H, Qiu L, et al. A macrophage migration inhibitory factor like gene from scallop *Chlamys farreri*: involvement in immune response and wound healing. *Dev Comp Immunol* 2011;**35**:62–71.
37. Cui S, Zhang D, Jiang S, Pu H, Hu Y, Guo H, et al. A macrophage migration inhibitory factor like oxidoreductase from pearl oyster *Pinctada fucata* involved in innate immune responses. *Fish Shellfish Immunol* 2011;**31**:173–81.
38. Kavaliers M. MIF-1 and Tyr-MIF-1 antagonize morphine and opioid but not non-opioid stress-induced analgesia in the snail, *Cepaea nemoralis*. *Peptides* 1987;**8**:1–5.
39. De Zoysa M, Nikapitiya C, Kim Y, Oh C, Kang DH, Whang I, et al. Allograft inflammatory factor-1 in disk abalone (*Haliotis discus discus*): molecular cloning, transcriptional regulation against immune challenge and tissue injury. *Fish Shellfish Immunol* 2010;**29**:319–26.
40. Zhang L, Zhao J, Li C, Su X, Chen A, Li T, et al. Cloning and characterization of allograft inflammatory factor-1 (AIF-1) from Manila clam *Venerupis philippinarum*. *Fish Shellfish Immunol* 2011;**30**:148–53.
41. Li J, Chen J, Zhang Y, Yu Z. Expression of allograft inflammatory factor-1 (AIF-1) in response to bacterial challenge and tissue injury in the pearl oyster, *Pinctada martensii*. *Fish Shellfish Immunol* 2013;**34**:365–71.
42. Wang J, Zhang H, Wang L, Qiu L, Yue F, Yang C, et al. Molecular cloning and transcriptional regulation of an allograft inflammatory factor-1 (AIF-1) in Zhikong scallop *Chlamys farreri*. *Gene* 2013;**530**:178–84.

43. Zhang Y, Li J, Yu F, He X, Yu Z. Allograft inflammatory factor-1 stimulates hemocyte immune activation by enhancing phagocytosis and expression of inflammatory cytokines in *Crassostrea gigas*. *Fish Shellfish Immunol* 2013;**34**:1071–7.

44. Xu T, Xie J, Zhu B, Liu X, Wu X. Allograft inflammatory factor 1 functions as a pro-inflammatory cytokine in the oyster, *Crassostrea ariakensis*. *PLoS One* 2014;**9**(4):e95859.

45. Martín-Gómez L, Villalba A, Carballal MJ, Abollo E. Molecular characterisation of TNF, AIF, dermatopontin and VAMP genes of the flat oyster *Ostrea edulis* and analysis of their modulation by diseases. *Gene* 2014;**533**:208–17.

46. Sun Y, Zhou Z, Wang L, Yang C, Jianga S, Song L. The immunomodulation of a novel tumor necrosis factor (CgTNF-1) in oyster *Crassostrea gigas*. *Dev Comp Immunol* 2014;**45**:291–9.

47. Zhang L, Li L, Guo X, Litman GW, Dishaw LJ, Zhang G. Massive expansion and functional divergence of innate immune genes in a protostome. *Sci Rep* 2015;**5**:8693.

48. Huang XD, Liu WG, Wang Q, Zhao M, Wu SZ, Guan YY, et al. Molecular characterization of interferon regulatory factor 2 (IRF-2) homolog in pearl oyster *Pinctada fucata*. *Fish Shellfish Immunol* 2013;**34**:1279–86.

49. Savan R, Ravichandran S, Collins JR, Sakai M, Young HA. Structural conservation of interferon gamma among vertebrates. *Cytokine Growth Factor Rev* 2009;**20**:115–24.

50. Canesi L, Betti M, Ciacci C, Citterio B, Pruzzo C, Gallo G. Tyrosine kinase-mediated cell signalling in the activation of *Mytilus* hemocytes: possible role of STAT-like proteins. *Biol Cell* 2003;**95**:603–13.

51. Zhang R, Liu R, Wang W, Xin L, Wang L, Li C, et al. Identification and functional analysis of a novel IFN-like protein (CgIFNLP) in *Crassostrea gigas*. *Fish Shellfish Immunol* 2015;**44**:547–54.

52. Green TJ, Raftos D, Speck P, Montagnani C. Antiviral immunity in marine molluscs. *J Gen Virol* 2015;**96**:2471–82.

53. Song L, Wang L, Zhang H, Wang M. The immune system and its modulation mechanism in scallop. *Fish Shellfish Immunol* 2015;**46**:65–78.

54. Allam B, Raftos D. Immune responses to infectious diseases in bivalves. *J Invertebr Pathol* 2015;**131**:121–36. http://dx.doi.org/10.1016/j.jip.2015.05.005.

55. Philipp EE, Kraemer L, Melzner F, Poustka AJ, Thieme S, Findeisen U, et al. Massively parallel RNA sequencing identifies a complex immune gene repertoire in the lophotrochozoan *Mytilus edulis*. *PLoS One* 2012;**7**:e33091.

56. Toubiana M, Gerdol M, Rosani U, Pallavicini A, Venier P, Roch P. Toll-like receptors and MyD88 adaptors in *Mytilus*: complete cds and gene expression levels. *Dev Comp Immunol* 2013;**40**:158–66.

57. Núñez-Acuña G, Gallardo-Escárate C. Identification of immune-related SNPs in the transcriptome of *Mytilus chilensis* through high-throughput sequencing. *Fish Shellfish Immunol* 2013;**35**:1899–905.

58. Toubiana M, Rosani U, Giambelluca S, Cammarata M, Gerdol M, Pallavicini A, et al. Toll signal transduction pathway in bivalves: complete cds of intermediate elements and related gene transcription levels in hemocytes of immune stimulated *Mytilus galloprovincialis*. *Dev Comp Immunol* 2014;**45**:300–12.

59. Bachère E, Rosa RD, Schmitt P, Poirier AC, Merou N, Charrière GM, et al. The new insights into the oyster antimicrobial defense: cellular, molecular and genetic view. *Fish Shellfish Immunol* 2015;**46**:50–64.

60. Canesi L, Gallo G, Gavioli M, Pruzzo C. Bacteria-hemocyte interactions and phagocytosis in marine bivalves. *Microsc Res Tech* 2002;**57**:469–76.

61. Hughes FM, Foster B, Grewal S, Sokolova IM. Apoptosis as a host defense mechanism in *Crassostrea virginica* and its modulation by *Perkinsus marinus*. *Fish Shellfish Immunol* 2010;**29**:247–57.
62. Soudant PE, Chu FL, Volety A. Host-parasite interactions: marine bivalve molluscs and protozoan parasites, *Perkinsus* species. *J Invertebr Pathol* 2013;**114**:196–216.
63. Garg AD, Dudek-Peric AM, Romano E, Agostinis P. Immunogenic cell death. *Int J Dev Biol* 2015;**59**:131–40.
64. Terahara K, Takahashi KG. Mechanisms and immunological roles of apoptosis in molluscs. *Curr Pharm Des* 2008;**14**:131–7.
65. Zmasek CM, Godzik A. Evolution of the animal apoptosis network. *Cold Spring Harb Perspect Biol* 2013;**5**:a008649.
66. Romero A, Novoa B, Figueras A. The complexity of apoptotic cell death in mollusks: an update. *Fish Shellfish Immunol* 2015;**46**:79–87.
67. Estévez-Calvar N, Romero A, Figueras A, Novoa B. Genes of the mitochondrial apoptotic pathway in *Mytilus galloprovincialis*. *PLoS One* 2013;**8**:e61502.
68. Richetta C, Faure M. Autophagy in antiviral innate immunity. *Cell Microbiol* 2013;**15**:368–76.
69. Moore MN. Autophagy as a second level protective process in conferring resistance to environmentally-induced oxidative stress. *Autophagy* 2008;**4**:254–6.
70. Rey-Jurado E, Riedel CA, González PA, Bueno SM, Kalergis AM. Contribution of autophagy to antiviral immunity. *FEBS Lett* 2015;**589**:3461–70. http://dx.doi.org/10.1016/j.febslet.2015.07.047.
71. Phillips T. Small non-coding RNA and gene expression. *Nat Educ* 2008;**1**:115. Available from: http://www.nature.com/scitable/topicpage/small-non-coding-rna-and-gene-expression-1078; NBCI. RNA Interference (RNAi), Available from: http://www.ncbi.nlm.nih.gov/genome/probe/doc/TechRnai.shtml.
72. Owens L, Malham S. Review of the RNA interference pathway in molluscs including some possibilities for use in bivalves in aquaculture. *J Mar Sci Eng* 2015;**3**:87–99.
73. Zhou Z, Wang L, Song L, Liu R, Zhang H, Huang M, et al. The identification and characteristics of immune-related microRNAs in haemocytes of oyster *Crassostrea gigas*. *PLoS One* 2014;**9**:e88397.
74. Chen G, Zhang C, Jiang F, Wang Y, Xu Z, Wang C. Bioinformatics analysis of hemocyte miRNAs of scallop *Chlamys farreri* against acute viral necrobiotic virus (AVNV). *Fish Shellfish Immunol* 2014;**37**:75–86.
75. Chan WL, Huang HD, Chang JG. lncRNAMap: a map of putative regulatory functions in the long non-coding transcriptome. *Comput Biol Chem* 2014;**50**:41–9.

Chapter 8

Crustacean Immunity: The Modulation of Stress Responses

Chiara Manfrin, Alberto Pallavicini, Silvia Battistella
University of Trieste, Trieste, Italy

Simonetta Lorenzon
OGS (National Institute of Oceanography and Experimental Geophysics), Sgonico (TS), Italy

Piero G. Giulianini
University of Trieste, Trieste, Italy

Stress is a vital mechanism that permits a physiological adjustment toward stressors. It includes molecular and biochemical modifications capable of restoring internal homeostasis or behavioral responses such as escape.

The stress responses may involve the immune system, depending on the effect of the stressors on animals. Behavioral responses are the first actions carried out in the presence of a stress, and they include simple reflex actions, such as avoidance, as well as complex feedback (aggression). The immune system in crustaceans is exclusively innate and, as in all invertebrates, is mainly based on three mechanisms: physical barriers, humoral mechanisms, and cellular defenses.[1–3] When escape is impossible and physical barriers prevent the disturbance played by stressors or pathogen entry, internal mechanisms are activated to face the situation and try to return to normal conditions.

SOURCES OF STRESS

Variables inducing stress may be mainly classified as external or inner variables. External variables include air exposure and changes in temperature, salinity, light, oxygen, and water pH (due to the increase of CO_2 and ocean acidification). Xenobiotic substances and, in general, pollution and anthropic activities may also modify environmental conditions and affect crustaceans' physiology, generating stress responses. In addition, the presence of conspecifics during particular stages of the life cycle (eg, reproductive or territorial competition) or competitors for food and space resources act as stress sources as well.

Lessons in Immunity: From Single-Cell Organisms to Mammals
http://dx.doi.org/10.1016/B978-0-12-803252-7.00008-4

107

Inner variables usually refer to gender, size, and exoskeleton hardness. Competition between adults and juveniles may result in cannibalism events, which are crucial density-dependence phenomena that control population dynamics. Moreover, crustaceans in the early postmolt stage are more vulnerable to injury; they modify their behavior, becoming solitary and staying to the ground until the exoskeleton hardens.

INDICATORS OF STRESS

Vitality/mortality estimation is the most direct indicator of health for all living organisms[4] and derives from direct observations of the animal itself. The three main stress indicators in evaluating the vitality/mortality state are (1) external visible injuries, (2) physiological stress measured in hemocytes or other tissues, and (3) behavioral indicators. "When reliable and consistent relationships can be established between metrics of stress (or vitality) and subsequent mortality for a broad range of operational conditions and different animal types, such as gender, size and molt-stage, the relationships can be used to predict mortality."[5] Whereas it is still difficult to find a thorough correlation between type and amount of injuries and mortality because lethal original causes and consequences are difficult to determine, plenty of studies have shown physiological stress responses in correlation to hemolymph chemistry.[6–8]

Stress responses have been classified as primary (short term), secondary, and tertiary (long term).[9] Primary responses stand for the initial neuroendocrine/endocrine reaction to the altered conditions. In crustaceans, this is represented by the rapid and consistent release of the crustacean hyperglycemic hormones (CHHs) from the sinus gland in the eyestalks, which primarily act in responding to the increasing demand for energy.[10] Secondary responses include the mobilization of intracellular glycogen and lactate/anaerobic production followed by an increase of the hemolymphatic glucose level, finally leading to metabolic acidosis.[11,12] The reduction in feeding, growth, reproduction, and disease resistance of animals represents tertiary responses.

STRESS RESPONSES MEDIATED BY NEUROPEPTIDES

Stress generally involves rapid mobilization from eyestalk neuroendocrine centers, and in crustaceans, the eyestalk X-organ/sinus gland (XO-SG) complex secretes hyperglycemic/steroidostatic hormones (CHH/MIH) under the control of biogenic amines and enkephalins.[13–15] This eyestalk complex is considered homoplastic to the hypothalamus–pituitary axis of vertebrates.[16] CHH has been described as the crustacean equivalent of cortisol or corticosterone, which is able to modulate immune functions.[11]

It is known, from several studies on crustaceans, that a variety of stressors, such as extreme temperature,[17] hypoxia,[18] organic and inorganic pollutants,[19,20] bacterial infection,[21] parasites,[22] and boat noise[23] induce hyperglycemia mediated by CHH release.[18,24,25]

Studies have led to an understanding of the effects of stress on biological activities, including metabolic control,[26,27] molting,[28] gonad maturation,[29–31] ionic and osmotic regulation,[32] and methyl farnesoate synthesis in mandibular glands.[33] Accordingly, the names CHH, and the structurally related peptides MIH (molt inhibiting hormone), GIH/VIH (gonad/vitellogenesis-inhibiting hormone), and MOIH (mandibular organ-inhibiting hormone) were conceived. Over time, numerous experiments evidenced that CHH is a pleiotropic neuropeptide. In fact, CHH not only controls metabolism and hyperglycemia, but it also plays an effect on the inhibition of ecdysteroid,[34] methyl farnesoate,[35] ovarian protein synthesis,[36,37] and other behavioral responses, such as aggression[38] and anxiety.[39]

The first evidence of neuropeptide involvement in the stress response dates back to 1944[27] when Abramowitz and colleagues found the presence of "diabetogenic factor," later named CHH, in the eyestalk of the decapod species. The aqueous extract from the eyestalk of *Uca pugilator* was injected in *Callinectes sapidus* inducing a dose-dependent hyperglycemia. Similarly, excessive handling or other forms of excitement cause hyperglycemic effects. Increasing levels of stress hormones, glucose, blood flow, and muscular activity help the animal to compensate for stress and eventually return to homeostasis, if possible.[5] It has been proved that hypoxia induces a CHH release in *Cancer pagurus*[18] and in *Homarus americanus*,[40] assessed by radioimmunoassay with an antiserum directed against HPLC-purified *C. pagurus* CHH and ELISA, respectively.

This neuropeptide belongs to a family of multifunctional peptides, all containing the same cysteine pattern (6 cys connected by three disulfide bridges), which can be divided, according to sequence and precursor structures, into two subfamilies, type-I and type-II.[41] The most evident difference characterizing the CHH type-I group is the presence of a CHH precursor related peptide (CPRP), usually 38 aa long between the signal peptide (26 aa long) and the mature peptide (about 76 aa) sequences.[42] Such a CPRP sequence is absent in the CHH type-II subgroup. The CHH type-I comprises the CHH *sensu stricto* and the ion transport peptide, whereas the CHH type-II includes MIH, GIH/VIH, and MOIH.[43,44]

UPSTREAM MODULATORS TRIGGERING CHHs

Biogenic amines and enkephalin modulate the release of neuropeptides from the crustacean neuroendocrine tissue[45] and are involved in stress responses.[46] In particular, serotonin (5-HT) possesses a potent hyperglycemic effect in numerous crustacean species,[47,48] while dopamine and enkephalin showed controversial results on different species. Enkephalins trigger hyperglycemic responses in intact *Squilla mantis* but not in eyestalkless specimens.[47] Dopamine decreases the glucose level within the hemolymph in *Palaemon elegans* and *S. mantis*,[47] but it has an opposite effect on intact *Procambarus clarkii*[49] and on *Macrobrachium malcolmsonii*.[50]

By means of high-performance liquid chromatography, brains of *P. clarkii* stressed by exposure to repetitive electrical fields that triggered tail-flips showed a significantly higher titer of 5-HT than untreated animals when chlordiazepoxide, a potent benzodiazepine with anxiolytic effects, which was abolished once, was administered to animals. These differences were not recorded in their thoracic and abdominal ganglia.[39] Interestingly, chlordiazepoxide, as benzodiazepine, functions on γ-aminobutyric acid (GABA) by increasing its sedative, anxiolytic, and muscle relaxant properties and revealing that GABA is also involved in suppressing activity of the XO-SG. In support of this, Polanco and colleagues demonstrated that GABA regulates both the electrical and secretory activity of the XO-SG system in *P. clarkii*.[51] Moreover, they reported that GABA receptors are present along the axon branches of the neuropil of the *medulla terminalis*, and they found colocalization of GABA and CHH-containing neurons putatively able to regulate another neuronal subset.

Through intracellular dye injection, double immunostaining, and confocal imaging it has been shown that 5-HT, octopamine, and CHH-immunoreactive neurons interact with each other in the neuronal somata located near branch points in the second thoracic nerve roots in the lobster nervous system.[46] In decapods, it is likely that multiple systems are active simultaneously, and they exhibit synergic effects, opening new paths on the modulation of neuronal function that regulate the release of eyestalk neuropeptides (Fig. 8.1).

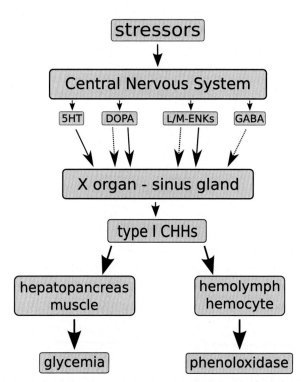

FIGURE 8.1 Cascade of systems and neuroregulators involved in the stress responses in decapod crustaceans. The *arrows with a solid line* indicate a positive modulation, and the *arrows with a dotted line* indicate a negative modulation. *5HT*, serotonin; *DOPA*, dopamine; *L/M-EnKs*, Leu-enkephalin/Met-enkephalin; *GABA*, γ-aminobutyric acid; *CHHs*, crustacean hyperglycemic hormones.

THE CRUSTACEAN HYPERGLYCEMIC HORMONE NEUROPEPTIDES

Different isoforms of CHH from those present in the XO-SG have been found in the pericardial organ in several crustacean species[52,53] and also in the epithelial endocrine cells of fore- and hindgut in *Carcinus maenas*.[54,55]

Based on the amino acid sequences, Kung et al.[56] identified hemocytes from *P. clarkii*, two CHH transcripts, namely CHH1 and CHH2, codified by two different genes. As reported by the authors, each gene encodes for two and three different alternative splicing forms, respectively (CHH1, CHH1-L, CHH2, CHH2-L, and tCHH2).

Consulting the eyestalk transcriptome[57] and the hemocytes transcriptome (unpublished data), both from *P. clarkii*, we confirm the existence of two different CHHs, and we found that CHH1 is about 6X more expressed than CHH2 in the eyestalk with 48.64 and 7.77 FPKM (fragments per kilobase of exon per million fragments mapped), respectively. Moreover, in the eyestalk the L-alternative splicing form is very poorly expressed (1 out of 1000 CHH1 transcripts and 1 out of 30 CHH2 transcripts), and the truncated form was observed in just one read. CHH1 and CHH2 genes have not been found expressed in our hemocytes transcriptome.

Another important aspect influencing the functionality of CHH is the amidation of the C-terminus, which strongly influences its biological activity.[58,59] In fact, a recombinant CHH with free carboxyl terminus evoked a weak hyperglycemic response compared to the recombinant peptide with an amidated C-terminus.[59]

Two different CHHs, CHH-A and CHH-B, were also determined from the sinus gland extracts from *H. americanus*[60]; each group contained two chiral variants (CHH and D-Phe[3] CHH). Diversity in the function of chiral variants (L- and D-isomerization) have been tested in *Pontastacus leptodactylus*,[61,62] in which the circulating glucose levels were much higher in response to the D-isoform than to the L-isoform 1 h postinjection. Similarly, the RNA-seq analysis confirmed a stronger effect on gene expression following the administration of D-CHH, while just limited alterations have been caused by the L-CHH.[61]

Moreover, the importance of amino acid residues has been investigated in *P. leptodactylus*.[63] The substitution of D-phenylalanine at position 3 (D-Phe[3] CHH) of the (N)-terminus with an alanine (D-Ala) was tested by in vivo biological assay. The mutated analogue was far less active than its wild-type counterparts, either in the D- (D-CHH) or L- (L-CHH) configuration, confirming that the N-terminus is also involved in binding with the receptor, and identifying in the Phe[3] a hot spot for the peptide–receptor binding.

On the contrary, very little is known about downstream CHH receptors; they appear to be a membrane (class II) guanylyl cyclase.[10,64] A model of the probable signaling pathways of CHH and MIH in Y-Organs has been proposed by Mykles and colleagues[65]: (1) cyclic adenosine monophosphate (cAMP) primarily inhibits constitutive synthesis, but it is also able to inhibit facultative synthesis, either directly or indirectly by way of cyclic guanosine monophosphate (cGMP); and (2) cGMP inhibits facultative synthesis but not constitutive synthesis.

PERSPECTIVES

Very recently, a few studies have demonstrated that the immune response is partly regulated by or involves bioactive neuropeptides in crustaceans,[66,67] since lipopolysaccharide (LPS), bacterial infections, and in general stress induce a hyperglycemia response.[24,68]

The scenario depicted in this chapter shows a complex system of a superfamily of bioactive neuropeptides, whose members are growing in number. In fact, different paralogs and sequence variants are reported by the emerging, increasingly applied next generation sequencing techniques. Moreover, chiral isoforms with specific and different activities and target tissues seem to expand the CHHs' universe described so far, leading to interesting developments in CHHs' function and mode of action. As far as immunology is concerned, recent data highlight that injections of CHH into shrimp (*Litopenaeus vannamei*) trigger phenoloxidase activity and lead to increasing resistance to a bacterial challenge (*Vibrio harveyi*).[67] A recent study focused on the suppression of the gene expression of the two main CHHs, CHH1 and CHH2,[57] from the eyestalk of *P. clarkii* through double-stranded CHH-RNA interference and reported osmotic deficits and mortality in specimens injected with CHH dsRNA. After 20 days, despite still being silenced for CHH, individuals that survived recovered a strong hyperglycemic response after a serotonin injection due to the compensatory effect of two peptides belonging to the crustacean neurohormone CHHs protein family. Moreover, one of the two new CHH-like transcripts, CHHip (CHH immune-related procambarus), significantly increases (18-fold) its expression in eyestalk following a 1 µg/animal (body weight 40 g) injection of LPS (unpublished data).

These findings open up the possibility of the existence of a broad CHH type-I family, involved in immune response and able to compensate for the lack of the most abundant CHHs normally allocated to the metabolism/homeostasis control.

REFERENCES

1. Boucias D, Pendland JC. *Principles of insect pathology*. Boston: Kluwer; 1998.
2. Giron-Perez MI. Relationships between innate immunity in bivalve molluscs and pollution. *Invertebr Surviv J* 2010;**7**:149–56.
3. Ellis RP, Parry H, Spicer JI, Hutchinson TH, Pipe RK, Widdicombe S. Immunological function in marine invertebrates: responses to environmental perturbation. *Fish Shellfish Immunol* 2011;**30**:1209–22.
4. Castillo LE, Pinnock M, Martinez E. Evaluation of a battery of toxicity tests for use in the assessment of water quality in a Costa Rican laboratory. *Environ Toxicol* 2000;**15**(4):312–21.
5. Stoner AW. Assessing stress and predicting mortality in economically significant Crustaceans. *Rev Fish Sci* 2012;**20**(3):111–35.
6. Lorenzon S, Giulianini PG, Libralato S, Martinis M, Ferrero EA. Stress effect of two different transport systems on the physiological profiles of the crab *Cancer pagurus*. *Aquaculture* 2008;**278**:156–63.

7. Fotedar S, Evans L. Health management during handling and live transport of crustaceans: a review. *J Invert Pathol* 2011;**106**:143–52.
8. Wei K, Yang J. Oxidative damage of hepatopancreas induced by pollution depresses humoral immunity response in the freshwater crayfish *Procambarus clarkii*. *Fish Shellfish Immunol* 2015;**43**(2):510–9.
9. Iwama GK, Vijayan MM, Morgan JD. The stress response in fish. In: Saksena DN, editor. *Ichthyology: recent research advances enfield*. Enfield, NH: Science Publisher; 1999. p. 44–57.
10. Fanjul-Moles ML. Biochemical and functional aspects of crustacean hyperglycemic hormone in decapod crustaceans: review and update. *Comp Biochem Physiol Part C Toxicol Pharmacol* 2006;**142**(3):390–400.
11. Elwood RW, Barr S, Patterson L. Pain and stress in crustaceans? *Appl Anim Behav Sci* 2009;**118**:128–36.
12. Lorenzon S, Giulianini PG, Martinis M, Ferrero EA. Stress effect of different temperatures and air exposure during transport on physiological profiles in the American lobster *Homarus americanus*. *Comp Biochem Physiol Part A Mol Integr Physiol* 2007;**147**(1):94–102.
13. Mattson MP, Spaziani E. Regulation of crab Y-organ steroidogenesis in vitro: evidence that ecdysteroid production increases through activation of cAMP-phosphodiesterase by calcium-calmodulin. *Mol Cell Endocrinol* 1986;**48**(2–3):135–51.
14. Lorenzon S, Edomi P, Giulianini PG, Mettulio R, Ferrero EA. Role of biogenic amines and cHH in the crustacean hyperglycemic stress response. *J Exp Biol* 2005;**208**(17):3341–7.
15. Lee CY, Yang PF, Zou HS. Serotonergic regulation of crustacean hyperglycemic hormone secretion in the crayfish, *Procambarus clarkii*. *Physiol Biochem Zool* 2001;**74**(3):376–82.
16. Hartenstein V. The neuroendocrine system of invertebrates: a developmental and evolutionary perspective. *J Endocrinol* 2006;**190**:555–70.
17. Chen R, Xu N, Zhao F, Wu Y, Huang Y, Yang Z. Temperature-dependent effect of food size on the reproductive performances of the small-sized cladoceran *Moina micrura*. *Biochem Syst Ecol* 2015;**59**:297–301.
18. Webster S. Measurement of crustacean hyperglycaemic hormone levels in the edible crab *Cancer pagurus* during emersion stress. *J Exp Biol* 1996;**199**(7):1579–85.
19. Singaram G, Harikrishnan T, Chen FY, Bo J, Giesy JP. Modulation of immune-associated parameters and antioxidant responses in the crab (*Scylla serrata*) exposed to mercury. *Chemosphere* 2013;**90**(3):917–28.
20. Sánchez-Bayo F. Comparative acute toxicity of organic pollutants and reference values for crustaceans. I. Branchiopoda, Copepoda and Ostracoda. *Environ Pollut* 2006;**139**(3): 385–420.
21. Yang Y, Bao C, Liu A, Ye H, Huang H, Li S. Immune responses of prophenoloxidase in the mud crab *Scylla paramamosain* against *Vibrio alginolyticus* infection: in vivo and in vitro gene silencing evidence. *Fish Shellfish Immunol* 2014;**39**(2):237–44.
22. Lynch SA, Darmody G, Laide C, Walsh D, Culloty SC. A preliminary health survey of the hermit crab, *Pagurus bernhardus*, on the southwest coast of Ireland. *J Invertebr Pathol* 2015;**127**:73–5.
23. Filiciotto F, Vazzana M, Celi M, Maccarrone V, Ceraulo M, Buffa G, et al. Behavioural and biochemical stress responses of *Palinurus elephas* after exposure to boat noise pollution in tank. *Mar Pollut Bull* 2014;**84**(1–2):104–14.
24. Lorenzon S, Giulianini PG, Ferrero EA. Lipopolysaccharide-induced hyperglycemia is mediated by CHH release in crustaceans. *General Comp Endocrinol* 1997;**108**(3):395–405.
25. Chang ES, Chang SA, Keller R, Reddy PS, Snyder MJ, Spees JL. Quantification of stress in lobsters: crustacean hyperglycemic hormone, stress proteins, and gene expression. *Am Zool* 1999;**39**(3):487–95.

26. Kegel G, Reichwein B, Weese S, Gaus G, Peter-Kataliníc J, Keller R. Amino acid sequence of the crustacean hyperglycemic hormone (CHH) from the shore crab, *Carcinus maenas*. *FEBS Lett* 1989;**255**(1):10–4.

27. Abramowitz AA, Hisaw FL, Papandrea DN. The occurrence of a diabetogenic factor in the eyestalks of crustaceans. *Biol Bull* 1944;**86**(1):1–5.

28. Webster SG. Amino acid sequence of putative moult-inhibiting hormone from the crab *Carcinus maenas*. *Proc R Soc Lond Ser B Biol Sci* 1991;**244**:247–52.

29. Yano I, editor. *Hormonal control of vitellogenesis in penaeid shrimp. Advances in shrimp biotechnology proceedings to the special session on shrimp biotechnology 5th Asian fisheries forum, November 11–14, 1998*. 1998. Bangkok, Chiengmai (Thailand).

30. Panouse JB. L'action de la glande du sinus sur l'ovaire chez la crevette Leander. *C.R. Acad Sci Paris* 1944;**218**:293–4.

31. Panouse JB. Influence de l'ablation du pedoncle oculaire sur Ia croissance de l'ovaire chez la crevette *Leander serratus*. *C.R. Acad Sci Paris* 1943;**217**:553–5.

32. Turner LM, Webster SG, Morris S. Roles of crustacean hyperglycaemic hormone in ionic and metabolic homeostasis in the christmas island blue crab, *Discoplax celeste*. *J Exp Biol* 2013;**216**(7):1191–201.

33. Wainwright G, Webster SG, Wilkinson MC, Chung JS, Rees HH. Structure and significance of mandibular organ-inhibiting hormone in the crab, *Cancer pagurus*. Involvement in multihormonal regulation of growth and reproduction. *J Biol Chem* 1996;**271**(22):12749–54.

34. Chung JS, Webster SG. Moult cycle-related changes in biological activity of moult-inhibiting hormone (MIH) and crustacean hyperglycaemic hormone (CHH) in the crab, *Carcinus maenas*: from target to transcript. *Eur J Biochem* 2003;**270**(15):3280–8.

35. Borst DW, Ogan J, Tsukimura B, Claerhout T, Holford KC. Regulation of the Crustacean mandibular organ. *Am Zool* 2001;**41**(3):430–41.

36. Khayat M, Yang WJ, Aida K, Nagasawa H, Tietz A, Funkenstein B, et al. Hyperglycaemic hormones inhibit protein and mRNA synthesis in in vitro- incubated ovarian fragments of the marine shrimp *Penaeus semisulcatus*. *Gen Comp Endocrinol* 1998;**110**(3):307–18.

37. Avarre JC, Khayat M, Michelis R, Nagasawa H, Tietz A, Lubzens E. Inhibition of de novo synthesis of a jelly layer precursor protein by crustacean hyperglycemic hormone family peptides and posttranscriptional regulation by sinus gland extracts in *Penaeus semisulcatus* ovaries. *Gen Comp Endocrinol* 2001;**124**(3):257–68.

38. Aquiloni L, Giulianini PG, Mosco A, Guarnaccia C, Ferrero EA, Gherardi F. Crustacean hyperglycemic hormone (cHH) as a modulator of aggression in Crustacean decapods. *PLoS One* 2012;**7**(11):e50047.

39. Fossat P, Bacqué-Cazenave J, De Deurwaerdère P, Delbecque JP, Cattaert D. Anxiety-like behavior in crayfish is controlled by serotonin. *Science* 2014;**344**:1293–7.

40. Chang ES, Keller R, Chang SA. Quantification of Crustacean hyperglycemic hormone by ELISA in hemolymph of the lobster, *Homarus americanus*, following various stresses. *Gen Comp Endocrinol* 1998;**111**(3):359–66.

41. Lacombe C, Grève P, Martin G. Overview on the sub-grouping of the crustacean hyperglycemic hormone family. *Neuropeptides* 1999;**33**(1):71–80.

42. Giulianini PG, Edomi P. Neuropeptides controlling reproduction and growth in Crustacea: a molecular approach. In: Satake H, editor. *Invertebrate neuropeptides and hormones: basic knowledge and recent advances*. Kerala, India: Transword Research Network; 2006. p. 225–52.

43. Webster SG, Keller R, Dircksen H. The CHH-superfamily of multifunctional peptide hormones controlling crustacean metabolism, osmoregulation, moulting, and reproduction. *Gen Comp Endocrinol* 2012;**175**(2):217–33.

44. Katayama H, Ohira T, Nagasawa H. Crustacean peptide hormones: structure, gene expression and function. *Aqua-BioScience Monogr* 2013;**6**(2):49–90.
45. Lorenzon S. Hyperglycemic stress response in Crustacea. *Invertebr Surviv J* 2005;**2**:132–41.
46. Basu AC, Kravitz EA. Morphology and monoaminergic modulation of Crustacean Hyperglycemic Hormone-like immunoreactive neurons in the lobster nervous system. *J Neurocytol* 2003;**32**(3):253–63.
47. Lorenzon S, Brezovec S, Ferrero EA. Species-specific effects on hemolymph glucose control by serotonin, dopamine, and L-enkephalin and their inhibitors in *Squilla mantis* and *Astacus leptodactylus* (Crustacea). *J Exp Zool A Comp Exp Biol* 2004;**301**(9):727–36.
48. Lorenzon S, Pasqual P, Ferrero EA. Biogenic amines control blood glucose level in shrimp *Palaemon elegans*. In: Schram FB, editor. *The biodiversity crisis and Crustacea*, vol. 12. Rotterdam: Balkema; 1999. p. 471–80.
49. Zou HS, Juan CC, Chen SC, Wang HY, Lee CY. Dopaminergic regulation of crustacean hyperglycemic hormone and glucose levels in the hemolymph of the crayfish *Procambarus clarkii*. *J Exp Zool A Comp Exp Biol* 2003;**298**(1):44–52.
50. Komali M, Kalarani V, Venkatrayulu CH, Reddy DCS. Hyperglycemic effects of 5-hydroxytryptamine and dopamine in the freshwater prawn *Macrobrachium malcolmsonii*. *J Exp Zool* 2005;**303**:448–55.
51. Pérez-Polanco P, Garduño J, Cebada J, Zarco N, Segovia J, Lamas M, et al. GABA and GAD expression in the X-organ sinus gland system of the *Procambarus clarkii* crayfish: inhibition mediated by GABA between X-organ neurons. *J Comp Physiol A Neuroethol Sens Neural Behav Physiol* 2011;**197**(9):923–38.
52. Chung JS, Zmora N, Katayama H, Tsutsui N. Crustacean hyperglycemic hormone (CHH) neuropeptides family: functions, titer, and binding to target tissues. *Gen Comp Endocrinol* 2010;**166**(3):447–54.
53. Jeon JM, Kim BK, Lee JH, Kim HJ, Kang CK, Mykles DL, et al. Two type I crustacean hyperglycemic hormone (CHH) genes in Morotoge shrimp (*Pandalopsis japonica*): cloning and expression of eyestalk and pericardial organ isoforms produced by alternative splicing and a novel type I CHH with predicted structure shared with type II CHH peptides. *Comp Biochem Physiol - B Biochem Mol Biol* 2012;**162**(4):88–99.
54. Chung JS, Dircksen H, Webster SG. A remarkable, precisely timed release of hyperglycemic hormone from endocrine cells in the gut is associated with ecdysis in the crab *Carcinus maenas*. *Proc Natl Acad Sci USA* 1999;**96**(23):13103–7.
55. Webster SG, Dircksen H, Chung JS. Endocrine cells in the gut of the shore crab *Carcinus maenas* immunoreactive to crustacean hyperglycaemic hormone and its precursor-related peptide. *Cell Tissue Res* 2000;**300**(1):193–205.
56. Kung PC, Wu SH, Nagaraju GPC, Tsai WS, Lee CY. Crustacean hyperglycemic hormone precursor transcripts in the hemocytes of the crayfish *Procambarus clarkii*: novel sequence characteristics relating to gene splicing pattern and transcript stability. *Gen Comp Endocrinol* 2013;**186**:80–4.
57. Manfrin C, Tom M, De Moro G, Gerdol M, Giulianini PG, Pallavicini A. The eyestalk transcriptome of red swamp crayfish *Procambarus clarkii*. *Gene* 2015;**557**(1):28–34.
58. Katayama H, Ohira T, Aida K, Nagasawa H. Significance of a carboxyl-terminal amide moiety in the folding and biological activity of crustacean hyperglycemic hormone. *Peptides* 2002;**23**(9):1537–46.
59. Mosco A, Edomi P, Guarnaccia C, Lorenzon S, Pongor S, Ferrero EA, et al. Functional aspects of cHH C-terminal amidation in crayfish species. *Regul Pept* 2008;**147**(1–3):88–95.
60. Ollivaux C, Vinh J, Soyez D, Toullec JY. Crustacean hyperglycemic and vitellogenesis-inhibiting hormones in the lobster *Homarus gammarus*: implications for structural and functional evolution of a neuropeptide family. *FEBS J* 2006;**273**(10):2151–60.

61. Manfrin C, Tom M, De Moro G, Gerdol M, Guarnaccia C, Mosco A, et al. Application of D-crustacean hyperglycemic hormone induces peptidases transcription and suppresses glycolysis-related transcripts in the hepatopancreas of the crayfish *Pontastacus leptodactylus* — results of a transcriptomic study. *PLoS One* 2013;**8**(6):e65176.

62. Lebaupain F, Boscameric M, Pilet E, Soyez D, Kamech N. Natural and synthetic chiral isoforms of crustacean hyperglycemic hormone from the crayfish *Astacus leptodactylus*: hyperglycemic activity and hemolymphatic clearance. *Peptides* 2012;**34**(1):66–73.

63. Mosco A, Zlatev V, Guarnaccia C, Giulianini PG. Functional analysis of a mutated analogue of the crustacean hyperglycaemic hormone from the crayfish *Pontastacus leptodactylus*. *J Exp Zool Part A Ecol Genet Physiol* 2015;**323**(2):121–7.

64. Chung JS, Webster SG. Binding sites of crustacean hyperglycemic hormone and its second messengers on gills and hindgut of the green shore crab, *Carcinus maenas*: a possible osmoregulatory role. *Gen Comp Endocrinol* 2006;**147**:206–13.

65. Mykles DL, Adams ME, Gäde G, Lange AB, Marco HG, Orchard I. Neuropeptide action in insects and crustaceans. *Physiol Biochem Zool* 2010;**83**(5):836–46.

66. Manfrin C, Peruzza L, Bonzi L, Pallavicini A, Giulianini P. Silencing two main isoforms of crustacean hyperglycemic hormone (CHH) induces compensatory expression of two CHH-like transcripts in the red swamp crayfish *Procambarus clarkii*. *Invertebr Surviv J* 2015;**12**:29–37.

67. Wanlem S, Supamattaya K, Tantikitti C, Prasertsan P, Graidist P. Expression and applications of recombinant crustacean hyperglycemic hormone from eyestalks of white shrimp (*Litopenaeus vannamei*) against bacterial infection. *Fish Shellfish Immunol* 2011;**30**:877–85.

68. Lorenzon S, de Guarrinia S, Smithb VJ, Ferrero EA. Effects of LPS injection on circulating haemocytes in crustaceans in vivo. *Fish Shellfish Immunol* 2004;**9**(1):31–50.

Chapter 9

How Insects Combat Infections

Małgorzata Cytryńska, Iwona Wojda, Teresa Jakubowicz
Maria Curie-Sklodowska University, Lublin, Poland

CHARACTERISTICS OF INSECT IMMUNE RESPONSE

Living in different habitats, insects are exposed to a wide range of infection agents, including bacteria, fungi, protists, or viruses. To protect themselves, they have developed a very fast and effective immune system based on cellular and humoral responses.

The cellular branch of immune response is mediated by hemocytes and comprises phagocytosis, nodulation, and encapsulation. During phagocytosis, a certain type of hemocytes, namely plasmatocytes and granulocytes, are engaged in the elimination of pathogenic microorganisms. Phagocytized particles are captured by hemocyte membrane-bound receptors, internalized, and ingested in phagolysosomes. Nodulation is characteristic only of insects and refers to the formation of nodules, ie, multicellular hemocyte aggregates that entrap a large number of bacterial and/or fungal cells. Encapsulation involves hemocyte aggregation around larger targets, such as nematodes or eggs of parasitic wasps.[1] The insect humoral response includes the activation of enzymatic cascades that regulate the coagulation and melanization of hemolymph, production of reactive oxygen and nitrogen species, and synthesis of defense molecules.[2] The key effector molecules of the humoral immune response, antimicrobial peptides (AMPs), synthesized mainly by fat body and hemocytes, are secreted into the hemolymph, enabling a systemic response to infection. In local reactions, AMPs produced by epithelial cells are involved.[3] These mostly cationic, amphipathic molecules interact with the microbial cell membrane, which leads to the disruption of membrane integrity, resulting in pathogen cell death. Some defense peptides enter the microbial cell, where they affect essential cellular processes, ie, replication, transcription, protein synthesis, and protein folding, which are lethal for a pathogen.[4–6]

Antibacterial and Antifungal Response

Recognition of Infection

Sensing the infection is mediated by pattern recognition receptors (PRRs) which recognize conserved motifs, called pathogen-associated molecular patterns

Lessons in Immunity: From Single-Cell Organisms to Mammals
http://dx.doi.org/10.1016/B978-0-12-803252-7.00009-6

(PAMPs), unique for microbes but absent in the host. In this chapter, we present characteristics of three major families of PRRs, namely, peptidoglycan recognition proteins (PGRPs), gram-negative bacteria binding proteins (GNBP)/β-1,3-glucan recognition proteins (β-GRP), and the Down syndrome cell adhesion molecule (Dscam), which are crucial for microbial recognition.

Peptidoglycan Recognition Protein Family

PGRP family members are able to distinguish structurally different peptidoglycans (PGNs) of bacterial cell walls. Bacterial PGNs important for immune system activation include lysine-type PGNs (Lys-PGN) characteristic for cell walls in the majority of gram-positive bacteria and *meso*-diaminopimelic acid-type PGNs (DAP-PGN) present in gram-negative bacteria and some gram-positive bacteria (*Bacillus* and *Clostridium*).[7,8] In *Drosophila melanogaster*, 13 genes encoding PGRPs have been described. They have a conserved PGRP domain in the C-terminal region, which exhibits similarity to bacterial amidases. Some members of the PGRPs family, not containing crucial amino acid residues essential for catalytic activity, are referred to as recognizing PGRPs. The PGRPs exhibiting enzymatic activity modulate various immune responses by processing PGNs to nonstimulatory fragments, thereby turning off the immune response.[9,10]

Drosophila PGRPs are also classified on the basis of molecular mass. The short forms of PGRPs, -SA, -SB, -SC, -SD, with molecular mass below 20 kDa, are secreted in the hemolymph. Among the long form proteins (30–90 kDa), PGRP-LA, -LC, -LD, and -LF are membrane-associated proteins, while others (PGRP-LB, -LE) are cytosolic or extracellular.[11] The *PGRP-LC* gene encodes three isomers, PGRP-LCa, -LCx, and -LCγ, from which heterodimers -LCa/-LCx recognize monomeric, while homodimers -LCx/-LCx polymeric PGNs. PGRP-SA and -SD, involved in the recognition of the Lys-PGN, and PGRP-LC and -LE, recognizing DAP-PGN, activate Toll and Imd signaling pathway, respectively. PGRP-LC interacts with PGRP-LE during the recognition. PGRP-LE is present in hemolymph and in the cytoplasm of immune-related cells such as the fat body, gut epithelium, and hemocytes. Extra- and intracellular PGRP-LE activates the Imd pathway dependently and independently of PGRP-LC, respectively.[9] *Drosophila* intestinal PGRP-LE is a master bacterial sensor, which controls balanced responses to microbial infections and immune tolerance to microbiota through the upregulation of Pirk protein and PGRP-LB, which negatively regulate the Imd pathway.[12] *Drosophila* PGPR-LE also plays an essential role in detecting DAP-PGN of the intracellular pathogenic bacteria *Listeria monocytogenes*, inducing autophagy as an alternative response independently of Toll and Imd signaling pathways.[13,14] Additionally, PGRP-LC plays a key role in phagocytosis of gram-negative bacteria, whereas PGRP-LE is involved in the activation of the prophenoloxidase (PPO) proteolytic cascade independently of Imd pathway activation.[9]

GNBP/β-GRP Family

The members of the GNBP/β-GRP family recognize fungal β-1,3-glucans, bacterial lipopolysaccharide, and lipoteichoic acid and may work in a complex with PGRPs in the detection of gram-positive bacteria.[15] In contrast to PGRPs present in both vertebrate and invertebrate organisms, GNBPs are characteristics of invertebrates. They contain a conserved C-terminal β-glucanase domain and an N-terminal domain binding β-1,3-glucans. In *Drosophila* three GNBPs, GNBP-1 to 3, have been discovered. Among these, GNBP-3 shows the greatest similarity to lepidopteran β-GRP, exhibits specificity in binding fungal β-1,3-glucans, and induces the Toll signaling pathway. Interestingly, *Drosophila* homologues of the GNBP, a receptor first identified in *Bombyx mori* hemolymph as *Enterobacter cloacae*-binding protein, are not involved in the recognition of gram-negative bacteria. Additionally, the interaction of *B. mori* and *Manduca sexta* β-GRPs with microbial polysaccharides promotes the assembly of β-GRP oligomers, which triggers the PPO proteolytic cascade.[16,17]

Down Syndrome Cell Adhesion Molecule

The Down syndrome cell adhesion molecule (Dscam) belongs to immunoglobulin-superfamily proteins that are important for neuronal development and microbial recognition. They are hypervariable receptors generated by alternative splicing potentially giving rise to tens of thousands (38,016 in *Drosophila*, 31,000 in *Anopheles gambiae*) different isoforms, which may be either secreted or membrane-bound molecules. Most of the diversity of membrane-bound Dscam isoforms lies in their extracellular part, which contains 10 Ig-like and 6 fibronectin type III domains. Various combinations of adhesive domains, facilitating specific interactions with particular microorganisms, would potentially lead to a directed immune response. In addition, soluble forms of Dscam present in insect hemolymph may function in binding microbes and stimulating phagocytosis (opsonization) thereof.[18,19]

Signaling Pathways

A hallmark of insect innate immunity is the rapid induction of AMPs genes, which is controlled by three major signaling pathways: Toll, Imd, and JAK/STAT, studied in detail in *D. melanogaster* and described in excellent reviews.[20-22] Each pathway induces the transcription of a specific set of immune-related genes. The Toll pathway is mainly responsible for the detection and response to gram-positive bacterial and fungal infections, whereas the Imd pathway is required for the response to gram-negative bacterial infections. The JAK/STAT pathway is activated by infection or septic injury detected by a variety of immunological receptors.

Toll and Imd Pathways

The activation of transmembrane receptors, Toll, and PGRP-LC initiates a series of intracellular events resulting in the activation of the transcription factors Dif/Dorsal and Relish, members of the Rel/NF-κB family. In the nucleus, they trigger the expression of AMPs genes and numerous other genes involved in the immune response.[23,24]

In the Toll pathway, recognition of bacterial Lys-PGN by PGRP-SA, PGRP-SD, and GNBP-1, or fungal β-1,3-glucan by GNBP-3, or a "danger signal" causes the activation of an adequate serine proteinase cascade in the hemolymph.[25–27] Consequently, the activated protease SPE converts pro-Spaetzle into the cytokine-like molecule Spaetzle, whose binding to Toll causes dimerization of the receptor.[28–30] Toll activation leads to the formation of a receptor–adaptor complex composed of dMyD88, Tube, and Pelle, eventually resulting in the release of the transcription factor Dif/Dorsal from the complex with its inhibitor cactus.[20]

Recognition of bacterial DAP-PGN by specific transmembrane PGRP-LC in cooperation with PGRP-LE receptors activates the Imd pathway in responding cells.[31–33] Ligand binding triggers receptor dimerization or multimerization, which leads to the recruitment of an adaptor protein, Imd. Then Imd recruits dFADD and a homologue of mammalian caspase-8, DREDD, which cleaves Imd preparing it to K63-polyubiquitination. This modification of Imd allows for further recruitment and activation of the protein kinase dTAK, responsible for the activation of two branches of the Imd pathway, ie, IKK/Relish and JNK. The NF-κB domain of Relish resulting from the precursor form after phosphorylation by the ird5 subunit of IKK and cleavage by DREDD translocates to the nucleus and initiates the expression of the target genes. *Drosophila* TAK1 signaling to JNK leads to the activation of the transcription factor AP-1, which was linked to the upregulation of stress response genes and wound repair. Involvement of the Imd/JNK branch in the regulation of AMPs genes expression has also been suggested.[21]

JAK/STAT Pathway

JAK/STAT in insects was characterized in terms of its role in embryonal development, hemocyte proliferation, and response to different types of stress. It also participates in the response to bacterial and viral infections by regulating the production of effector molecules, including AMPs. This pathway is activated in a paracrine fashion through the binding of secreted ligands UPD (unpaired) produced as a consequence of nonself recognition. Ligand binding to the receptor Dome (Domeless) activates the tyrosine kinase HOP (the receptor-associated Janus Kinase), which then phosphorylates Dome, creating docking sites for binding and phosphorylation of STAT transcription factors. Phosphorylated STATs dimerize and translocate to the nucleus where they activate the expression of effector genes. Complement-like thioester containing proteins expressed after bacterial infection, or antiviral protein vir1 produced after viral infection, are, among others, under the control of the JAK/STAT pathway.[34,35]

Antiviral Response

Insects are susceptible to diverse families of DNA and RNA viruses. Studies performed mainly on *D. melanogaster* and mosquitos revealed two types of innate immune responses to viral infections: a constitutive response based on the degradation of viral RNA by the RNA interference mechanism (RNAi) and an inducible immune response that prevents infection by virus-induced antiviral gene expression. In both mechanisms, a clue role is played by the multifunctional DExD/H-box containing helicase Dicer-2, which acts as PRR in recognition of dsRNA that functions as PAMP.[36]

RNA interference is a major mechanism of insect defense against viruses in which Dicer-2 restricts viral infection by generating small interfering RNAs (siRNAs) leading to recognition and targeting viral RNA for degradation and hence inhibition of viral replication.

The inducible immune response also involves Dicer-2, which activates in a dsRNA-dependent manner, the transcription, and then the synthesis of the secreted peptide Vago (CuVago in *Culex*), which can restrict viral infection by the activation of the JAK/STAT pathway in a paracrine way, similarly to the action of interferons in mammals.[34,35]

Autophagy has been proposed as an alternative antiviral mechanism that is independent of the Imd, Toll, JAK/STAT, and RNAi pathways. Probably, vesicular stomatitis virus (VSV) induces autophagy in *Drosophila* through the envelope glycoprotein VSV-G acting as a PAMP. Additionally, it has been discovered that the *Drosophila* Toll-7 receptor functions as PRR recognizing VSV and elicits antiviral autophagy independently of the classic Toll pathway. The signaling of autophagy is mediated through the phosphoinositide 3-kinase (PI3K)-AKT-dTOR pathway.[14,37]

Specificity of Immune Response, Memory, and Immune Priming

Innate immunity pathways have been well characterized in *Drosophila* and a number of mosquito species. The system of acquired immunity based on B and T lymphocytes, typical for vertebrates, does not exist in insects. Despite the lack of acquired immunity, the insect immune system produces a relatively specific response to detected pathogens by employing alternative mechanisms.[38,39]

As early as 1997, it was documented that *D. melanogaster* AMP genes were diversely expressed depending on the class of the pathogen, providing evidence of immune response specificity in insects.[40] An impressive example of the enormous capabilities of specific interactions is represented by the high variety of isoforms of the Dscam receptor.[18,19] The infection signals, initially diversified by recognition by PRRs, are further diversified at the level of signaling pathways. Once inside a cell, the signal can be tuned accordingly by combining Dif, Dorsal, and Relish in homodimers and heterodimers differing in affinity to κB sites within the gene promoters.[41,42]

Growing evidence indicates that priming-based immune memory functions in insects. Immune priming is usually defined as an improved response to a pathogen upon the second contact. Various pathogens, from viruses to parasites, can induce priming in a single insect.[43] Within and transgeneration immune priming was demonstrated to be pathogen specific in insects, implying that a lack of acquired immunity does not exclude the development of response specificity and immunological memory.[44,45] Studies on *Periplaneta americana* cockroaches performed more than 30 years ago indicated that they possessed immunological memory. The cockroaches injected with killed bacteria mounted a two-step reaction with a nonspecific first phase and a highly specific second phase response resembling acquired immunity.[46,47] *Bombus terrestris* bumblebees prechallenged with different bacteria were protected for up to 22 days against subsequent infection only in a homologous configuration.[48] Immunological memory resulting from the preinjection of sublethal doses of *Streptococcus pneumoniae* was also implicated in *D. melanogaster* protection against lethal doses of only these bacteria. The Toll pathway and phagocytes expressing selected isoforms of Dscam activated during the first contact with the pathogen were suggested to play an essential role in this process.[49] It is also worth mentioning that abiotic factors like mechanical or heat stress may influence the immune response and prime immune system in nonspecific ways.[50–52]

Antimicrobial pathways must communicate to form an integrated and pathogen-specific immune response. Recent evidence has demonstrated that the insect immune system can coordinate different defense mechanisms by switching between humoral and cellular immune response. Activation of the vascular endothelial growth factor receptor (Pvr) mediated by the growth-blocking peptide (GBP) in *Drosophila* plasmatocytes led to the stimulation of cell spreading, enabling the initiation of cellular response reactions, simultaneously inhibiting humoral immune responses.[53]

INTERACTION BETWEEN INSECT HOST AND PATHOGEN

Both insects and entomopathogens undergo antagonist coevolution; while insects develop a protective mechanism, entomopathogens evolve strategies to break protective barriers. Insects are protected against surrounding microbes by the cuticle as well as the structure and internal conditions of the digestive tract and trachea, which make a barrier for microorganisms. In parallel, natural insect pathogens possess mechanisms that allow them to force the insect anatomic barriers and establish a biotope inside the infected body where they can proliferate. Virulence strategies used by entomopathogens can be divided into active and passive. The active strategy is to produce and secrete virulence factors whose role may inter alia be (1) to destroy the insect tissue, (2) to inhibit the expression or activity of the host defense molecules, and (3) to degrade the immune-relevant molecules of the infected host. The passive strategy is to avoid detection by "hiding" immune elicitors (PAMPs) on the cell surface, changing the composition of the cell wall to increase resistance to insect defense molecules, and to colonize places of poorer access of hemocytes.

Getting Into the Insect Body

The main route of insect infection by entomopathogenic bacteria is ingestion. Some bacteria like *Photorhabdus* and *Xenorhabdus* can access the hemocoel inside entomophagous hosts, eg, nematodes.[54,55] Other pathogens, like most fungi, have developed mechanisms allowing them to force the insect cuticle. Because it is not possible to mention all insects and their pathogens in this short chapter, as an example, we will describe very briefly two different ways of infection: the oral one, used by *Bacillus thuringiensis*, and the infection via cuticle, used by the fungus *Beauveria bassiana*. Both species or their toxins are used for biological pest control. *Bacillus thuringiensis* is a gram-positive bacterium living naturally in the soil. During spore formation, it produces parasporal inclusions containing Cry and Cyt toxins encoded by plasmid genes, which allow bacteria to break the gut anatomical barrier. Cry toxins are highly specific for particular insect species, while Cyt toxins are present in a lower number of strains and are less specific. The death of many insect species can be caused by the action of toxins alone (toxemia), while for others the presence of bacterial cells is required.[56] Ingested parasporal crystal inclusions are solubilized in the insect gut and activated by gut digestive proteases. Afterward, they cross the peritrophic barrier and bind to different classes of midgut receptors, which results in the formation of pores. This interferes with the natural functioning of the intestine and can be already lethal in the case of species highly sensitive to the particular toxin. The next step of *B. thuringiensis* invasion is the germination of spores and vegetative growth. Bacterial cells reach the hemocoel via a perforated gut and proliferate in the body of the infected insect, causing septicemia.[57,58]

Most entomopathogenic fungi infect through the insect cuticle. *Beauveria bassiana* is a natural pathogen of many insects and other invertebrates causing the so-called *white muscardine disease*. The infection process consists of several steps: (1) adsorption of fungal cells to the cuticular surface, (2) adhesion or consolidation of the interface between pregerminant propagules and the epicuticle, (3) germination and development at the insect cuticular surface until the appearance of the appressorium, and (4) development of the penetration peg, which exerts physical pressure on host covers of the body. The fungus forces the cuticle and gets to the hemocoel. During these steps, the intruder produces enzymes like proteases, chitinases, esterases, and lipases, which digest the main components of the insect cuticle.[59]

Inside the Hemocoel

After forcing the host anatomic barriers, the fierce fight between the insect and the pathogen enters the next phase, in which different strategies are used by both parties. In order to protect itself, the pathogen may change its surface. For example, in the *Bacillus* species, alanylation of teichoic acids of the cell wall occurs, which neutralizes their negative charge, thereby preventing an attack by AMPs, and increases resistance to lysozyme.[60] In *B. bassiana*, in turn, a significant difference in the cell wall composition between cells growing in vitro and inside the insect host has been demonstrated. In the hemocoel, *Beauveria* grows in the form of yeast-like cells, having a considerably thinner cell wall than cells growing in vitro. The differences in cell wall thinness have been correlated with transcriptional regulation of chitin and glucan synthases, which are downregulated inside the host.[61] Additionally, in the virulent state of the fungus, there are no detectable galactose residues in the cell wall.[62] All these changes in the cell wall structure reduce the number of surface epitopes recognized by the host immune system as nonself. While growing, the fungus secretes many bioactive metabolites such as beauvericin, bassianolide, and oosporein, which are toxic to the host, and some of them prevent the growth of other organisms that may antagonize the growth and compete for nutrient resources.[63] *Beauveria bassiana* colonizes the insect fat body, the main organ producing defense molecules, and proliferates in the host. Inside the body of the infected host, a significant role is played by proteases secreted by the invading organism. Interestingly, these enzymes and their degradation products may act as signals inducing the host defense mechanisms.[64,65] On the other hand, some insects, eg, the greater wax moth *Galleria mellonella*, produce inducible proteinases inhibitors, among which the most interesting is IMPI (*inducible metalloproteinase inhibitor*), which represents the first peptidic inhibitor of metalloproteinases identified in invertebrates.[66] The infecting pathogen may also reduce the host cellular immune response. For example, hemolysin HlyII of *B. thuringiensis* was found to induce apoptosis of hemocytes.[67] The insect infected by the entomopathogen dies as a result of mechanical injury and the toxic action of the intruder's toxins.

The other side of the fight between the insect and its intruder is the competition for iron. The host strategy is to deprive the intruder of iron sources to limit its growth, while the pathogen possesses factors involved in iron acquisition. For example, expression of the transferrin gene is upregulated in the infected insect host like *G. mellonella* in order to bind iron and create an environment low in free iron that impedes bacterial survival inside the infected host.[68] On the other hand, the pathogen possesses factors involved in iron acquisition like the IlsA protein produced by the *Bacillus cereus* group, which is involved in iron uptake from ferritin, and its gene is specifically transcribed in the insect hemocoel. The *ilsA* mutant has decreased virulence toward *G. mellonella*.[69]

It is worth mentioning that insects are good models for studying the virulence mechanisms of human pathogens. Their low cost, simplicity of use, and short life span make insect models ideal candidates for in vivo experiments. The course of infection caused by human pathogens, such as *Pseudomonas aeruginosa*, *Enterococcus faecalis*, *Staphylococcus aureus*, or *Candida albicans*, can be studied first in insect models, facilitating identification of their virulence factors and testing their mode of action.[70–72]

REFERENCES

1. Strand MR. The insect cellular immune response. *Insect Sci* 2008;**15**:1–14.
2. Lemaitre B, Hoffmann J. The host defense in *Drosophila melanogaster*. *Annu Rev Immunol* 2007;**25**:697–743.

3. Davis MM, Engström Y. Immune response in the barrier epithelia: lessons from the fruit fly *Drosophila melanogaster*. *J Innate Immun* 2012;**4**:273–83.
4. Bulet P, Stöcklin R. Insect antimicrobial peptides: structures, properties and gene regulation. *Protein Pept Lett* 2005;**12**:3–11.
5. Nguyen LT, Haney EF, Vogel HJ. The expanding scope of antimicrobial peptide structures and their modes of action. *Trends Biotechnol* 2011;**29**:464–72.
6. Scocchi M, Tossi A, Gennaro R. Proline-rich antimicrobial peptides: converging to a non-lytic mechanism of action. *Cell Mol Life Sci* 2011;**68**:2317–30.
7. Dziarski R. Peptidoglycan recognition proteins (PGRPs). *Mol Immunol* 2004;**40**:877–86.
8. Steiner H. Peptidoglycan recognition proteins: on and off switches for innate immunity. *Immunol Rev* 2004;**198**:83–96.
9. Kurata S. Peptidoglycan recognition proteins in *Drosophila* immunity. *Dev Comp Immunol* 2014;**42**:36–41.
10. Werner T, Liu G, Kang D, Ekengren S, Steinerh, Hultmark D. A family of peptidoglycan recognition proteins in the fruit fly *Drosophila melanogaster*. *Proc Natl Acad Sci USA* 2000;**97**:13772–7.
11. Kurata S. Extracellular and intracellular pathogen recognition by *Drosophila* PGRP-LE and PGRP-LC. *Int Immunol* 2010;**22**:143–8.
12. Bosco-Drayon V, Poidevin M, Boneca IG, Narbonne-Reveau K, Royet J, Charroux B. Peptidoglycan sensing by the receptor PGRP-LE in *Drosophila* gut induces immune responses to infectious bacteria and tolerance to microbiota. *Cell Host Microbe* 2012;**12**:153–65.
13. Yano T, Mita S, Ohmori H, Oshima Y, Fujimoto Y, Ueda R, et al. Autophagic control of *Listeria* through intracellular innate immune recognition in *Drosophila*. *Nat Immunol* 2008; **9**:908–16.
14. Ryan HM, Cherry S. Antimicrobial autophagy: a conserved innate immune response in *Drosophila*. *J Innate Immun* 2013;**5**:444–55.
15. Royet J. Infectious non-self recognition in invertebrates: lessons from *Drosophila* and other insect models. *Mol Immunol* 2004;**41**:1063–75.
16. Barillas-Mury C, Paskewitz S, Kanost MR. Immune response of vectors. In: Marquardt WC, Black WC, Freier J, Hagedorn H, Hemingway J, Higgs S, et al., editors. *The biology of disease vectors*. Elsevier/Academic Press; 2005. p. 363–76.
17. Takahashi D, Dai H, Hiromasa Y, Krishnamoorthi R, Kanost MR. Self-association of an insect β-1,3-glucan recognition protein upon binding laminarin stimulates prophenoloxidase activation as an immune response. *J Biol Chem* 2014;**289**:28399–410.
18. Cherry S, Silverman N. Host-pathogen interactions in *Drosophila*: new tricks from an old friend. *Nat Immunol* 2006;**7**:911–7.
19. Dong Y, Taylor HE, Dimopoulos G. AgDscam, a hypervariable immunoglobulin domain-containing receptor of the *Anopheles gambiae* innate immune system. *PLoS Biol* 2006; **4**:1137–46.e229.
20. Lindsay SA, Wasserman SA. Conventional and non-conventional *Drosophila* Toll signaling. *Dev Comp Immunol* 2014;**42**:16–24.
21. Kleino A, Silverman N. The *Drosophila* IMD pathway in the activation of the humoral immune response. *Dev Comp Immunol* 2014;**42**:25–35.
22. Imler JL. Overview of *Drosophila* immunity: a historical perspective. *Dev Comp Immunol* 2014;**42**:3–15.
23. Hayden M, Ghosh S. Signaling to NF-κB. *Genes Dev* 2004;**18**:2195–224.
24. Minakhina S, Steward R. Nuclear factor-kappa B pathways in *Drosophila*. *Oncogene* 2006;**25**:6749–57.

25. Gottar M, Gobert V, Matskevich AA, Reichhart JM, Wang C, Butt TM, et al. Dual detection of fungal infections in *Drosophila* via recognition of glucans and sensing of virulence factors. *Cell* 2006;**127**:1425–37.

26. Kambris Z, Brun S, Jang IH, Nam HJ, Romeo Y, Takahashi K, et al. *Drosophila* immunity: a large-scale *in vivo* RNAi screen identifies five serine proteases required for Toll activation. *Curr Biol* 2006;**6**:808–13.

27. Krautz R, Arefin B, Theopold U. Damage signals in the insect immune response. *Front Plant Sci* 2014;**5**:342.

28. Weber AN, Tauszig-Delamasure S, Hoffmann JA, Lelievre E, Gascan H, Ray KP, et al. Binding of the *Drosophila* cytokine Spatzle to Toll is direct and establishes signaling. *Nat Immunol* 2003;**4**:794–800.

29. Hu X, Yagi Y, Tanji T, Zhou S, Ip YT. Multimerization and interaction of Toll and Spätzle in *Drosophila*. *Proc Natl Acad Sci USA* 2004;**101**:9369–74.

30. Jang IH, Chosa N, Kim SH, Nam HJ, Lemaitre B, Ochiai M, et al. A Spätzle-processing enzyme required for Toll signaling activation in *Drosophila* innate immunity. *Dev Cell* 2006;**10**:45–55.

31. Gottar M, Gobert V, Michel T, Belvin M, Duyk G, Hoffmann JA, et al. The *Drosophila* immune response against Gram-negative bacteria is mediated by a peptidoglycan recognition protein. *Nature* 2002;**416**:640–4.

32. Stenbak CR, Ryu JH, Leulier F, Pili-Floury S, Parquet C, Herve M, et al. Peptidoglycan molecular requirements allowing detection by the *Drosophila* immune deficiency pathway. *J Immunol* 2004;**173**:7339–48.

33. Werner T, Borge-Renberg K, Mellroth P, Steiner H, Hultmark D. Functional diversity of the *Drosophila PGRP-LC* gene cluster in the response to lipopolysaccharide and peptidoglycan. *J Biol Chem* 2003;**278**:26319–22.

34. Paradkar PN, Trinidad L, Voysey R, Duchemin JB, Walker PJ. Secreted Vago restrict West Nile Virus infection in *Culex* mosquito cells by activating the Jak-STAT pathway. *Proc Natl Acad Sci USA* 2012;**109**:18915–20.

35. Kingslover MB, Huang Z, Hardy RW. Insect antiviral innate immunity: pathways, effectors, and connections. *J Mol Biol* 2013;**425**:4921–36.

36. Deddouche S, Matt N, Budd A, Mueller S, Kemp C, Galiana-Arnoux D, et al. The DExD/H-box helicase Dicer-2 mediates the induction of antiviral activity in *Drosophila*. *Nat Immunol* 2008;**9**:1425–32.

37. Lamiable O, Imler JL. Induced antiviral innate immunity in *Drosophila*. *Curr Opin Microbiol* 2014;**20**:62–8.

38. Armitage SA, Peuß R, Kurtz J. Dscam and pancrustacean immune memory - a review of the evidence. *Dev Comp Immunol* 2015;**48**:315–23.

39. Ng TH, Chiang YA, Yeh YC, Wang HC. Review of Dscam-mediated immunity in shrimp and other arthropods. *Dev Comp Immunol* 2014;**46**:129–38.

40. Lemaitre B, Reichhart JM, Hoffmann JA. *Drosophila* host defense: differential induction of antimicrobial peptide genes after infection by various classes of microorganisms. *Proc Natl Acad Sci USA* 1997;**94**:14614–9.

41. Pal S, Wu J, Wu LP. Microarray analyses reveal distinct roles for Rel proteins in the *Drosophila* immune response. *Dev Comp Immunol* 2008;**32**:50–60.

42. Tanji T, Hu X, Weber ANR, Ip YT. Toll and IMD pathways synergistically activate an immune response in *Drosophila melanogaster*. *Mol Cell Biol* 2007;**27**:4578–88.

43. Chambers MC, Schneider DS. Pioneering immunology: insect style. *Curr Opin Immunol* 2012;**24**:10–4.

44. Freitak D, Schmidtberg H, Dickel F, Lochnit G, Vogel H, Vilcinskas A. The maternal transfer of bacteria can mediate trans-generational immune priming in insects. *Virulence* 2014;**5**:547–54.
45. Tidbury HJ, Pedersen AB, Boots M. Within and transgenerational immune priming in an insect to a DNA virus. *Proc Biol Sci* 2011;**278**:871–6.
46. Rheins LA, Karp RD, Butz A. Induction of specific humoral immunity to soluble proteins in the American cockroach (*Periplaneta americana*). I. Nature of the primary response. *Dev Comp Immunol* 1980;**4**:447–58.
47. Karp RD, Rheins LA. Induction of specific humoral immunity to soluble proteins in the American cockroach (*Periplaneta americana*). II. Nature of the secondary response. *Dev Comp Immunol* 1980;**4**:629–39.
48. Sadd BM, Schmid-Hempel P. Insect immunity shows specificity in protection upon secondary pathogen exposure. *Curr Biol* 2006;**16**:1206–10.
49. Pham LN, Dionne MS, Shirasu-Hiza M, Schneider DS. A specific primed immune response in *Drosophila* is dependent on phagocytes. *PLoS Pathog* 2007;**3**:e26.
50. Linder JE, Owers KA, Promislow DE. The effects of temperature on host-pathogen interactions in *D. melanogaster*: who benefits? *J Insect Physiol* 2008;**54**:297–308.
51. Mowlds P, Barron A, Kavanagh K. Physical stress primes the immune response of *Galleria mellonella* larvae to infection by *Candida albicans*. *Microbes Infect* 2008;**10**:628–34.
52. Wojda I, Taszłow P. Heat shock affects host-pathogen interaction in *Galleria mellonella* infected with *Bacillus thuringiensis*. *J Insect Physiol* 2013;**59**:894–905.
53. Tsuzuki S, Matsumoto H, Furihata S, Ryuda M, Tanaka H, Sung EJ, et al. Switching between humoral and cellular immune responses in *Drosophila* is guided by the cytokine GBP. *Nat Commun* 2014;**5**:4628.
54. Forst S, Dowds B, Boemare N, Stackebrandt E. *Xenorhabdus* and *Photorhabdus* spp.: bugs that kill bugs. *Annu Rev Microbiol* 1997;**51**:47–72.
55. Nielsen-LeRoux C, Gaudriault S, Ramarao N, Lereclus D, Givaudan A. How the insect pathogen bacteria *Bacillus thuringiensis* and *Xenorhabdus/Photorhabdus* occupy their hosts. *Curr Opin Microbiol* 2012;**15**:220–31.
56. Li RS, Jarrett P, Burges HD. Importance of spores, crystals, and δ-endotoxins in the pathogenicity of different varieties of *Bacillus thuringiensis* in *Galleria mellonella* and *Pieris brassicae*. *J Invertebr Pathol* 1987;**50**:277–84.
57. Raymond B, Johnston PR, Nielsen-LeRoux C, Lereclus D, Crickmore N. *Bacillus thuringiensis*: an impotent pathogen? *Trends Microbiol* 2010;**18**:189–94.
58. Vachon V, Laprade R, Schwartz JL. Current models of the mode of action of *Bacillus thuringiensis* insecticidal crystal proteins: a critical review. *J Invertebr Pathol* 2012;**111**:1–12.
59. Pedrini N, Crespo R, Juárez MP. Biochemistry of insect epicuticle degradation by entomopathogenic fungi. *Comp Biochem Physiol C Toxicol Pharmacol* 2007;**146**:124–37.
60. Abi Khattar Z, Rejasse A, Destoumieux-Garzon D, Escoubas JM, Sanchis V, Lereclus D, et al. The dlt operon of *Bacillus cereus* is required for resistance to cationic antimicrobial peptides and for virulence in insects. *J Bacteriol* 2009;**22**:7063–73.
61. Tartar A, Shapiro AM, Scharf DW, Boucias DG. Differential expression of chitin synthase (CHS) and glucan synthase (FKS) genes correlates with the formation of a modified, thinner cell wall in *in vivo*-produced *Beauveria bassiana* cells. *Mycopathologia* 2005;**160**:303–14.
62. Pendland JC, Hung SY, Boucias DG. Evasion of host defense by *in vivo*-produced protoplast-like cells of the insect mycopathogen *Beauveria bassiana*. *J Bacteriol* 1993;**175**:5962–9.
63. Gibson DM, Donzelli BG, Krasnoff SB, Keyhani NO. Discovering the secondary metabolite potential encoded within entomopathogenic fungi. *Nat Prod Rep* 2014;**31**:1287–305.

64. Griesch J, Wedde M, Vilcinskas A. Recognition and regulation of metalloproteinase activity in the haemolymph of *Galleria mellonella*: a new pathway mediating induction of humoral immune responses. *Insect Biochem Mol Biol* 2000;**30**:461–72.

65. Altincicek B, Linder M, Linder D, Preissner KT, Vilcinskas A. Microbial metalloproteinases mediate sensing of invading pathogens and activate innate immune responses in the lepidopteran model host *Galleria mellonella*. *Infect Immun* 2007;**75**:175–83.

66. Wedde M, Weise C, Nuck R, Altincicek B, Vilcinskas A. The insect metalloproteinase inhibitor gene of the lepidopteran *Galleria mellonella* encodes two distinct inhibitors. *Biol Chem* 2007;**88**:119–27.

67. Tran SL, Guillemet E, Ngo-Camus M, Clybouw C, Puhar A, Moris A, et al. Haemolysin II is a *Bacillus cereus* virulence factor that induces apoptosis of macrophages. *Cell Microbiol* 2011;**13**:92–108.

68. Seitz V, Clermont A, Wedde M, Hummel M, Vilcinskas A, Schlatterer K, et al. Identification of immunorelevant genes from greater wax moth (*Galleria mellonella*) by subtractive hybridization approach. *Dev Comp Immunol* 2003;**27**:207–15.

69. Daou N, Buisson C, Gohar M, Vidic J, Bierne H, Kallassy M, et al. IlsA, a unique surface protein of *Bacillus cereus* required for iron acquisition from heme, hemoglobin and ferritin. *PLoS Pathog* 2009;**5**:e1000675.

70. Junqueira JC. *Galleria mellonella* as a model host for human pathogens: recent studies and new perspectives. *Virulence* 2012;**3**:474–6.

71. Arvanitis M, Glavis-Bloom J, Mylonakis E. Invertebrate models of fungal infection. *Biochim Biophys Acta* 2013;**1832**:1378–83.

72. Cook SM, McArthur JD. Developing *Galleria mellonella* as a model host for human pathogens. *Virulence* 2013;**4**:350–3.

Chapter 10

Aedes aegypti Immune Responses to Dengue Virus

Cole Schonhofer[a], Heather Coatsworth[a]
Simon Fraser University, Burnaby, BC, Canada

Paola Caicedo, Clara Ocampo
CIDEIM, Cali, Valle del Cauca, Colombia

Carl Lowenberger
Simon Fraser University, Burnaby, BC, Canada

INTRODUCTION

Dengue fever (DF), colloquially known as "break-bone fever," is a mosquito-borne viral disease that affects 50–400 million people each year[1] and is characterized by muscle and joint pain, fever, headaches, nausea, and rashes. Despite significant effort, there are no vaccines or Dengue-specific drugs currently available.[2] There are four established serotypes of Dengue (DENv), and most infected people recover completely 5–12 days after the initial infection.[2] A primary infection with one DENv serotype provides lifelong protection to subsequent infections with that same serotype. Subsequent infection with a different serotype, however, may result in severe Dengue (SD), also called Dengue hemorrhagic fever (DHF) or Dengue shock syndrome (DSS), which causes approximately 25,000 deaths annually. SD is linked to a previous DENv exposure[3] that results in a phenomenon known as antibody-dependant enhancement.[4] The immune responses and the life-threatening potential problems associated with DHF and DSS have challenged the development of a tetravalent vaccine that must protect equally well against all four serotypes at once.[5] With 2–4 billion people around the world at risk of the disease, DENv is currently the world's most significant arthropod-borne virus (arbovirus).

---

a. These authors have contributed equally and should be considered the first coauthors.

Lessons in Immunity: From Single-Cell Organisms to Mammals
http://dx.doi.org/10.1016/B978-0-12-803252-7.00010-2

TRANSMISSION TO HUMAN HOSTS: VECTORS

DENv is transmitted by adult female mosquitoes of the genus *Aedes*, primarily *Aedes aegypti*, and, to a lesser extent, *Aedes albopictus*. Both species breed in small water-filled containers around human habitation and are extremely well adapted to urban human environments.[6] Female *A. aegypti* and *A. albopictus* bite during the daytime, and Dengue control measures have emphasized vector control programs to eradicate or reduce mosquito populations and therefore transmission. The ease and speed of international commerce and human travel between endemic and nonendemic regions have contributed directly to the spread of mosquito vectors and the constant circulation of multiple DENv serotypes; there are now areas where all four serotypes occur, increasing the prevalence and incidence of SD.

An adult female *A. aegypti* feeds on human blood to obtain the proteins required to develop and lays a batch of eggs. DENv ingested with the blood meal leaves the blood bolus to infect and replicate within midgut epithelial cells. Two to three days postinfection (dpi), DENv exits midgut cells and disseminates throughout the vector via the hemolymph, infecting and replicating within cells of the fat body, trachea, and nervous tissues.[7,8] Although DENv can be found in the salivary glands as early as 4 dpi, there is an extrinsic incubation period (EIP) of 7–14 days during which the virus disseminates throughout the mosquito, infects the salivary gland, and replicates to a high enough titer in the salivary glands to infect humans during a subsequent blood meal.[7,8]

Vector competence (VC), the intrinsic ability of a vector to transmit a pathogen, is determined by the dynamics between DENv and the vector. Different mosquito species and strains show different responses to DENv infection in terms of susceptibility and infection rate.[7] A competent or susceptible vector will allow viral infection, dissemination, and transmission, as described previously, whereas a refractory vector will not. There are four established immune-related barriers to virus development[9] (Fig. 10.1). If DENv is unable to infect midgut cells or cannot replicate within them, the mosquito is considered refractory via a midgut infection barrier (MIB), and if the midgut is infected, but the virus is unable to disseminate into the hemocoel, a midgut escape barrier (MEB) is present. Additional barriers may exist in the salivary glands, in which the virus escapes the midgut but cannot enter the salivary glands, a salivary gland infection barrier (SIB), or is unable to disseminate into the salivary gland lumen, a salivary gland escape barrier (SEB).[10,11] These barriers represent selective pressures for DENv to overcome, and their presence in some mosquito strains, and their absence in others, is genetically predetermined.

DENGUE VIRUS IN THE VECTOR: INNATE IMMUNE RESPONSES

There are other processes and factors that also contribute to VC,[12] such as the inducible immune responses of individual mosquitoes.[10] Mosquitoes, like all invertebrates, rely exclusively on their innate immune system to eliminate pathogens. In order to initiate classical innate immune responses, pattern

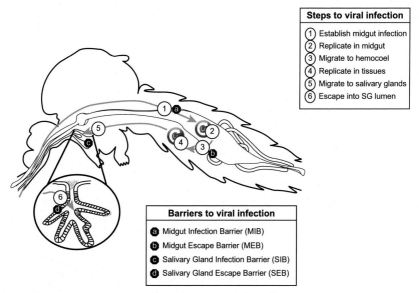

FIGURE 10.1 Development of Dengue viruses in *Aedes aegypti* and the locations on natural infection barriers that prevent virus development, replication, or transmission.

recognition receptors (PRRs)[13] must recognize conserved pathogen-associated molecular patterns (PAMPs) on the outer surfaces of pathogens. Subsequently, components of the humoral and cellular responses are activated via multiple signaling cascades, including the Toll, immune deficiency (IMD), RNA Interference (RNAi), JNK, and Janus Kinase—signal transducer and activator of transcription (JAK-STAT) pathways (Fig. 10.2).[14] These responses culminate in numerous effector mechanisms, including phagocytosis, encapsulation, melanization, and the expression of reactive oxygen intermediates,[15,16] along with the expression of multiple antimicrobial peptides (AMPs) that target and kill microorganisms.[17–19] The strongest immune responses are expressed in the hemocoel of insects,[18] but many AMPs also are expressed in the gastrointestinal tracts of insects to eliminate or prevent the overproliferation of nondesirable symbionts.[19] DENv, however, is an intracellular pathogen and, as such, is not exposed to classic extracellular insect immune responses. Nonetheless, DENv infection in mosquitoes results in the activation of multiple pathways, including Toll, IMD, JAK-STAT, RNAi, autophagy, and apoptosis. These pathways have been reported to control, regulate, or modulate DENv success in mosquitoes and are described in more detail below.

Toll Pathway

The Toll pathway, first described in *Drosophila melanogaster* in the innate immune defense against gram-positive bacteria and fungi, also is activated during DENv infection in *A. aegypti*.[20] In response to microbes, PRRs at the cell

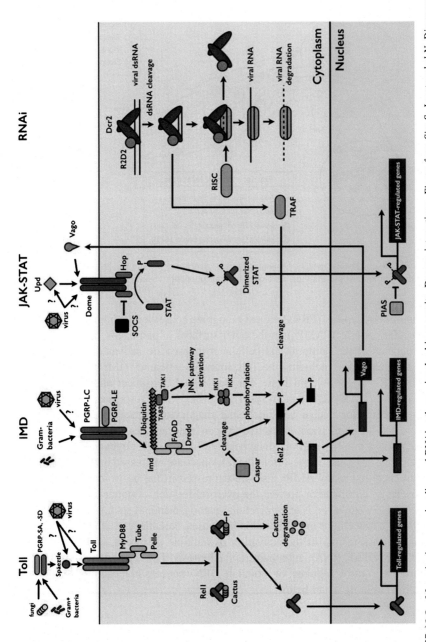

FIGURE 10.2 Mosquito immune signaling and RNAi pathways involved in mosquito–Dengue interactions. *Figure from Sim S, Jupatanakul N, Dimopoulos G. Mosquito immunity against arboviruses. Viruses 2014;6:4479–504. Reproduced with permission.*

surface recognize PAMPs and initiate an intracellular signaling cascade that leads to the eventual activation of Rel proteins via degradation of the inhibitory binding protein Cactus. Activated Rel is an NF-kB transcription factor that enters the cell nucleus and initiates transcription of multiple effector AMP genes, such as Drosomycin and Defensins.[21] Transcriptional profiling of DENv-2 infected *A. aegypti* midguts and carcasses revealed increased expression of genes linked to the Toll pathway, including *Toll*, *Spatzle*, and *Rel1A*, as well as a decrease in transcription of the negative regulator Cactus.[20] Additionally, targeted RNAi silencing of *Cactus* resulted in a decreased midgut viral load, while RNAi silencing of *MYD88*, an activator of the Toll pathway, resulted in an increased midgut viral load.[20] Consistent results were obtained when the experiment was performed 3–7 dpi using different mosquito and viral serotypes.[22] Although Toll pathway-mediated responses are activated in DENv-infected mosquitoes, DENv transmission is not eliminated.

Immune Deficiency Pathway

The IMD pathway is often considered the principal immune response against gram-negative bacteria and also results in the activation of an NF-kB transcription factor, Rel2. The IMD pathway is initiated by different PRR–PAMP interactions, involves different signaling cascades, and activates a variety of effector AMPs. In *A. aegypti*, Rel2 is held inactive in the cytosol by Caspar, which is degraded during IMD signal transduction, allowing Rel2 to be translocated to the nucleus, leading to the transcription of several AMPs.

Although IMD activation in *D. melanogaster* protects against viral infection,[23] similar IMD-mediated protection against DENv infection in *A. aegypti* is unclear. RNAi silencing of *Caspar* in DENv-2 infected mosquitoes had no effect on viral titers in midgut or carcass tissues.[20] RNAi silencing of *IMD* in two strains of *A. aegypti* significantly increased midgut DENv-2 titers whereas RNAi silencing of *Caspar* did not reduce viral titers significantly,[10] possibly because the IMD pathway is already fully activated.[10] As was the case with Toll, activation of the IMD pathway and the expression of IMD-induced AMPs do not eliminate DENv from infected mosquitoes.

Janus Kinase—Signal Transducer and Activator of Transcription Pathway

The JAK-STAT pathway is a signaling pathway involved in development, immunity, and multiple other processes. Activation of the pathway begins with the extracellular binding of the unpaired ligand (Upd) to the Domeless receptor (Dome), which leads to the self-phosphorylation of JAKs (Hop) and the creation of binding sites on Dome. These sites induce dimerization of STATs, which then translocate to the nucleus and affect the expression of target genes.[24]

Although the JAK-STAT pathway has been studied predominately in *D. melanogaster*, *A. aegypti* possesses orthologs of key JAK-STAT pathway molecules that likely function in a similar manner.[21] The JAK-STAT pathway is intricately integrated into multiple pathways, and relatively few of the genes directly induced by JAK-STAT are involved directly in immunity,[25] suggesting that their contributions to immune responses are possibly indirect.[26] The JAK-STAT pathway, however, is activated during DENv infection in *A. aegypti*, as measured by the upregulation of pathway genes such as *Dome* and *Hop*, among others, in midguts and carcasses at 3 h, 18 h, and 7 dpi.[20,27] Inhibition of the pathway via RNAi silencing of either *Hop* or *Dome* resulted in increased midgut DENv titers in infected *A. aegypti* at 3 and 7 dpi, respectively.[25] Additionally, RNAi depletion of *PIAS*, a JAK-STAT inhibitor, led to decreased midgut titers. These effects were consistent across several *A. aegypti* strains and led to the identification of two putative anti-Dengue restriction factors (DVRFs) regulated by the JAK-STAT pathway.[25] While the JAK-STAT pathway is initiated during DENv infection, and DENv titers may be modulated, the virus is not eliminated.

RNA Interference

RNAi is considered the predominant antiviral immune response used by insects.[24] In contrast to classic extracellular signaling pathways, RNAi acts as an intracellular defense mechanism against foreign RNA. RNA viruses such as DENv form double stranded RNA (dsRNA) structures during replication, although dsRNA can also be generated via the creation of intrastrand secondary structures. Long dsRNA structures are recognized by Dicer proteins and are cleaved to generate small interfering RNAs (siRNAs) of 20–23 nucleotides.[28] These siRNAs occur in a relatively equal ratio of positive and negative sense strands, suggesting that Dicer-2 targets replicative dsRNA.[29] Once generated, these siRNAs are loaded onto the RNA-induced silencing complex (RISC) by the R2D2 protein and are then unwound. One siRNA strand is degraded via the RNAse activity of one of RISC's constitutive proteins, Argonaute-2, while the other is used to target complementary viral RNA for degradation.[24]

Specific siRNAs are generated in *A. aegypti* midguts during DENv infection, confirming that RNAi is activated.[29,30] Cells with nonfunctioning Dicer-2 are extremely susceptible to DENv,[29] and RNAi inhibition of key pathway genes such as *Dicer-2*, *Argonaute-2*, and *R2D2* leads to increased viral replication and a decreased EIP in infected mosquitoes.[30] However, RNAi does not eliminate DENv-2 completely, suggesting that DENv suppresses or evades RNAi in some manner. Indirect evidence suggests that West Nile virus has RNAi-suppressing properties within its subgenomic RNA, a property that might be conserved in other flaviviruses such as Dengue virus.[31] It should also be noted that the DENv-2 protein NS4B can suppress RNAi in mammalian and nonmosquito insect cell lines.[32] However, these responses have not been reported in DENv infections of *Aedes* sp. and thus remain conjecture.

The siRNA pathway is not the only pathway within mosquito cells that utilizes RNAi machinery. The micro RNA (miRNA) pathway uses RNAi to influence gene expression at the translational level.[28] Although miRNA levels are modified during and following DENv infection of *A. aegypti*, their role in infection dynamics is unclear. PIWI-interacting RNAs (piRNAs) are longer than siRNAs and are generated independently of Dicer-2.[28] They are generated in *A. aegypti* in response to DENv infection.[28] However, their potential role in antiviral defenses is also unclear.

Autophagy

Autophagy involves the creation of an autophagosome that encloses cellular components targeted for degradation, which then fuses with lysosomes in order to destroy the contents. Autophagy is used to recycle molecules, especially during times of nutritional starvation, and can destroy nonfunctioning entities such as damaged organelles and malfunctioning proteins. Numerous autophagy regulators and factors (ATG proteins) also coordinate with components of the innate immune response, such as Toll-like receptors, to target intracellular pathogens.[33] Under the regulation of the phosphatidylinositol 3-kinase-Akt pathway, autophagy is activated and prevents viral infection in *D. melanogaster*, while the inhibition of autophagy leads to increased viral replication.[34]

Some viruses manipulate the autophagy pathway to facilitate viral replication, and DENv relies on autophagy to replicate efficiently within mammalian cells. Autophagosomes generated during DENv infection target lipid droplets, leading to the release of stored triglycerides and energy generation via β-oxidation.[35] The proviral role of autophagy during DENv infection can be replicated in autophagy-deficient cells by adding exogenous fatty acids.[35] Although these processes have not been demonstrated in whole mosquitoes, a potential role of autophagy against Chikungunya virus in mosquito cells has been reported,[36] and as ATG proteins are conserved among metazoans, these processes also may occur in DENv-infected *A. aegypti*.

Apoptosis

Apoptosis is a highly regulated process responsible for the destruction of abnormal or infected cells. It can be triggered by intracellular signals such as DNA replication failure, DNA or mitochondrial damage, or a host of other catastrophic events including viral infection.[37] Virus replication causes large changes within the cell, many of which can trigger apoptosis at various stages of infection. Early apoptosis can eliminate infected cells before the virus can replicate and thus can be protective for the host. Apoptosis is carried out by a series of caspases; initiator caspases initiate apoptosis, while effector caspases are the executioners and work toward the organized degradation of cellular components.[37] Finally, the resulting cell fragments are recognized and removed by phagocytic cells.

Although much of our knowledge of apoptosis in the invertebrate immune response has been derived from studies with *D. melanogaster*, the apoptotic machinery is highly conserved in mosquitoes. Several studies have characterized caspases in *A. aegypti*, including the initiator caspases Dronc and Dredd.[38,39] Additionally, several studies have demonstrated that apoptotic genes are upregulated in DENv-infected cells in refractory, but not in susceptible mosquitoes, suggesting that apoptosis contributes to the refractory phenotype.[20,27,40,41] Furthermore, RNAi knockdown of the proapoptotic caspases, *dronc*, and *caspase-16*, in a refractory strain of *A. aegypti*, significantly increased susceptibility to DENv-2.[41] In general, apoptosis of virus-infected cells is detrimental to virus replication and represents an effective method of eliminating DENv-infected cells. Many viruses, however, encode factors that block or arrest host apoptotic machinery and thus avoid destruction,[37] while some viruses such as Sindbis virus appear to require some level of apoptosis for efficient dissemination in *A. aegypti*.[42] There is still much to be elucidated regarding the role of apoptosis in mosquito immune responses to DENv infection.

Interactions Among Pathways

DENv infection in mosquitoes activates the Toll, IMD, JAK-STAT, RNAi, autophagy, and apoptosis pathways through means that are not well understood. Although most studies have been conducted on individual pathways, it is apparent that the immune pathways do not act completely independently of one another. The interactions between pathways and the mechanisms driving these interactions are varied, complex, and largely uncharacterized.

Activation of the JAK-STAT pathway in the midguts of DENv-infected *A. aegypti* was linked to the downregulation of NF-kB-responsive genes and the transcriptional repression of several AMPs.[25] There is intriguing evidence that DENv may actively repress AMP production. DENv-infected *A. aegypti* cells produce lower levels of cecropin and defensin when challenged with either gram-positive or gram-negative bacteria than do uninfected cells,[43] suggesting that DENv can suppress both the Toll and IMD pathway antibacterial responses and that this repression is in some way beneficial to the virus. Why a virus would repress the antibacterial response of its host and make it susceptible to microbial infection is unclear.

The apoptosis and IMD signaling pathways also interact through a shared molecule, Fadd. As an upstream regulator of Rel2, Fadd is necessary for IMD function and the expression of cecropin and defensin during bacterial challenges.[44] Fadd also serves as an adapter required by the initiator caspase Dredd for apoptosis. Knockdown of *Fadd* stops *Dredd* activity and also renders the insect incapable of eliminating bacterial infections.[44] It is difficult to determine if a specific measured response has been induced directly by DENv or whether it is an indirect consequence of activating a shared molecule that then activates downstream events in multiple pathways. Teasing apart the timing and control of these responses is complex and challenging.

Dengue Virus in the Vector: Midgut Microbes

The makeup of an insect's midgut microbiome has variable effects on multiple physiological parameters including the innate immune system responses to pathogens[45] that ultimately determine the VC of mosquitoes to specific pathogens. Whereas some insects maintain obligate intestinal symbionts, the role and contribution of most microbes in the intestinal tracts of insects is unknown. There are, however, differences in the makeup and abundance of midgut microbial communities between strains of *A. aegypti* that are susceptible or refractory to DENv,[45] and eliminating midgut bacteria using antibiotics can reduce AMP expression and increase midgut DENv titers.[20] Additionally, specific strains of bacteria have been linked to an increased or decreased susceptibility to DENv.[46] How bacteria and viruses interact, and whether they compete directly in the midgut for resources or space or indirectly through immune system modulation, is unknown but has become an exciting area of current research.

Vector Competence: Refractory and Susceptible A. aegypti Phenotypes

Strains of *A. aegypti* differ in their susceptibility to DENv, producing high, medium, low, or zero DENv titers in the salivary glands. This is due, in part, to the immune responses and barriers described previously. This discrepancy in VC among strains is affected by interacting genetic loci, age, size, larval conditions, and environmental factors.[47,48] Undoubtedly, variation in immune responses also impacts VC directly. Understanding the physiological basis of VC will allow a greater understanding of innate immune responses and might identify targets for novel control measures. These complex interactions between DENv and *A. aegypti* also may be affected by specific genotype-by-genotype interactions[49] and influenced by genetic–environmental interactions that combine to contribute to the VC.[48]

Refractory A. aegypti

Laboratory strains of *A. aegypti* have been selected specifically to generate DENv-refractory phenotypes. The Moyo-S and Moyo-R strains, selected from the original Moyo-D strain, are 53.60% and 19% susceptible to DENv-2, respectively.[27] These two strains differ significantly in expression levels of several immune-related genes when exposed to DENv-2.[50] Compared with the MOYO-S strain, MOYO-R mosquitoes demonstrated an elevated expression of genes related to the JAK-STAT and apoptotic pathways,[27] suggesting that the refractory phenotype was related to the expression of specific immune related genes.

A separate laboratory selection process generated the *A. aegypti* D2S3 strain that features a weak MIB and MEB, thus generating high midgut infection and dissemination rates.[51] Subsequently, a D2MEB strain was selected with a weak MIB and a strong MEB, proving that these phenotypes could be selected and manipulated independently.[51] These strains were crossed, and the progeny were mapped to identify quantitative trait loci that contribute to the phenotype, as has been done for the MIB in other *A. aegypti* strains.[47] The gene expression patterns of all these strains have been compared.[50] Although mosquito strains respond to infection differently, there seems to be a core set of genes that undergo a similar expression change in refractory and susceptible mosquitoes that may be required for DENv development.

The studies cited above represent long-established laboratory strains used to select specific phenotypes. There are, however, feral strains of *A. aegypti* that are naturally refractory to DENv. In Cali, Colombia, approximately 30% of feral *A. aegypti* are refractory to DENv.[40,52] Subsequent analysis and selection identified both MIB and MEB factors in the feral populations[40,53] and differential gene expression in the midguts and carcasses of these different phenotypes.[40,41] Both anti- and proapoptotic genes were activated in both strains, suggesting that the phenotype may be a result of competing pro- and antiapoptotic responses, as well as manipulation of host apoptosis factors by DENv to facilitate viral dissemination. Many differentially expressed genes were identified and characterized and subsequently assigned to an immune function. Nonimmune-related genes, including a trypsin inhibitor gene, were differentially expressed in the MIB strain.[40] Trypsin inhibition has been shown to reduce both DENv titers and dissemination rates[12] and, as such, trypsin may represent a nonimmune-related contributor to the refractory phenotype.

The expression levels of selected apoptosis-related genes (Caspase-16, dronc, dredd, and inhibitor of apoptosis (IAP1)) and one RNAi-related gene (Argonaut-2) were compared in the midguts and fat body tissues of Cali-S (susceptible), Cali-MIB, and Cali-MEB 12–48h after an initial dengue infection.[41,53] The proapoptotic caspases, dronc, dredd, and Caspase-16, were upregulated in midgut tissues 24–48h postinfection in the Cali-MIB strain. The authors proposed that upon infection, infected mosquito cells initiated apoptosis, but DENv subsequently induced the expression of IAP1 to stop apoptosis. In the Cali-S strain, IAP1 prevented apoptosis whereas in the Cali-MIB strain the overexpression of proapoptotic caspases could not be regulated by low levels of IAP1. Knocking down dronc and Caspase-16 in the Cali-MIB strain using RNAi increased the proportion of Cali-MIB mosquitoes that was susceptible to DENv-2. Although these studies demonstrate that apoptosis contributes to the refractory phenotype, it is clear that there are other, yet unidentified, factors that also contribute to this phenotype.[41]

Feral Cali-S, Cali-MIB, and Cali-MEB strains were selected to generate phenotypically consistent strains. While the Cali-S strain became 99% susceptible, the prevalence of the refractory individuals never exceeded 50% in the Cali-MIB or Cali-MEB strains.[53] Refractory mosquitoes were slightly smaller, had a slightly reduced life span, and produced slightly fewer eggs than Cali-S. It is generally assumed that trade-offs will evolve when the cost of having a pathogen exceeds the costs of eliminating the pathogen. The effects of DENv on *Aedes* spp. are not universal; several studies have indicated no detrimental effects,[11] while others have demonstrated a shorter life span, reduced fecundity, increased locomotion, and lower feeding efficiencies,[54] but DENv-2 infection appears to present no significant or measurable costs to Cali-S mosquitoes. It is unclear from an evolutionary perspective why a Cali-MIB phenotype would evolve and be maintained if there is a trade-off with overall fitness in the refractory phenotype, especially when no observable fitness effects seem to exist in Cali-S mosquitoes in the presence or absence of DENv.[53]

MITIGATING DENGUE: CONTROL MEASURES

DF represents an enormous economic cost to endemic areas and countries. Accordingly, there are many efforts underway to curb the spread of both DENv and its mosquito vectors, including vaccine development and vector control using insecticides, sterile insect techniques, and the release of insects carrying a dominant lethal strategy.

Other ecologically stable approaches have focused on reducing VC for DENv rather than eliminating the vector itself. Population replacement by mosquitoes that are refractory to DENv would reduce the VC of the population and reduce transmission. One such approach uses bacterial symbionts to reduce longevity and VC of *A. aegypti* that acts through interactions with the immune system of the vectors. The intracellular bacterium *Wolbachia pipientis* is a natural endosymbiont of arthropods that induces cytoplasmic incompatibility and is transmitted vertically from mother to progeny, resulting in very fast rates of infection of entire populations.[55] In fact, *W. pipientis* manipulates the gene expression, including miRNAs, of its *A. aegypti* hosts to facilitate the establishment and colonization of the bacterium.[56] Different strains of *W. pipientis* shorten mosquito life spans, which ultimately should reduce DENv transmission[57] or reduce DENv replication in *A. aegypti*, thus reducing VC.[58] *Wolbachia*-mediated protection against DENv appears to be density dependant, as higher *W. pipientis* infections provide greater resistance.[55] The exact means by which *W. pipientis* reduces the life span of *A. aegypti* and reduces DENv replication is not well understood but appears to be mediated through components of the immune system and gene regulation.[55] Current field trials of *W. pipientis*-infected mosquitoes will provide data on the ability to use such paratransgenic mosquitoes to reduce or eliminate DENv transmission.

CONCLUSION

The interactions between Dengue viruses, humans, and their principal vector, *A. aegypti,* are complex and intricate. There is substantial variation in VC between strains of virus and vector, based on genetic compatibility and environmental factors. Dengue and other arboviruses represent a huge burden on global society and affect billions of people. The interplay between vector and virus, especially regarding how mosquito vectors recognize DENv, antiviral immune mechanisms used by the vectors, as well as strategies used by DENv to circumvent vector immune responses determine VC. It is becoming increasingly clear that the innate immune system of insects acts in a directed manner to specific types of pathogens rather than a general overall response to all infections. Multiple immune pathways work in concert rather than in isolation to eliminate pathogens. Our detailed understanding of DENv-vector interactions is a relatively new, but rapidly evolving, field of research that is expanding from molecular interactions between vector and virus to understanding the effects of climate change on vector-virus-human interactions. Until an effective tetravalent vaccine is available worldwide, species specific, immune-related, vector control strategies to limit DENv development or to reduce the VC of feral vectors will continue to rely on an in-depth knowledge and understanding of the innate immune responses in these vectors.

REFERENCES

1. Messina JP, Brady OJ, Pigott DM, Golding N, Kraemer MUG, Scott TW, et al. The many projected futures of dengue. *Nat Rev Microbiol* 2015;**13**:230–9.
2. Srikiatkhachorn A. Plasma leakage in dengue haemorrhagic fever. *Thromb Haemost* 2009;**102**:1042–9.
3. Guzman MG, Alvarez M, Halstead SB. Secondary infection as a risk factor for dengue hemorrhagic fever/dengue shock syndrome: an historical perspective and role of antibody-dependent enhancement of infection. *Arch Virol* 2013;**158**:1445–59.
4. Whitehead SS, Blaney JE, Durbin AP, Murphy BR. Prospects for a dengue virus vaccine. *Nat Rev Microbiol* 2007;**5**:518–28.
5. Thomas SJ. Developing a dengue vaccine: progress and future challenges. *Ann NY Acad Sci* 2014;**1323**:140–59.
6. David MR, Lourenço-de-Oliveira R, de Freitas RM. Container productivity, daily survival rates and dispersal of *Aedes aegypti* mosquitoes in a high income dengue epidemic neighbourhood of Rio de Janeiro: presumed influence of differential urban structure on mosquito biology. *Mem Inst Oswaldo Cruz* 2009;**104**:927–32.
7. Salazar MI, Richardson JH, Sánchez-Vargas I, Olson KE, Beaty BJ. Dengue virus type 2: replication and tropisms in orally infected *Aedes aegypti* mosquitoes. *BMC Microbiol* 2007;**7**:9.
8. Sim S, Jupatanakul N, Dimopoulos G. Mosquito immunity against arboviruses. *Viruses* 2014;**6**:4479–504.
9. Black WC, Bennett KE, Gorrochótegui-escalante N, Barillas-mury CV, Fernández-salas I, Muñoz DL, et al. Flavivirus susceptibility in *Aedes aegypti*. *Arch Med Res* 2002;**33**:379–88.
10. Sim S, Jupatanakul N, Ramirez JL, Kang S, Romero-Vivas CM, Mohammed H, et al. Transcriptomic profiling of diverse *Aedes aegypti* strains reveals increased basal-level immune activation in dengue virus-refractory populations and identifies novel virus-vector molecular interactions. *PLoS NTD* 2013;**7**:e2295.
11. Sim S, Ramirez JL, Dimopoulos G. Dengue virus infection of the *Aedes aegypti* salivary gland and chemosensory apparatus induces genes that modulate infection and blood-feeding behavior. *PLoS Pathog* 2012;**8**.

12. Molina-Cruz A, Gupta L, Richardson J, Bennett KF, Black W, Barillas-Mury C. Effect of mosquito midgut trypsin activity on dengue-2 virus infection and dissemination in *Aedes aegypti*. *Am J Trop Med Hyg* 2005;**72**:631–7.
13. Medzhitov R, Janeway CA. Innate immunity: impact on the adaptive immune response. *Curr Opin Immunol* 1997;**9**:4–9.
14. Tsakas S, Marmaras V. Insect immunity and its signalling: an overview. *Invert Surv J* 2010: 228–38.
15. Christensen BM, Li J, Chen C-C, Nappi AJ. Melanization immune responses in mosquito vectors. *Trends Parasitol* 2005;**21**:192–9.
16. Lemaitre B, Hoffmann J. The host defense of *Drosophila melanogaster*. *Annu Rev Immunol* 2007;**25**:697–743.
17. Bulet P, Hetru C, Dimarcq JL, Hoffmann D. Antimicrobial peptides in insects; structure and function. *Dev Comp Immunol* 1999;**23**:329–44.
18. Lowenberger C. Innate immune response of *Aedes aegypti*. *Insect Biochem Mol Biol* 2001;**31**:219–29.
19. Ursic-Bedoya R, Buchhop J, Joy JB, Durvasula R, Lowenberger C. Prolixicin: a novel antimicrobial peptide isolated from *Rhodnius prolixus* with differential activity against bacteria and *Trypanosoma cruzi*. *Insect Mol Biol* 2011;**20**:775–86.
20. Xi Z, Ramirez JL, Dimopoulos G. The *Aedes aegypti* toll pathway controls dengue virus infection. *PLoS Pathog* 2008;**4**:e1000098.
21. Waterhouse RM, Kriventseva EV, Meister S, Xi Z, Alvarez KS, Bartholomay LC, et al. Evolutionary dynamics of immune-related genes and pathways in disease-vector mosquitoes. *Science* 2007;**316**:1738–43.
22. Ramirez JL, Dimopoulos G. The Toll immune signaling pathway control conserved anti-dengue defenses across diverse *Ae. aegypti* strains and against multiple dengue virus serotypes. *Dev Comp Immunol* 2010;**34**:625–9.
23. Costa A, Jan E, Sarnow P, Schneider D. The Imd pathway is involved in antiviral immune responses in Drosophila. *PLoS One* 2009;**4**:e7436.
24. Kingsolver MB, Huang Z, Hardy RW. Insect antiviral innate immunity: pathways, effectors, and connections. *J Mol Biol* 2013;**425**:4921–36.
25. Souza-Neto J, Sim S, Dimopoulos G. An evolutionary conserved function of the JAK-STAT pathway in anti-dengue defense. *Proc Natl Acad Sci USA* 2009;**106**:17841–6.
26. Dostert C, Jouanguy E, Irving P, Troxler L, Galiana-Arnoux D, Hetru C, et al. The Jak-STAT signaling pathway is required but not sufficient for the antiviral response of drosophila. *Nat Immunol* 2005;**6**:946–53.
27. Behura SK, Gomez-Machorro C, Harker BW, deBruyn B, Lovin DD, Hemme RR, et al. Global cross-talk of genes of the mosquito *Aedes aegypti* in response to dengue virus infection. *PLoS NTD* 2011;**5**:e1385.
28. Blair CD, Olson KE. The role of RNA interference (RNAi) in arbovirus-vector interactions. *Viruses* 2015;**7**:820–43.
29. Scott JC, Brackney DE, Campbell CL, Bondu-Hawkins V, Hjelle B, Ebel GD, et al. Comparison of dengue virus type 2-specific small RNAs from RNA interference-competent and -incompetent mosquito cells. *PLoS NTD* 2010;**4**:e848.
30. Sánchez-Vargas I, Scott JC, Poole-Smith BK, Franz AWE, Barbosa-Solomieu V, Wilusz J, et al. Dengue virus type 2 infections of *Aedes aegypti* are modulated by the mosquito's RNA interference pathway. *PLoS Pathog* 2009;**5**:e1000299.
31. Schnettler E, Sterken MG, Leung JY, Metz SW, Geertsema C, Goldbach RW, et al. Noncoding flavivirus RNA displays RNA interference suppressor activity in insect and mammalian cells. *J Virol* 2012;**86**:13486–500.

32. Kakumani PK, Ponia SS, Rajgokul SK, Sood V, Chinnappan M, Banerjea AC, et al. Role of RNA interference (RNAi) in dengue virus replication and identification of NS4B as an RNAi suppressor. *J Virol* 2013;**87**:8870–83.

33. Nakamoto M, Moy RH, Xu J, Bambina S, Yasunaga A, Shelly SS, et al. Virus recognition by Toll-7 activates antiviral autophagy in Drosophila. *Immunity* 2012;**36**:658–67.

34. Shelly S, Lukinova N, Bambina S, Berman A, Cherry S. Autophagy is an essential component of Drosophila immunity against vesicular stomatitis virus. *Immunity* 2009;**30**:588–98.

35. Heaton NS, Randall G. Dengue virus-induced autophagy regulates lipid metabolism. *Cell Host Microbe* 2010;**8**:422–32.

36. Raquin V, Moro CV, Bernardin C, Tran F-H, Van VT, Potier P, et al. Potential role of autophagy during Wolbachia antiviral interference against chikungunya virus in mosquito cells. *Conference Proccedings, 5th European Congress of Virology, Lyon, France* 2013.

37. Clarke TE, Clem RJ. Insect defenses against virus infection: the role of apoptosis. *Int J Mol Sci* 2003;**22**:401–24.

38. Cooper DM, Pio F, Thi EP, Theilmann D, Lowenberger C. Characterization of Aedes Dredd: a novel initiator caspase from the yellow fever mosquito, *Aedes aegypti*. *Insect Biochem Mol Biol* 2007;**37**:559–69.

39. Cooper DM, Thi EP, Chamberlain CM, Pio F, Lowenberger C. Aedes Dronc: a novel ecdysone-inducible caspase in the yellow fever mosquito, *Aedes aegypti*. *Insect Mol Biol* 2007;**16**:563–72.

40. Barón OL, Ursic-Bedoya RJ, Lowenberger CA, Ocampo CB. Differential gene expression from midguts of refractory and susceptible lines of the mosquito, *Aedes aegypti*, infected with Dengue-2 virus. *J Insect Sci (Online)* 2010;**10**:41.

41. Ocampo CB, Caicedo PA, Jaramillo G, Ursic Bedoya R, Baron O, Serrato IM, et al. Differential expression of apoptosis related genes in selected strains of *Aedes aegypti* with different susceptibilities to dengue virus. *PLoS One* 2013;**8**:e61187.

42. Wang H, Gort T, Boyle DL, Clem RJ. Effects of manipulating apoptosis on sindbis virus infection of *Aedes aegypti* mosquitoes. *J Virol* 2012;**86**:6546–54.

43. Sim S, Dimopoulos G. Dengue virus inhibits immune responses in *Aedes aegypti* cells. *PLoS One* 2010;**5**:e10678.

44. Cooper DM, Chamberlain CM, Lowenberger C. Aedes FADD: a novel death domain-containing protein required for antibacterial immunity in the yellow fever mosquito, *Aedes aegypti*. *Insect Biochem Mol Biol* 2009;**39**:47–54.

45. Charan SS, Pawar KD, Severson DW, Patole MS, Shouche YS. Comparative analysis of midgut bacterial communities of *Aedes aegypti* mosquito strains varying in vector competence to dengue virus. *Parasitol Res* 2013;**112**:2627–37.

46. Ramirez JL, Souza-Neto J, Torres Cosme R, Rovira J, Ortiz A, Pascale JM, et al. Reciprocal tripartite interactions between the *Aedes aegypti* midgut microbiota, innate immune system and dengue virus influences vector competence. *PLoS NTD* 2012;**6**:e1561.

47. Bosio CF, Fulton RE, Salasek ML, Beaty BJ, Black WC. Quantitative trait loci that control vector competence for dengue-2 virus in the mosquito *Aedes aegypti*. *Genetics* 2000;**156**:687–98.

48. Schneider JR, Chadee DD, Mori A, Romero-Severson J, Severson DW. Heritability and adaptive phenotypic plasticity of adult body size in the mosquito *Aedes aegypti* with implications for dengue vector competence. *Infect Genet Evol* 2011;**11**:11–6.

49. Lambrechts L. Quantitative genetics of *Aedes aegypti* vector competence for dengue viruses: towards a new paradigm? *Trends Parasitol* 2011;**27**:111–4.

50. Chauhan C, Behura SK, Debruyn B, Lovin DD, Harker BW, Gomez-Machorro C, et al. Comparative expression profiles of midgut genes in dengue virus refractory and susceptible *Aedes aegypti* across critical period for virus infection. *PLoS One* 2012;**7**:e47350.

51. Bennett KE, Beaty BJ, Black WC. Selection of D2S3, an *Aedes aegypti* (Diptera: Culicidae) strain with high oral susceptibility to Dengue 2 virus and D2MEB, a strain with a midgut barrier to Dengue 2 escape. *J Med Entomol* 2005;**42**:110–9.

52. Ocampo CB, Wesson DM. Population dynamics of *Aedes aegypti* from a dengue hyperendemic urban setting in Colombia. *Am J Trop Med Hyg* 2004;**71**:506–13.

53. Caicedo P, Barón OL, Pérez M, Alexander N, Lowenberger C, Ocampo CB. Selection of *Aedes aegypti* (Diptera: Culicidae) strains that are susceptible or refractory to Dengue-2 virus. *Can Entomol* 2013;**145**:273–82.

54. Maciel-de-Freitas R, Koella JC, Lourenço-de-Oliveira R. Lower survival rate, longevity and fecundity of *Aedes aegypti* (Diptera: Culicidae) females orally challenged with dengue virus serotype 2. *Trans R Soc Trop Med Hyg* 2011;**105**:452–8.

55. Rainey SM, Shah P, Kohl A, Dietrich I. Understanding the Wolbachia-mediated inhibition of arboviruses in mosquitoes: progress and challenges. *J Gen Virol* 2014;**95**:517–30.

56. Hussain M, Frentiu FD, Moreira LA, O'Neill SL, Asgari S. Wolbachia uses host microRNAs to manipulate host gene expression and facilitate colonization of the dengue vector *Aedes aegypti*. *Proc Natl Acad Sci USA* 2011;**108**:9250–5.

57. McMeniman C, Lana R, Cass B, Fong A, Sidhu M, Wang Y-F, et al. Stable introduction of a life-shortening Wolbachia infection into the mosquito *Aedes aegypti*. *Science* 2009;**323**:141–4.

58. Sinkins SP. Wolbachia and arbovirus inhibition in mosquitoes. *Fut Microbiol* 2013;**8**:1249–56.

Chapter 11

Protective Responses in Invertebrates

Magda de Eguileor, Annalisa Grimaldi, Gianluca Tettamanti
University of Insubria, Varese, Italy

BACKGROUND

Foreign molecules from bacteria (lipopolysaccharide (LPS)) and fungi phorbol 12-myristate 13-acetate (PMA), parasites, and chemical toxins are omnipresent in the environment and are in close contact with organisms threatening their fitness. Invertebrates and vertebrates, even if constantly exposed, are able to protect themselves and live successfully because of their ability to distinguish self from nonself, danger from nondanger, and to activate protective responses, timely and intensively modulated.

All the different types of interactions mentioned before can be responsible for serious, eventually strong and lasting, stress stimuli perturbing the extremely complicated internal equilibrium that is the *conditio sine qua non* required for survival.

The broad spectrum of stressful stimuli is capable of inducing an extraordinary amount of protective responses, often resulting from a mix of interconnected immune and neuroendocrine processes conserved and enhanced during evolution.

When external intruders enter the organisms, breaking their physical protective barriers, multiple and complex humoral and cellular defense reactions, controlled by soluble molecules and different types of cells moving freely in the body cavities, in the circulating fluid, or migrating in the connective tissue are activated.

MEDIATORS OF IMMUNE RESPONSES

The "oldest" innate immunity, involved in rapid and nonspecific events, is a shared character of both vertebrates and invertebrates, which elicits sophisticated immune and neuroendocrine responses. Innate immunity is responsible for discriminating between self and nonself using sensors represented by the pattern-recognition receptors (PRRs) that detect conserved pathogen-associated molecular patterns (PAMPs) present in microbes or linked to cellular stress as well as danger-associated molecular pattern molecules (DAMPs) associated to cell endogenous damage that constitute a danger signal alerting the immune system. Among the innate receptors able to detect microbial products or extracellular and endosomal molecules, there are the Toll-like receptors (TLRs) (the most important group), retinoic acid-inducible gene I [RIG-I]-like receptors (RLRs), AIM2-like receptors (ARLs), and NACH-leucine-rich repeat receptors (NLRs). The molecular sensors, once recognized by the foreign presences, initiate signal transduction pathways playing as activators of a plethora of intracellular signaling cascades, involving immune adaptors that can work as regulators, intracellular kinases, and transcription factors, inducing the expression of genes involved in inflammatory responses.[1–3]

An extensive literature has been produced clarifying not only every single mechanism but also the intermingled actions involved in invertebrate innate immunity.

Some representative examples: in *Drosophila* hemocytes, the innate immune recognition of microorganisms is mediated by signaling through TLRs that are also present in mammalian immune cells.[4,5] Peptidoglycan recognition proteins (PGRPs) are able to recognize the peptidoglycan, one of the major components of the bacteria cell wall. PGRPs are well conserved in invertebrates such as molluscs, insects, echinoderms, and mammals, even if they have acquired different functions in invertebrates and vertebrates.[6] The mosquito *Anopheles gambiae* secretes a thioester-containing protein (TEP), aTEP1 with an antiparasitic effect, which is related to vertebrate complement factors and a_2-macroglobulins.[7]

Intriguingly, abiotic material can also be recognized by invertebrate immunocytes, suggesting that these cells are able to detect a wide range of alien molecules due to the presence of receptors with promiscuous capacities.[8]

The detection of PAMPs as well as DAMPs by mediators of innate immunity regulates multiple immune responses. For instance, activated macrophages secrete cytokines, a class of phylogenetically ancient immunomodulatory molecules that communicate via cell receptors to induce specific cell activities. Molecules like interleukin (IL)-1 and IL-8, TNF-like molecules, transforming growth factor-β (TGF-β), etc. mediate and finely regulate several regeneration processes, such as angiogenesis or fibroplasia, in protostomes (such as annelids, molluscs, arthropods) and in deuterostomes (such as echinoderms and urochordates)[9] and can be considered functional analogues of mammalian inflammatory cytokines. It is important to emphasize that the functional similarities between invertebrate cytokines and their vertebrate counterparts can be due to molecular convergence related to structural similarity of the lectin-like recognition domain rather than a true homology.[10,11] In addition, cytokines released by cells involved in the innate activity can influence the responses of adaptive immunity. Among the soluble mediators, there are initiators of the complement system that, despite the lack of specificity, selectively recognize foreign pathogens and damaged self-cells, using the recognition molecules of classic and alternative pathways.

Lectins produced by different types of activated cells of invertebrates are localized on the cell surface, functioning as primitive recognition molecules detecting and binding carbohydrates. Intracellular lectins are present in invertebrates and vertebrates but with various functions in different groups of animals. In invertebrates, their ability to opsonize and agglutinate foreign cells supplies the phagocytosis or encapsulation of invaders.[12] The fight against nonself in invertebrates such as annelids, molluscs, arthropods, and urochordates is also sustained by numerous antimicrobial peptides (AMPs) that can be present constitutively in the organisms, synthesized ex novo after nonself contact, or transported by mobile cells into the area of invasion.[13–15] This large group of AMPs (about 900) comprises molecules that are quite different, but all of them share clusters of hydrophobic and cationic amino acids that allow (1) the attachment to negatively charged bacterial membranes; (2) the integration with the cell membrane to form pores; and (3) the destruction of plasma membrane.[16]

DEGREE OF INTERCELLULAR REACTIVE OXYGEN SPECIES LEVELS AND IMMUNE RESPONSES

The killing of pathogens involves oxygen-dependent mechanisms. Reactive oxygen species (ROS) are produced by all metazoan, from invertebrates up to man. ROS include hydrogen peroxide (H_2O_2), nitric oxide (NO), superoxide anion $(O_2 \cdot)$, hydrochlorous acid (HOCl), and hydroxyl radical (OH$\cdot$). If ROS signal intensity, site of production, and chemical identity are tightly controlled, ROS serve as signaling molecules to coordinate a wide range of processes. Sponges produce superoxide as an agent to fight bacteria.[17] Molluscs and arthropod hemocytes produce superoxide in response to specific stimulators[18] during immune responses.[19–22] The increased formation of ROS can also be linked to the presence of abiotic stressors.

Even if the involvement of ROS can play important protective roles during organism immunity or wound processes or in regulating, by temporal and spatial coordination, many biological events, its overproduction can generate a chronic oxidative stress that leads to the damage of cell components (proteins/lipids/nucleic acids). Detrimental ROS, produced in the intracellular compartments, generate protective responses such as upregulation of antioxidants, superoxide dismutase, catalase, glutathione peroxidase, and glutathione that convert dangerous free radicals to harmless molecules (ie, water), autophagy, adrenocorticotropin hormone (ACTH)/alpha MSH loop activation, and synthesis of melanin.[23]

PROPHENOL OXIDASE SYSTEM ACTIVATION

Among the various potent weapons typical of an innate defense, there is the prophenol oxidase (pro-PO) system activation.[24–31] The pro-PO system is active in many invertebrates,[32–34] and independently from their phylogenetic position, animals produce melanin both in body fluids and/or in cells, and its biosynthesis is due to the activation of the pro-PO system. The pro-PO system is well known in the crayfish *Pacifasticus leniusculus*,[24] the silkworm *Bombyx mori*,[25,35] the fly *Drosophila melanogaster*,[27,28] echinoderms such as *Holoturia tubulosa*,[26] ascidians,[30,31,33] and cephalochordates.[29] Melanization is a widespread immune response fundamental in isolating and inactivating any type of nonself at the injury site and/or on the surface of foreign invaders. The biosynthesis of the melanin and the precursors of pigment are essential in those invertebrates where invaders such as parasites or fungi are rapidly isolated and sequestered in capsules formed by pigment and circulating cells.[30,31,36–40]

In relation to invasions of pathogens or any kind of stressors in sea fan corals (cnidarians), a localized melanization in the tissues is due to amoebocyte melanosome and pro-PO activities.[41,42] In oligochaets and polychaets (annelids), there is an efficient activation of the pro-PO cascade in coelomic fluid and in a subpopulation of granulocytes.[43–48] In molluscs, melanization is reported as a humoral and cellular response.[49–51] In arthropods,[4,24,25,52,53] melanin is derived from humoral and cellular activity. In deuterostomes, such as echinoderms (sea urchin, holoturians)[54] and tunicates (sea squirts),[30,31,55–57] morula cells are able to recognize foreign molecules and release phenol oxidase (PO), which induces melanin formation.[31,56,58]

CELLULAR RESPONSES

Animal immune systems react to the presence of foreign antigens with the production of a large amount of molecules, synergistically sustained by the action of a wide variety of cellular responses. Activated cells can combat intruders in different ways in relation to the size of the nonself and according to the adopted repertoire. Agglutination, phagocytosis, nodulation, and encapsulation can occur. Phagocytosis, the cell's ability to engulf foreign material, is a nonspecific event having the ultimate function of freeing organisms from unwanted, eventually pathogenic agents.[44,59–65] Phagocytosis is a performance of the activated circulating immune cells that are considered the main effectors of the invertebrate defense system showing the functional characteristics of vertebrate macrophages. These typology of cells in invertebrates are variously named: amoebocytes (in animals without the coelom), hemocytes, and coelomocytes (in animals that have the coelom along with a vascular system), plasmatocytes, and macrophage-like cells (involved in the ingestion or encapsulation of pathogens as well as in the removal of apoptotic cells, etc.[66]). The general term of phagocytes can be used to describe these cells that are performing the same immune functions and possessing very similar morphology.

In invertebrate immunocytes, all signal transduction pathways that modulate phagocytosis are complex and well-conserved events: at the plasma membrane level, TLRs trigger phagocytosis and the production of agents toxic to the phagocytosed nonself. The last phase, characterized by the formation of phagosomes, and subsequent lysosomal fusion, also promotes killing.

Encapsulation, a different type of response, is utilized by all invertebrates when the foreign antigen is too cumbersome to be phagocytosed.[32,44,65,67] For instance, in insects,[68] encapsulation is considered an efficient system for immobilizing parasites, fungi, and large protozoans that escape the phagocytic activity of the single immunocyte. The event that can be followed by melanization is very efficient against living organisms while it is weak against abiotic material. A multicellular sheath made of granular cells and plasmatocytes surrounds the encapsulated material. The first event is the contact of the immunocytes with foreign material followed by degranulation. The material released from granules adheres to foreign surfaces and activates the plasmatocytes that participate, as main actors, in the formation of the capsule. Insects are a good model for studying elaborated intermingled series of events leading to encapsulation. In *Drosophila*, injuries evoke a response that consists of the release of clotting factors stored in hemocyte granules and in cellular aggregation. Plasma coagulation is followed by the formation of cellular capsules surrounding the foreign bodies (eggs of parasites deposited in the host body cavity) while PO is involved in the clotting as well as the encapsulation of pathogens.

EMERGING CONCEPTS ABOUT NEW PLAYERS INVOLVED IN PROTECTIVE RESPONSES

Above, we have proposed a summary of the events characterizing protective responses of cells, tissues, or organisms since there is an abundance of data describing the modulated responses activated according to the cellular needs, the type of tissue/organ, the specific lifetime, or developmental stage. In this section, we will focus on emerging concepts regarding several solutions that cells, tissues, or organisms can set up during the first phase of immune response as well as in recognition of danger signals. A new player involved in different protective responses is "functional amyloidogenesis." Even if amyloid fibril production is generally interpreted as a sign of diseases, growing evidences suggest that their synthesis contributes to normal physiology, accomplishing various important functions.[69–71] Amyloidogenesis is not only involved in pigment synthesis and in capsule formation but also in salvific processes.[70,71] Even if the encapsulation event is well known, there is a phase of the process that is still neglected. We have demonstrated that induced melanization/encapsulation against nonself, studied in the insect host/parasitoid model (*Heliothis virescens/Toxoneuron nigriceps*),[70–73] is based on the synthesis of the pigment that occurs, as in vertebrates. Fowler and coworkers[74] suggested that melanin is packaged in vertebrate melanocytes due to the production of large amounts of amyloid fibrils. Invertebrates share with vertebrates these linked events: amyloid fibrils template and accelerate the formation of pigment. Both in vertebrate and invertebrate, melanogenesis and amyloid fibril formation are physiologically associated,[70,71,73,74] and the cross-beta sheet structure of amyloid fibrils is always necessary for providing a template for melanin deposition.

We showed, in parasitized insects, that the amyloid fibrils promote the polymerization of toxic quinone precursors and melanin deposition around the encapsulated target, suggesting a role for fibrils in coordinating humoral and cellular defense responses (Fig. 11.1). The key differences in insects with respect to vertebrates is that, while in vertebrates melanin and amyloid fibrils are produced in organules of the same cell,[74] in insects, the two processes are disjoined. Even if a modest production of melanin is also visible in the cytoplasm of hemocytes, melanization largely occurs in the hemocoel in which the exocytosed amyloid fibrils package the large amount of pigment resulting from the humoral pro-PO system[72,75] (Fig. 11.1). PO is the enzyme for the massive melanin synthesis that occurs around the nonself invader which is, at least physically, isolated within a rigid capsule (Fig. 11.1). The confined pro-PO system

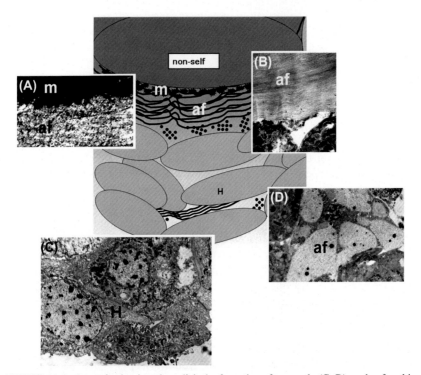

FIGURE 11.1 Large foreign intruders elicit the formation of a capsule (C, D) made of multi-layered hemocytes (H) that degranulate due to the nonself recognition. The surface of the nonself (A, B) is coated by a layer of amyloid fibrils (af) that act as a molecular scaffold templating the deposition of melanin (m). The af interspersed among the hemocytes (D) "glue" the cell layers and package any pigment precursors to avoid diffuse melanin biosynthesis.

action (ie, melanin synthesis) close to the nonself invader presumably avoids systemic melanization and may be attributable to the large amount of amyloid fibrils discharged from granulocytes. Thus these fibrils may have a dual function: to enable pigment polymerization and, because of their intrinsic adhesiveness,[76,77] to "fix" the pigment to the nonself surface (Fig. 11.1).

In several invertebrates, as previously described for insects, melanin is massively produced in the body cavity, especially as a pro-PO system product, while amyloid fibrils are due to exocytosis of circulating cells (named granulocytes or amoebocytes) that are able to produce a huge amount of amyloid fibrils that adhere to the nonself, driving the pigment accumulation close to the invaders[70–73] (Fig. 11.2).

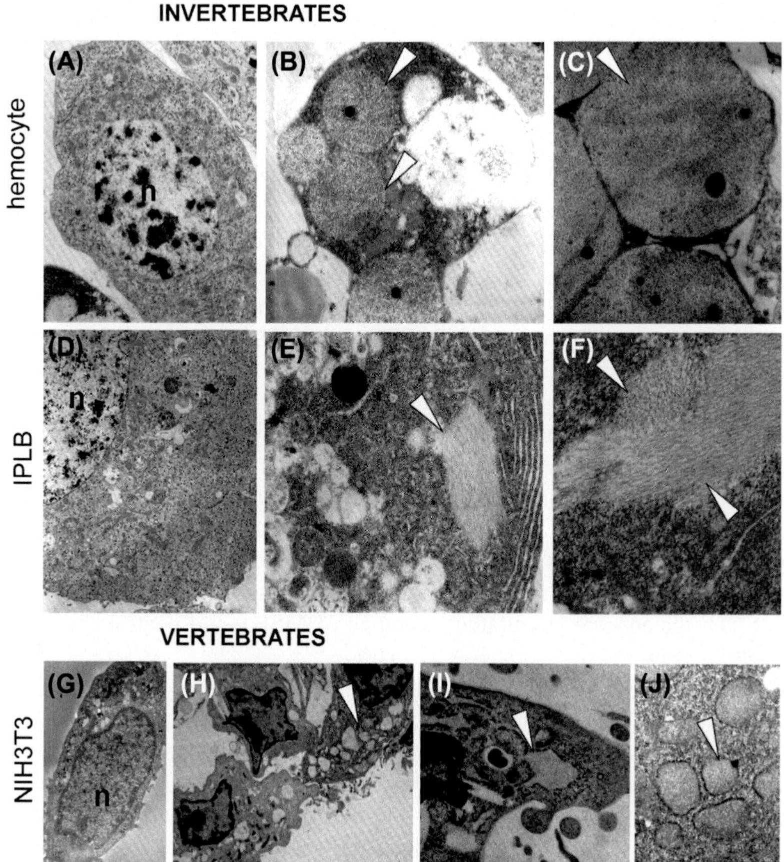

FIGURE 11.2 Thin sections of unstimulated and activated cells from invertebrates (insects: hemocytes and IPLB-LdF, cell line derived from the fat body of *Lymanthria dispar*) and vertebrates (mouse: embryonic fibroblast cells) (A–J) showing that, at a short time from nonself recognition (lipopolysaccharide incubation), significant morphological changes at the cytoplasmic level occur. Activated cells (B, C, E, F, H–J) lose the shape typical of control (A, D, G) and acquire irregular profiles. These cells exhibit the presence of dilated reticulum cisternae filled with fibrillar material (*arrowheads*).

In other invertebrates, as well as in vertebrates, there is a coupled productive system (melanin/amyloid fibrils) concentrated in a specific cell type, where melanin on amyloid fibrils is stocked in organules. Summarizing, it is interesting to highlight that melanin synthesis is always coupled, from invertebrates up to man, with a physiological production of amyloid fibrils. The trade-off in utilizing the coupled system amyloid/melanin may shift from the possibility of having two separated producers (a humoral pro-PO system for melanin and granulocytes for amyloid fibrils), as recorded in insects, echinoderms, and ascidians, with the following assemblage of the two products, up to a single cellular producer of both products (pigment and amyloid fibrils) as in coelenterates, annelids, molluscs, and vertebrates. An additional striking aspect refers to the cells involved in amyloid/melanin synthesis. These cells, belonging to freely circulating hemocytes, show the same phenotype with a nucleus localized in the central position, surrounded by large reticulum cisternae filled with fibrillar material, spatially organized in respect to a central electron-dense core.[23]

The processes involved in amyloid fibrils/melanin synthesis in phylogenetically distant animals (viz., cnidaria, molluscs, annelids, insects, ascidians, and vertebrates) can be interpreted as evolutionarily conserved. These shared innate immune responses in invertebrates are basic events, considered as an integral component of immunity, independently deriving from a mix of cellular and humoral or from exclusive cellular responses, while in vertebrates are modest and restricted events of innate immunity masked by the multiple and multifaceted responses belonging to acquired immunity.

Another aspect that must be considered is that the massive amyloid fibril formation is an ancient physiological cell response harmonically integrated with the stress response. During invertebrate pigment synthesis, the amyloidogenesis is sustained by the cross talk between the immune and endocrine systems,[78,79] the redox status/cytoplasmic pH modification, and the cleavage of proprotein precursors. The amyloid fibril formation is accompanied by the overexpression of ACTH, melanocyte-stimulating hormone (α-MSH), and neutral endopeptidase[70,71,73] (Fig. 11.3).

Summarizing, in invertebrates, the presence of an ancestral defense, based on the combined immune-neuroendocrine responses, generates a large, variable, complex, and efficient repertoire of reactions in response to a few recognition units (always responsible of cytoplasmic variations of ROS, the real key player in stress signaling). Any type of stress condition generates a transient or persistent increase of ROS that, functioning as a variable electrical resistor, regulates and defines the type of protective responses both in invertebrates and vertebrates. One of the most intriguing responses is amyloidogenesis. The synthesized amyloid fibril functions as (1) a scaffold to package melanin and (2) a method to strive ROS overproduction for avoiding severe damages ending with cell death.

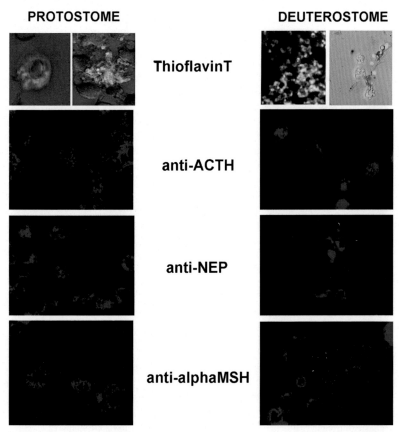

FIGURE 11.3 Immunocytochemical evidence of amyloid fibrils, detected with thioflavin T (yellow-green brightly fluorescence), in stimulated cells of protostome (insect hemocytes) and deuterostome (ascidian circulating cells). Nuclei can be stained with DAPI and marked in brilliant blue. Immunocytochemical characterizations for adrenocorticotropin hormone (ACTH), neutral endopeptidase (NEP), and alpha melanocyte-stimulating hormone (α-MSH) expression. Oxidative stress is responsible for a series of an integrated network of events starting with ACTH overproduction. The inactivation of ACTH, by the conversion in α-MSH, is due to the NEP degrading enzyme.

REFERENCES

1. Medzhitov R, Janeway C. Innate immune recognition: mechanisms and pathways. *Immunol Rev* 2000;**173**:89–97.
2. Tang D, Kang R, Coyne CB, Zeh HJ, Lotze MT. PAMPs and DAMPs: signal 0s that spur autophagy and immunity. *Immunol Rev* 2012;**249**:158–75.
3. Zhang L, Li L, Guo X, Litman GW, Dishaw LJ, Zhang G. Massive expansion and functional divergence of innate immune genes in a protostome. *Sci Rep* 2015;**5**:8693.
4. Hoffmann JA. The immune response of Drosophila. *Nature* 2003;**426**:33–8.
5. Takeda K, Kaisho T, Akira S. Toll-like receptors. *Annu Rev Immunol* 2003;**21**:335–76.

6. Dziarski R. Peptidoglycan recognition proteins (PGRPs). *Mol Immunol* 2004;**40**:877–86.

7. Yassine H, Osta MA. *Anopheles gambiae* innate immunity. *Cell Microbiol* 2010;**12**:1–9.

8. Lavine MD, Strand MR. Insect hemocytes and their role in immunity. *Insect Biochem Mol Biol* 2002;**32**:1295–309.

9. Beschin A, Bilej M, Torreele E, De Baetselier P. On the existence of cytokines in invertebrates. *Cell Mol Life Sci* 2001;**58**:801–14.

10. Tettamanti G, Malagoli D, Benelli R, Albini A, Grimaldi A, Perletti G, et al. Growth factors and chemokines: a comparative functional approach between invertebrates and vertebrates. *Curr Med Chem* 2006;**13**:2737–50.

11. Malagoli D, Conklin D, Sacchi S, Mandrioli M, Ottaviani E. A putative helical cytokine functioning in innate immune signalling in *Drosophila melanogaster*. *Biochim Biophys Acta* 2007;**1770**:974–8.

12. Dodd RB, Drickamer K. Lectin-like proteins in model organisms: implications for evolution of carbohydrate-binding activity. *Glycobiology* 2001;**11**:71R–9R.

13. Salzet M, Tasiemski A, Cooper E. Innate immunity in lophotrochozoans: the annelids. *Curr Pharm Des* 2006;**12**:3043–50.

14. Hancock REW, Brown KL, Mookherjee N. Host defence peptides from invertebrates–emerging antimicrobial strategies. *Immunobiology* 2006;**211**:315–22.

15. Danilova N. The evolution of immune mechanisms. *J Exp Zool B Mol Dev Evol* 2006;**306**: 496–520.

16. Brogden KA. Antimicrobial peptides: pore formers or metabolic inhibitors in bacteria? *Nat Rev Microbiol* 2005;**3**:238–50.

17. Peskin AV, Labas YA, Tikhonov AN. Superoxide radical production by sponges *Sycon* sp. *FEBS Lett* 1998;**434**:201–4.

18. García-García E, Prado-Álvarez M, Novoa B, Figueras A, Rosales C. Immune responses of mussel hemocyte subpopulations are differentially regulated by enzymes of the PI 3-K, PKC, and ERK kinase families. *Dev Comp Immunol* 2008;**32**:637–53.

19. Pereira LS, Oliveira PL, Barja-Fidalgo C, Daffre S. Production of reactive oxygen species by hemocytes from the cattle tick *Boophilus microplus*. *Exp Parasitol* 2001;**99**:66–72.

20. Whitten MMA, Ratcliffe NA. In vitro superoxide activity in the haemolymph of the West Indian leaf cockroach, *Blaberus discoidalis*. *J Insect Physiol* 1999;**45**:667–75.

21. Luckhart S, Vodovotz Y, Cui L, Rosenberg R. The mosquito *Anopheles stephensi* limits malaria parasite development with inducible synthesis of nitric oxide. *Proc Natl Acad Sci USA* 1998;**95**:5700–5.

22. Nappi AJ, Vass E, Frey F, Carton Y. Nitric oxide involvement in Drosophila immunity. *Nitric Oxide* 2000;**4**:423–30.

23. Grimaldi A, Tettamanti G, Girardello R, Pulze L, Valvassori R, Malagoli D, et al. Functional amyloid formation in LPS activated cells from invertebrates to vertebrates. *Invertebr Surviv J* 2014;**11**:286–97.

24. Söderhäll K, Smith VJ. The prophenoloxidase activating system: the biochemistry of its activation and role in arthropod cellular immunity, with special reference to Crustaceans. In: Brehélin M, editor. *Immunity in invertebrates*. Berlin, Heidelberg: Springer Berlin Heidelberg; 1986. p. 208–23.

25. Ashida M, Yoshida H. Biochemistry of the phenoloxidase system in insects: with special reference to its activation. In: Ohnishi E, Ishizaki H, editors. *Molting and metamorphosis*. Japan Scientific Societies Press; 1990. p. 239–65.

26. Roch P, Canicatti C, Sammarco S. Tetrameric structure of the active phenoloxidase evidenced in the coelomocytes of the echinoderm *Holothuria tubulosa*. *Comp Biochem Physiol Part B Comp Biochem* 1992;**102**:349–55.

27. Nappi AJ, Vass E. Melanogenesis and the generation of cytotoxic molecules during insect cellular immune reactions. *Pigment Cell Res* 1993;**6**:117–26.
28. Fujimoto K, Okino N, Kawabata S, Iwanaga S, Ohnishi E. Nucleotide sequence of the cDNA encoding the proenzyme of phenol oxidase A1 of *Drosophila melanogaster*. *Proc Natl Acad Sci USA* 1995;**92**:7769–73.
29. Pang Q, Zhang S, Wang C, Shi X, Sun Y. Presence of prophenoloxidase in the humoral fluid of amphioxus *Branchiostoma belcheri tsingtauense*. *Fish Shellfish Immunol* 2004;**17**:477–87.
30. Cammarata M, Parrinello N. The ascidian prophenoloxidase activating system. *Invertebr Surviv J* 2009;**6**:67–76.
31. Ballarin L. Ascidian cytotoxic cells: state of the art and research perspectives. *Invertebr Blood Cells* 2012;**9**:1–6.
32. Söderhäll K. Prophenoloxidase activating system and melanization - a recognition mechanism of arthropods? A review. *Dev Comp Immunol* 1982;**6**:601–11.
33. Johansson MW, Soderhall K. Cellular immunity in crustaceans and the proPO system. *Parasitol Today* 1989;**5**:171–6.
34. Söderhäll K, Cerenius L, Johansson MW. The prophenoloxidase activating system and its role in invertebrate defence. *Ann NY Acad Sci* 1994;**712**:155–61.
35. Yasuhara Y, Koizumi Y, Katagiri C, Ashida M. Reexamination of properties of prophenoloxidase isolated from larval hemolymph of the silkworm *Bombyx mori*. *Arch Biochem Biophys* 1995;**320**:14–23.
36. Smith VJ, Söderhäll K. A comparison of phenoloxidase activity in the blood of marine invertebrates. *Dev Comp Immunol* 1991;**15**:251–61.
37. Nappi AJ, Ottaviani E. Cytotoxicity and cytotoxic molecules in invertebrates. *Bioessays* 2000;**22**:469–80.
38. Cerenius L, Söderhäll K. The prophenoloxidase-activating system in invertebrates. *Immunol Rev* 2004;**198**:116–26.
39. Carton Y, Poirié M, Nappi AJ. Insect immune resistance to parasitoids. *Insect Sci* 2008;**15**:67–87.
40. Cerenius L, Lee BL, Söderhäll K. The proPO-system: pros and cons for its role in invertebrate immunity. *Trends Immunol* 2008;**29**:263–71.
41. Petes LE, Harvell CD, Peters EC, Webb MAH, Mullen KM. Pathogens compromise reproduction and induce melanization in Caribbean sea fans. *Mar Ecol Prog Ser* 2003;**264**:167–71.
42. Mydlarz LD, Holthouse SF, Peters EC, Harvell CD. Cellular responses in sea fan corals: granular amoebocytes react to pathogen and climate stressors. *PLoS One* 2008;**3**:e1811.
43. Valembois P, Roch P, Lassegues M. Evidence of plasma clotting system in earthworms. *J Invertebr Pathol* 1988;**51**:221–8.
44. Porchet-Henneré E, Vernet G. Cellular immunity in an annelid (*Nereis diversicolor*, Polychaeta): production of melanin by a subpopulation of granulocytes. *Cell Tissue Res* 1992;**269**:167–74.
45. Beschin a, Bilej M, Hanssens F, Raymakers J, Van Dyck E, Revets H, et al. Identification and cloning of a glucan-and lipopolysaccharide-binding protein from *Eisenia foetida* earthworm involved in the activation of prophenoloxidase cascade. *J Biol Chem* 1998;**273**:24948.
46. Fyffe WE, Kronz JD, Edmonds PA, Donndelinger TM. Effect of high-level oxygen exposure on the peroxidase activity and the neuromelanin-like pigment content of the nerve net in the earthworm, *Lumbricus terrestris*. *Cell Tissue Res* 1999;**295**:349–54.
47. Adamowicz A. Morphology and ultrastructure of the earthworm *Dendrobaena veneta* (Lumbricidae) coelomocytes. *Tissue Cell* 2005;**37**:125–33.
48. Procházková P, Silerová M, Stijlemans B, Dieu M, Halada P, Josková R, et al. Evidence for proteins involved in prophenoloxidase cascade *Eisenia fetida* earthworms. *J Comp Physiol B* 2006;**176**:581–7.

49. Ottaviani E, Cossarizza A. Immunocytochemical evidence of vertebrate bioactive peptide-like molecules in the immuno cell types of the freshwater snail *Plianorbarius corneus* (L.) (Gastropoda, Pulmonata). *FEBS Lett* 1990;**267**:250–2.

50. Ottaviani E. Molluscan immunorecognition. *Invertebr Surviv J* 2006;**3**:50–63.

51. Venier P, Varotto L, Rosani U, Millino C, Celegato B, Bernante F, et al. Insights into the innate immunity of the Mediterranean mussel *Mytilus galloprovincialis*. *BMC Genomics* 2011;**12**:69.

52. Martin GG, Oakes CT, Tousignant HR, Crabtree H, Yamakawa R. Structure and function of haemocytes in two marine gastropods, *Megathura crenulata* and *Aplysia californica*. *J Molluscan Stud* 2007;**73**:355–65.

53. Gallo C, Schiavon F, Ballarin L. Insight on cellular and humoral components of innate immunity in *Squilla mantis* (Crustacea, Stomatopoda). *Fish Shellfish Immunol* 2011;**31**:423–31.

54. Canicatti C, Seymour J. Evidence for phenoloxidase activity in *Holothuria tubulosa* (Echinodermata) brown bodies and cells. *Parasitol Res* 1991;**77**:50–3.

55. Shirae M, Ballarin L, Frizzo A, Saito Y, Hirose E. Involvement of quinones and phenoloxidase in the allorejection reaction in a colonial ascidian, *Botrylloides simodensis*: histochemical and immunohistochemical study. *Mar Biol* 2002;**141**:659–65.

56. Hirose E. Colonial allorecognition, hemolytic rejection, and viviparity in botryllid ascidians. *Zool Sci* 2003;**20**:387–94.

57. Ballarin L. Immunobiology of compound ascidians, with particular reference to *Botryllus schlosseri*: state of art. *Invertebr Surviv J* 2008;**5**:54–74.

58. Ballarin L, Menin A, Franchi N, Bertoloni G, Cima F. Morula cells and non-self recognition in the compound ascidian *Botryllus schlosseri*. *Invertebr Surviv J* 2005;**2**:1–5.

59. Cooper EL. Phylogeny of cytotoxicity. *Endeavour* 1980;**4**:160–5.

60. Cooper EL, Mansour MH, Negm HI. Marine invertebrate immunodefense responses: molecular and cellular approaches in tunicates. *Annu Rev Fish Dis* 1996;**6**:133–49.

61. Porchet-Hennere E, Nejmeddine A, Baert JL, Dhainaut-Courtois N. Selective immunostaining of type 1 granulocytes of the polychaete annelid *Nereis diversicolor* by a monoclonal antibody against a cadmium-binding protein (MP II). *Biol Cell* 1987;**60**:259–61.

62. Bilej M, Brys L, Beschin A, Lucas R, Vercauteren E, Hanusová R, et al. Identification of a cytolytic protein in the coelomic fluid of Eisenia foetida earthworms. *Immunol Lett* 1995;**45**:123–8.

63. Blanco GA, Escalada AM, Alvarez E, Hajos S. LPS-induced stimulation of phagocytosis in the sipunculan worm *Themiste petricola*: possible involvement of human CD14, CD11B and CD11C cross-reactive molecules. *Dev Comp Immunol* 1997;**21**:349–62.

64. Ottaviani E, Franceschi C. The invertebrate phagocytic immunocyte: clues to a common evolution of immune and neuroendocrine systems. *Immunol Today* 1997;**18**:169–74.

65. De Eguileor M, Grimaldi A, Tettamanti G, Valvassori R, Cooper EL, Lanzavecchia G. Different types of response to foreign antigens by leech leukocytes. *Tissue Cell* 2000;**32**:40–8.

66. Buchmann K. Evolution of innate immunity: clues from invertebrates via fish to mammals. *Front Immunol* 2014;**5**:459.

67. Ratcliffe NA, Rowley AF, Fitzgerald SW, Rhodes CP. Invertebrate immunity: basic concepts and recent advances. *Int Rev Cytol* 1985;**97**:183–350.

68. Rowley AF, Ratcliffe NA. Insects. In: Ratcliffe NA, Rowley AF, editors. *Invertebrate blood cells*. 1981. p. 471–90.

69. Maury CPJ. The emerging concept of functional amyloid. *J Intern Med* 2009;**265**:329–34.

70. Grimaldi A, Tettamanti G, Congiu T, Girardello R, Malagoli D, Falabella P, et al. The main actors involved in parasitization of *Heliothis virescens* larva. *Cell Tissue Res* 2012;**350**:491–502.

71. Grimaldi A, Girardello R, Malagoli D, Falabella P, Tettamanti G, Valvassori R, et al. Amyloid/melanin distinctive mark in invertebrate immunity. *ISJ* 2012;**9**:153–62.

72. Ferrarese R, Brivio M, Congiu T, Falabella P, Grimaldi A, Mastore M, et al. Early suppression of immune response in *Heliothis virescens* larvae by the endophagous. *Invertebr Surviv J* 2005;**2**:60–8.

73. Falabella P, Riviello L, Pascale M, Di Lelio I, Tettamanti G, Grimaldi A, et al. Functional amyloids in insect immune response. *Insect Biochem Mol Biol* 2012;**42**:203–11.

74. Fowler DM, Koulov AV, Alory-Jost C, Marks MS, Balch WE, Kelly JW. Functional amyloid formation within mammalian tissue. *PLoS Biol* 2006;**4**:0100–7.

75. Schmidt O, Theopold U, Strand M. Innate immunity and its evasion and suppression by hymenopteran endoparasitoids. *Bioessays* 2001;**23**:344–51.

76. Mostaert AS, Higgins MJ, Fukuma T, Rindi F, Jarvis SP. Nanoscale mechanical characterisation of amyloid fibrils discovered in a natural adhesive. *J Biol Phys* 2006;**32**:393–401.

77. Mostaert AS, Jarvis SP. Beneficial characteristics of mechanically functional amyloid fibrils evolutionarily preserved in natural adhesives. *Nanotechnology* 2007;**18**:044010.

78. Ottaviani E, Franchini A, Genedani S. ACTH and its role in immune-neuroendocrine functions. A comparative study. *Curr Pharm Des* 1999;**5**:673–81.

79. Ottaviani E, Malagoli D, Franceschi C. Common evolutionary origin of the immune and neuro-endocrine systems: from morphological and functional evidence to in silico approaches. *Trends Immunol* 2007;**28**:497–502.

Chapter 12

Echinoderm Antimicrobial Peptides: The Ancient Arms of the Deuterostome Innate Immune System

Vincenzo Arizza, Domenico Schillaci
University of Palermo, Palermo, Italy

INTRODUCTION

The deuterostomes, of which echinoderms, hemichordates, tunicates, and all higher chordates are the major extant groups, constitute a separate branch of the animal kingdom.[1,2] During the early Precambrian period, these animals split into two main groups: protostomes and deuterostomes. In the protostomes, the blastopore differentiates into the mouth. In the deuterostomes, the blastopore can differentiate into the anus, while the mouth can develop from another embryonic area. The echinoderms and the chordates are deuterostomes, while all other invertebrates are protostomes. Due to the abundance and calcareous shells of echinoderms, these organisms have been well preserved as fossils. It has been suggested that the echinoderms diverged from a common vertebrate ancestor before the beginning of the Cambrian period, over 600 million years ago. The phylum of Echinodermata, comprising approximately 6000 extant species,[3] is an ancient group formed of benthic marine animals that live in both intertidal and deep sea benthos. Currently, echinoderms are divided into five major classes: the **Asteroidea** (Fig. 12.1A), commonly known as starfish or sea stars, typically possessing five arms, each of which contains gonads and part of the digestive tract; the **Ophiuroidea** (Fig. 12.1B), or brittle stars, with slender arms sharply set off from the central disc without lobes of the alimentary tract; the **Echinoidea** (Fig. 12.1C), commonly known as flat sand dollars and spherical sea urchins, lacking arms but possessing a typical pentamerous plan of echinoderms in five ambulacral areas; the **Crinoidea** (Fig. 12.1D), nearly exclusively comprising sessile animals, such as sea lilies and feather stars (sea lilies have a flower-shaped body, while feather stars have long arms with many branches);

Lessons in Immunity: From Single-Cell Organisms to Mammals
http://dx.doi.org/10.1016/B978-0-12-803252-7.00012-6

159

Phylum Echinodermata

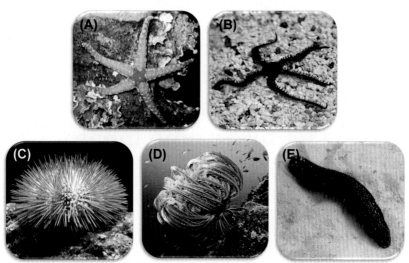

FIGURE 12.1 The different classes of phylum Echinodermata: (A) Asteroidea, (B) Ophiuroidea, (C) Echinoidea, (D) Crinoidea, and (E) Holothuroidea .

and the **Holothuroidea** (Fig. 12.1E), commonly known as sea cucumbers, with a body plan significantly extended in the oral–aboral axis and lacking arms.

ECHINODERM IMMUNITY

Hildemann and colleagues first demonstrated a functioning immune system in echinoderms, showing that sea cucumbers and sea stars reject allograft and accept autograft.[4,5] These experiments demonstrated that echinoderms, and other invertebrates, possess an innate immune system. The major immunological activity of echinoderms, comprising cellular and humoral components, is primarily detected in the coelomic fluid. Different types of coelomocytes[6–10] were observed in the fluid of the coelomic cavity, and these cells mediate echinoderm immunity. Metchnikoff[11] first recognized the coelomocyte immune function when he inserted rose thorns, glass shards, or bacteria into the blastocoel of larval sea stars and observed that the blastocoelar cells, the larval equivalents of coelomocytes, can perform either encapsulation or phagocytosis. In echinoderms, there are four classes of coelomocytes: phagocytes, colorless spherulocytes, vibratile cells, and red spherule cells.[8,9,12] Asteroidea and Ophiuroidea lack red spherule cells, and Crinoidea lack vibratile cells.[13] Phagocytes possess different morphotypes that vary in size and shape.[14–16] These cells represent the most abundant coelomocyte type in the coelomic fluid.[8] The spherule cells include colorless spherulocytes and red spherules containing echinochrome A, a pigment that has antibacterial and antifungal activity.[17–20]

Matranga et al.[21] showed that the number of coelomocytes in *Paracentrotus lividus* changes according to the environmental stress conditions. Vibratile cells use a flagellum for movement, showing great motility, and these cells may be involved in clotting reactions.[10,22] Only the holothurians seem to have the crystal cells with regular geometric morphology and a crystal inclusion in the cytoplasm.[23] The role of these cells is not completely understood but may be associated with osmoregulation.[24] Coelomocytes mediate several immune functions, such as phagocytosis and the encapsulation and degranulation of echinochrome A from red spherule cells in response to bacterial contact[10] and injury.[25] Phagocytes contain antimicrobial peptides (AMPs) but do not release them in coelomic fluid. They can adhere to bacteria, after their phagocytosis, participating in the clearance of bacteria within the phagolysosome.[26] Coelomocytes release complement C3 homologue from a subset of discoidal cells,[8,27] and cytolytic activity is released from colorless spherulocytes.[9] Several humoral factors, such as hemolysin, lectin, agglutinin, phenoloxidase, and reactive oxygen intermediates, are involved in defense processes, such as clotting, opsonization, encapsulation, cell lysis, and wound healing.[12] Cytotoxic activity was detected in the coelomic fluid of the sea star, *Asterias forbesi*,[28] several sea urchin species,[29,30] and the holothuroid, *Holothuria polii*.[31] In echinoderms, lectins may play important roles in defense, as these proteins may be involved in opsonization and lytic functions, clot formation, and wound repair. Calcium- and magnesium-dependant agglutinins were identified in three sea urchin species[32]: the sea star, *Asterina pectinifera*,[33] and *H. polii*.[31] The hemagglutinin in *P. lividus*, a heterotrimeric complex that binds rabbit red blood cells, enhances the adhesive properties of autologous coelomocytes and may be involved in cell–cell and cell–matrix interactions, such as clotting, wound repair, opsonization, and encapsulation.[34] Two different C-type (Ca^{2+}-dependent) lectins were identified in the holothurian, *Stichopus japonicus*,[35] and three lectins were identified in the sea star *A. pectinifera*, exhibiting different binding abilities: one lectin preferentially agglutinates rabbit erythrocytes, while another lectin binds human erythrocytes, and the third lectin agglutinates bacteria.[33] Giga et al.[36] showed that the sea urchin *Anthocidaris crassispina* possessed Echinoidin, a C-type lectin that contains an RGD sequence (a tripeptide that contains Arg-Gly-Asp), which binds integrin and mediates cell adhesion and cell–cell recognition.[37–39] CEL-III is another C-type lectin, from the holothurian *Cucumaria echinata*, which lyses rabbit and human erythrocytes through a new pore-forming mechanism and may be toxic to microbes.[40] Sodergren et al.[41] sequenced the genome of *Strongylocentrotus purpuratus*, revealing a complex immune gene repertoire, indicating that sea urchins have an astonishingly high diversity of immune molecules.[42,43] The genome sequence revealed 253 Toll-like receptor genes,[44] more than 200 NACHT domain-LRR genes, and 218 scavenger receptor genes.[43] Another large putative immune response gene family encodes the Sp185/333 protein family identified from Lipopolysaccharides (LPS)-challenged sea urchins.[45,46] Furthermore, Smith et al.[47] identified the first complement components in an invertebrate, showing that the *S. purpuratus* genome contained sequences homologous to vertebrate complement protein C3 and factor B, called *Sp*C3 and *Sp*Bf, respectively. LPS challenge upregulated the expression of *Sp*C3,[48] which binds to both methylamine and yeast, functioning as an opsonin with typical C3 functions.[49] In addition, two transcripts from *S. purpuratus* encode putative complement proteins with domains that are also present in C6 and C7.[50] The deduced proteins may participate as complement regulatory proteins or act in the terminal complement pathway.

ANTIMICROBIAL PEPTIDES

AMPs are molecules with small molecular masses of less than 10 kDa, comprising more or less than 100 amino acids.[51,52] Based on the amino acid composition, these peptides significantly differ in structural conformation and function. The molecular arrangement of AMPs, reflecting the relative abundance of hydrophobic and hydrophilic domains, could form an amphipathic structure with a hydrophilic polar face opposing a hydrophobic nonpolar face.[53,54] Therefore, the AMPs can show different structural features: (1) The α-helical, including magainin from the African clawed frog, *Xenopus laevis*,[55] and cecropin from giant silk moth, *Hyalophora cecropia*,[56] constitutes a typical class of AMPs that are the most well established in structure–activity relationships. In particular, the α-helical AMPs are usually unstructured in aqueous solution and form amphipathic helices in membranes or membrane-mimicking environments. Most α-helical AMPs disrupt bacterial membranes, and several mechanisms of action employed by various AMPs have been proposed.[57,58] The characteristics possessed by the AMPs allow them to be both water soluble and able to interact with the hydrophobic layer of the microbial membranes,[53,59] which are also negatively charged, as they are composed of phosphatidylglycerol, cardiolipin, or phosphatidylserine.[60] (2) β-sheet peptides as human defensins are peptides with 29–40 amino acid residues and three intramolecular cysteine-disulfide bonds, which have no regular secondary structure elements. The defensins, from the insect *Phormia terraenovae*, can penetrate both anionic and zwitterionic phospholipids monolayers[61] and can form, with phospholipid, lipid–immiscible complexes at a ratio of 1:4 that may be responsible for antimicrobial activity. (3) The linear AMPs do not show activity against the microbial membranes, but they can realize their antimicrobial activities by penetrating across the membranes and interacting with bacterial proteins inside.[62] The linear peptides, such as indolicidin from bovine neutrophils, a tryptophan/proline-rich peptide,[63] or Bac5 and Bac7 from bovine neutrophils, a proline-/arginine-rich peptide,[64] use their membrane affinity property for entering the cytoplasm and exert their antibacterial activity by attacking other targets.[65,66] (4) The loop AMPs, including bactenecin, from bovine neutrophils form one disulfide bond, making it a cyclic molecule.[67] Little is known about its antimicrobial mechanism and whether it shares the common killing mechanism of other AMPs or if it has a distinct mode of action due to its unique compact structure.

MODE OF ACTION

The characteristics of AMPs confer both water solubility and the ability to interact with the hydrophobic layer of the microbial membranes.[53,59] In general, studies on the antimicrobial activity of AMPs show that the recruitment and interaction of AMPs with bacterial membranes is an electrostatic attraction between the cationic portion of the AMPs and the negatively charged microbial membrane containing phosphatidylglycerol, cardiolipin, or phosphatidylserine.[60,68,69] When the peptide/lipid ratio increases, AMPs self-associate on the surface of the bacterial membrane and fit perpendicularly into the lipid bilayer, forming a toroidal pore, a barrel stave, or a carpet model. In the toroidal pore, the peptides inserted perpendicularly in the membrane bilayer induce a local membrane curvature, and the pore lumen is partly covered by peptides and phospholipid head groups.[70] In the barrel-stave pore, the peptides are perpendicularly oriented and inserted into the bilayer, where these molecules combine in multimers to form a pore. In this model, the peptides are aligned to the axis of the pore parallel to the phospholipid chain and do not change orientation with respect to the membrane plane.[71,72] Moreover, in the carpet mechanism, the peptides are adsorbed in parallel with the bilayer and, when a sufficient concentration is reached, these peptides destabilize the membrane, which is subsequently disintegrated. AMPs also act as multifunctional microbicides that kill bacteria, simultaneously targeting the cell membrane or reacting with intracellular targets, interfering with essential metabolic functions, such as protein, DNA, or cell membrane synthesis.[53,73,74] AMPs can be produced constitutively or in response to contact with microorganisms; moreover, some AMPs can protect the organisms through multiple activities. Indeed, these proteins confer protection not only through antimicrobial function, but it has also been demonstrated that AMPs exhibit antitumor and mitogenic activities and can modulate the immune mechanisms through controlling signal transduction and chemokine production and/or release.[75–78]

ANTIMICROBIAL PEPTIDES IN ECHINODERMS

Studies conducted by the late 1970s showed that echinoderms possess many different AMPs (Table 12.1). Beauregard et al.[79] identified AMPs in the coelomic fluid of holothuroid *Cucumaria frondosa*, and these proteins had a molecular weight of <6 kDa and exhibited activity against gram-positive and gram-negative bacteria. Since then, several other AMPs have been identified in other echinoderms. Maltseva et al.[80] identified a number of partial peptide sequences with antimicrobial activity in an extract from the coelomocytes of

TABLE 12.1 Antimicrobial Peptides in Echinoderms

Class and Genus	Origins	AMPs	Molecular Mass (kDa)	Target	Charge	References
Asteroidea						
Asterias rubens	C, CF, GO, E, BW		~20	Gram (−) Gram (+)	n.d.	87
	C	Fragments of actin, histone H2A, and filamin A	1.8–2.4 2.6–4.7	Gram (−) Gram (+) Fungi	Cationic	80
Echinoidea						
Strongylocentrotus droebachiensis	C	Strongylocins 1	5.6	Gram (−)	Cationic	84
	C	Strongylocins 2	5.8	Gram (+)	Cationic	
Strongylocentrotus purpuratus	C	SpStrongylocins 1	5.6	Gram (−)	Cationic	85
	C	SpStrongylocins 2	6.0	Gram (+)	Cationic	
S. droebachiensis	C	Centrocins 1	4.4	Fungi	Cationic	86
	C	Centrocins 2	4.5	Gram (+) Gram (−)		

				Gram (+) / Gram (−) / Fungus		
Paracentrotus lividus	C	Paracentrin 1	1.2	Gram (+) / Gram (−) / Fungus	Cationic	88,89
Holothuroidea						
Cucumaria frondosa		–	~6	Gram (−) / Gram (+)	n.d.	79
Cucumaria echinata	WB	–	4.2	Gram (+)	–	90
Holothuria tubulosa	C	Holothuroidin 1	1.4	Gram (+)	Cationic	91
	C	Holothuroidin 2	1.5	Gram (−)		
Apostichopus japonicus	ENT	A3	6.5	Gram (−) / Gram (+)	–	92

C, coelomocites; *CF*, coelomic fluid; *GO*, gastrointestinal organs; *E*, eggs; *BW*, body wall; *WB*, whole body; *ENT*, enteron; *AMP*, antimicrobial peptides; *n.d.*, not determined; *Sp*Strongylocins, Strongylocins of *Strongylocentrotus purpuratus*.

the sea star *Asterias rubens*, including fragments of histone H2A, actin, and filamin A. Gowda et al.[81] showed that the sea cucumber *Holothuria scabra* possesses an agglutinin that can agglutinate and kill gram-positive and gram-negative bacteria in vivo and in vitro. Ng et al.[82] isolated defensin-like peptides from *Strongylocentrotus droebachiensis*. Hatakeyama et al.[83] demonstrated that a synthetic peptide, corresponding to the α-helical region of CEL-III, a lectin isolated from the sea cucumber *C. echinata*, shows strong antibacterial activity against *Staphylococcus aureus* and *Bacillus subtilis*. Although these preliminary investigations only involve a few echinoderm species, the findings suggest that echinoderms deserve more attention to discover new active compounds. From the analysis of the purple sea urchin *S. droebachiensis* genome, Li et al.[84] obtained cDNAs encoding two cystein-rich AMPs. This family of peptides includes two native members named *Sd*Strongylocins 1 and 2 (Strongylocins of Strongylocentrotus droebachiensis), and each peptide has putative isoforms (*Sd*Strongylocins1b and 2b). The *Sd*Strongylocins display potent activity against both gram-positive and gram-negative bacteria at minimal inhibitory concentrations (MIC) of 1.3–2.5 μM. *Listonella anguillarum*, a marine fish and shellfish pathogen, is particularly susceptible to *Sd*Strongylocin 2. Homologous peptides of *Sd*Strongylocin are also expressed in the purple sea urchin, *S. purpuratus*, referred to as *Sp*Strongylocins 1 and 2 (Strongylocins of Strongylocentrotus purpuratus).[85] Recombinant *Sp*Strongylocins (r*Sp*Strongylocins) are active against both gram-positive and gram-negative bacteria; however, membrane integrity studies showed that r*Sp*Strongylocins 1 and 2 do not enhance the permeability of the bacterial membrane.[85] This evidence suggests that the microbicidal activity of *Sp*Strongylocins may involve intracellular targets, or microbial killing might be achieved through other mechanisms. Another set of AMPs, namely Centrocins 1 and 2, with potent activities against gram-positive and gram-negative bacteria, have been identified from the coelomocytes of *S. droebachiensis*.[86] They are similar heterodimeric cationic peptides: Centrocin 1 consists of 119 amino acids (4.5 kDa), whereas Centrocin 2 consists of 118 amino acids (4.4 kDa). Their structure consists of a heavy chain (30 aa) and a light chain (12 aa) that are linked by an internal disulfide bond. Centrocins 1 and 2 are present both in adult coelomocyte and in pluteus stages, indicating a crucial role in immunity not only in adult sea urchins but also in larvae.[26]

ANTIMICROBIAL BIOFILM PEPTIDES IN ECHINODERMS

The most common bacterial form of growth is the biofilm, a sessile multistratified community embedded in a matrix of extracellular polymeric substances (EPS) comprising a variety of organic substances, such as polysaccharides, proteins, lipids, and extracellular DNA.[93] Almost all gram-negative and gram-positive bacteria show biofilm formation, and in this form, many of these microorganisms can be highly pathogenic toward animals and humans (Fig. 12.2).

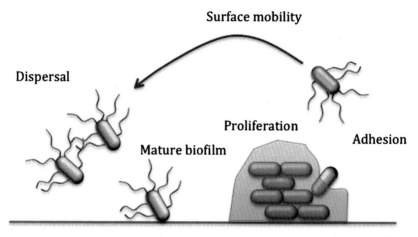

FIGURE 12.2 A model for biofilm development. Planktonic bacterial cells use flagella to approach and swim on a surface. Upon interacting with the substrate, the cells attach irreversibly. The attached cells begin to create extracellular polymeric substances and start to grow. The biofilm grows, and in response to environmental and/or physiological clues the cells may be released from the matrix and return to the planktonic state, dispersing and thus completing the development cycle.

Although antibiotics are effective against pathogenic bacteria in planktonic (free-living) form, these compounds are not effective against bacteria organized in biofilms, showing increased resistance of approximately 1000 times.[94] The antibiotic resistance in bacterial biofilm formation is based on multifactorial mechanisms that involve physical and/or chemical and biological features of the biofilm structure.[95]

EPS offer a mechanical shield, preventing or suppressing the targeting of antibiotics to target structures, such as the bacterial membrane, or intracellular target processes, such as metabolic functions. Moreover, biofilm formation is associated with the physiological status of the biofilm-embedded cells, with slow growth and low metabolic activity of bacterial cells in the internal layer of the community and the expression of stress genes, making these structures naturally resistant to conventional antibiotics that act on dividing and metabolically active cells.

Biofilm formation is typically initiated when planktonic bacteria adhere to biotic or abiotic surfaces through the sedimentation and Brownian motion of microbial cells, convection currents within bulk liquid transporting bacteria to the surface, the active movements of flagellated bacteria, or electrostatic forces and physical interactions between the bacterial membrane and surface.[96] The attachment of bacteria onto the surface initiates a cascade of changes. Indeed, it has been shown that a different set of genes responsible for the biofilm phenotype are triggered in response to cell attachment.[97,98] Other planktonic bacteria are recruited through EPS.[99] The maturation of the biofilm structure involves cell growth (and potential reproduction) within a given microenvironment, as determined based on exopolysaccharide substances, neighboring cells, and the proximity to water channels.[100] Finally, bacteria can be detached from the biofilm through external forces, as a part of a wavelike migrating physical movement,[101] or even as a self-induced process to disseminate into the environment.

During biofilm formation, bacteria communicate through a quorum sensing (QS) system. The QS is a system of cell–cell communication based on small molecules that facilitate information sharing, such as cell density, among bacteria, resulting in the adjustment of gene expression accordingly. The effects influence behaviors, such as bioluminescence, virulence factor production, and biofilm formation.[102–104] The AMPs are candidates of molecules for fighting biofilm formation, as these molecules kill the bacteria comprising the biofilm because their main mechanism of action is based on their ability to generate pores within bacterial membranes. However, unlike conventional antibiotics, these molecules can act on bacterial cells that grow slowly and show low metabolic activity. AMPs also interfere with the formation of the biofilm through different mechanisms that affect the various stages of biofilm formation. Indeed, by altering the adhesive properties of the abiotic surface, binding to the membrane of the bacteria through electrostatic interactions, or killing bacterial cells that first colonize the surface, AMPs counteract the initial adhesion of bacterial cells. It is demonstrated that cationic AMPs can bind extracellular DNA, an important biofilm component,[105] involved in *Pseudomonas aeruginosa*, cell–cell attachment, and biofilm developments,[106] and due to the high affinity of cationic AMPs for DNA,[107] it may be presumed that this binding might facilitate the detachment or disruption of the otherwise stable biofilm structures. Moreover, AMPs may prevent the maturation of the biofilm through the inhibition of the molecules required for QS. It has also been suggested that bacterial resistance to AMPs is less probable because most of these molecules rapidly kill bacteria through pore formation or membrane perturbation, which includes the entire membrane, or function through complex mechanisms.[108]

Recently, Arizza and Schillaci examined the immune systems of echinoderms and identified novel cationic peptides with antibiofilm activity in the sea urchin *P. lividus* and sea cucumber *Holothuria tubulosa*.[88,109,110] This activity can inhibit the pathogens responsible for human and animal infectious diseases, such as *S. aureus*, *Staphylococcus epidermidis*, or *P. aeruginosa*.[88,91,109] Antimicrobial activity was detected in the acid extract of coelomocytes lysate in a protein fraction at a low molecular weight of <5 kDa. Paracentrin 1 is an AMP extracted from the sea urchin *P. lividus*. This molecule is an 11-amino acid peptide with a molecular weight of 1.251 kDa that possesses the same amino acid sequence of the 9–19 fragments of *P. lividus* β-thymosin. The β-thymosin is a peptide that exerts numerous biological effects, such as the induction of chemotaxis, angiogenesis, metalloproteinases, and inhibition of inflammation[111] and is one of the AMPs of platelets from animals, including human beings.[112] Two AMPs have been identified in *H. tubulosa*, Holothuroidin 1 (H1) and Holothuroidin

2 (H2), with molecular weights of 1.389 and 1.547 kDa, respectively.[91] The peptides of both species share similarity with other AMPs present in several organisms. Paracentrin 1 shares 38.46% amino acid sequence similarity with Jelleine-III, a short AMP present in the royal jelly of *Apis mellifera* worker bees, exhibiting activity against yeasts and gram-positive and gram-negative bacteria.[113] Both Holothuroidin 1 and Holothuroidin 2 show ≥35% similarity, respectively, with protonectins, AMPs in the venom of the neotropical social wasp *Agelaia pallipes*, exhibiting activity against both gram-positive and gram-negative bacteria,[114] and signiferins, a naturally occurring cationic AMP present in the frog *Crinia signifera*, exhibiting activity against a wide spectrum of gram-positive and gram-negative bacterial strains, including *Bacillus cereus*, *Enterococcus faecalis*, *Lactobacillus lactis*, *Lactobacillus innocua*, *Micrococcus luteus*, *Staphylococcus aureus*, *Staphylococcus epidermidis*, and *Streptococcus uberis*.[115] Molecular dynamics analysis showed that structurally Paracentrin 1 significantly differs from other echinoderm AMPs.[89,91] Indeed, the asymmetrical arrangement of the polar charged and hydrophobic residues contributes to a protein with a hydrophobic core with a binding site for the bacterial membrane flanked at both ends by cationic and polar residues that solubilize the peptides in aqueous solution.[110] The two AMPs of *H. tubulosa* possess the features of many AMPs, as these cationic peptides comprise approximately 30% hydrophobic residues. The molecular dynamics analysis showed that the protein structure might contain α-helices with an unbalanced arrangement of the hydrophobic and hydrophilic residues arranged in an amphipathic molecule with a hydrophilic face opposing a hydrophobic face. For interactions with bacterial membranes, this characteristic H1 and H2 folding facilitates the interaction of nonpolar surfaces with the hydrophobic core of the lipids and engages the hydrophilic face with the polar side of membrane lipids.[91] Although the AMPs from *P. lividus* and *H. tubulosa* differ in structure, these compounds share the same chemical/physical features, as these molecules have cationic features. The use of synthetic AMPs, assembled according to the sequences specified through the MS/MS analysis, showed that synthetic peptides are active against both planktonic gram-positive and gram-negative bacterial strains, such as *S. aureus*, *S. epidermidis*, and *P. aeruginosa*, and at sub-MIC concentrations, these molecules inhibit biofilm formation. Particularly, Paracentrin 1 inhibits either early (6-h old) or mature (24-h old) biofilm formation for *S. epidermidis* 1457.[88] The AMPs from *H. tubulosa* inhibit the biofilm growth of two staphylococcal strains, such as *S. aureus* ATCC25923 and *S. epidermidis* ATCC 35984.[91] Using rabbit erythrocytes as target cells, Schillaci and colleagues observed that synthetic Paracentrin 1, H1, and H2 do not show hemolytic activity, confirming a role for these molecules in the specific toxicity of bacterial cells.[91,110] Thus these AMPs could be classified as peptide antibiotics.[116]

CONCLUSION

As part of the innate immune system, AMPs are defensive molecules that appeared early in the evolution of organisms. The ubiquitous distribution of these molecules in all kingdoms, within both unicellular and multicellular organisms, suggests that AMPs play an important and essential role in the biology of organisms that likely evolved through positive selection.[117–119]

AMPs from marine invertebrates can fight bacterial infections, which can often escape and even suppress the host immune system through complex life cycles.[120] AMPs from marine invertebrates can also be applied in biotechnology and medicine. These natural compounds constitute potential candidates for the development of alternative strategies to prevent and treat bacterial infections, including those associated with the biofilm formation of bacteria intrinsically resistant to conventional antibiotics as these developed on medical devices. Indeed, some AMPs are used to impregnate the medical device surfaces by functionalized coatings that allow a localized antimicrobial delivery.[121–123] In general, the identification of novel AMPs from any marine/aquatic invertebrate suggests an innovative approach for the design of new synthetic derivatives with modified chemical–physical properties to improve antimicrobial activity against pathogens and the pharmaceutical potential of these molecules.[104,124]

REFERENCES

1. Schaeffer B. Deuterostome monophyly and phylogeny. In: Hecht M, Wallace B, Prance G, editors. *Evolutionary biology*. New York: Plenum Press; 1987. p. 179–235.
2. Hyman LH. *The invertebrates: smaller coelomate groups chaetognatha, hemichordata, pogonophora, phoronida, ectoprocta, brachipoda, sipunculida, the coelomate bilateria*. New York: McGraw-Hill; 1959.
3. Ruppert E, Barnes R. *Invertebrate zoology*. 6th ed. New York: Saunders College Publishing; 1994.
4. Hildemann W, Dix TG. Transplantation reactions of tropical Australian echinoderms. *Transplantation* 1972;**14**:624–33.
5. Karp RD, Hildemann W. Specific allograft reactivity in the sea star *Dermasterias imbricata*. *Transplantation* 1976;**22**:434–9.
6. Boolootian RA, Giese AC. Coelomic corpuscles of echinoderms. *Biol Bull* 1958;**115**:53–63.
7. Smith VJ. The echinoderms. In: Ratcliffe N, Rowley AF, editors. *Invertebrate blood cells*, vol. 2. New York Academic Press; 1981. p. 50.
8. Smith LC, Ghosh J, Buckley KM, Clow LA, Dheilly NM, Haug T, et al. Echinoderm immunity. *Invertebr Immun* 2010;**708**:260–301.
9. Arizza V, Giaramita FT, Parrinello D, Cammarata M, Parrinello N. Cell cooperation in coelomocyte cytotoxic activity of *Paracentrotus lividus* coelomocytes. *Comp Biochem Physiol A Mol Integr Physiol* 2007;**147**:389–94.
10. Johnson PT. The coelomic elements of sea urchins (Strongylocentrotus) I. The normal coelomocytes; their morphology and dynamics in hanging drops. *J Invert Pathol* 1969;**13**:25–41.
11. Metchnikoff E. *Lectures on the comparative pathology of inflammation: delivered at the Pasteur Institute in 1891*. Kegan, P., Trench, T.; 1893.

12. Gross PS, Al-Sharif WZ, Clow LA, Smith LC. Echinoderm immunity and the evolution of the complement system. *Dev Comp Immunol* 1999;**23**:429–42.

13. Ramirez-Gomez F, Garcia-Arraras JE. Echinoderm immunity. *Invert Surviv J* 2010;**7**:211–20.

14. Henson JH, Svitkina TM, Burns AR, Hughes HE, MacPartland KJ, Nazarian R, et al. Two components of actin-based retrograde flow in sea urchin coelomocytes. *Mol Biol Cell* 1999;**10**:4075–90.

15. Henson JH, Nesbitt D, Wright BD, Scholey JM. Immunolocalization of kinesin in sea urchin coelomocytes. Association of kinesin with intracellular organelles. *J Cell Sci* 1992;**103**: 309–20.

16. Edds KT. Cell biology of echinoid coelomocytes: I. Diversity and characterization of cell types. *J Invert Pathol* 1993;**61**:173–8.

17. Separation of coelomocytes of *Echinus esculentus* by density gradient centrifugation. In: Messer L, Wardlaw A, editors. *Proceedings of the European Colloquium on Echinoderms*. A.A. Balkema, Rotterdam; 1980.

18. Service M, Wardlaw AC. Echinochrome-A as a bactericidal substance in the coelomic fluid of *Echinus esculentus* (L.). *Comp Biochem Physiol Part B Comp Biochem* 1984;**79**:161–5.

19. Calestani C, Rast JP, Davidson EH. Isolation of pigment cell specific genes in the sea urchin embryo by differential macroarray screening. *Development* 2003;**130**:4587–96.

20. Johnson PT. The coelomic elements of sea urchins (Strongylocentrotus and Centrostephanus). VI. Cellulose-acetate membrane electrophoresis. *Comp Biochem Physiol* 1970;**37**:289–300.

21. Matranga V, Pinsino A, Celi M, Di Bella G, Natoli A. Impacts of UV-B radiation on short-term cultures of sea urchin coelomocytes. *Mar Biol* 2006;**149**:25–34.

22. Bertheussen K, Seljelid R. Echinoid phagocytes in vitro. *Exp Cell Res* 1978;**111**:401–12.

23. Endean R. The coelomocytes and the coelomic fluids. In: Boolootian RA, editor. *Physiology of echinodermata*. London and New York: Wiley, J.; 1966.

24. Xing K, Yang HS, Chen MY. Morphological and ultrastructural characterization of the coelomocytes in *Apostichopus japonicus*. *Aquat Biol* 2008;**2**:85–92.

25. Coffaro KA, Hinegardner RT. Immune response in the sea urchin *Lytechinus pictus*. *Science* 1977;**197**:1389–90.

26. Li C, Blencke H-M, Haug T, Jørgensen Ø, Stensvåg K. Expression of antimicrobial peptides in coelomocytes and embryos of the green sea urchin (*Strongylocentrotus droebachiensis*). *Dev Comp Immunol* 2014;**43**:106–13.

27. Gross PS, Clow LA, Smith LC. SpC3, the complement homologue from the purple sea urchin, *Strongylocentrotus purpuratus*, is expressed in two subpopulations of the phagocytic coelomocytes. *Immunogenetics* 2000;**51**:1034–44.

28. Leonard LA, Strandberg JD, Winkelstein JA. Complement-like activity in the sea star, *Asterias forbesi*. *Dev Comp Immunol* 1990;**14**:19–30.

29. Stabili L, Pagliara P, Metrangolo M, Canicatti C. Comparative aspects of echinoidea cytolysins: the cytolytic activity of *Spherechinus granularis* (Echinoidea) celomic fluid. *Comp Biochem Physiol A Physiol* 1992;**101**:553–6.

30. Ryoyama K. Studies on the biological properties of coelomic fluid of sea urchin. I. Naturally occurring hemolysin in sea urchin. *Biochim Biophys Acta* 1973;**320**:157–65.

31. Canicatti C, Parrinello N. Hemagglutinin and hemolysin levels in the coelomic fluid from *Holothuria polii* (Echinodermata) following sheep erythrocyte injection. *Biol Bull* 1985;**168**:175–82.

32. Ryoyama K. Studies on the biological properties of coelomic fluid of sea urchin. II. Naturally occurring hemagglutinin in sea urchin. *Biol Bull* 1974;**146**:404–14.

33. Kamiya H, Muramoto K, Goto R, Sakai M. Lectins in the hemolymph of a starfish, *Asterina pectinifera*: purification and characterization. *Dev Comp Immunol* 1992;**16**:243–50.

34. Canicatti C, Pagliara P, Stabili L. Sea urchin coelomic fluid agglutinin mediates coelomocyte adhesion. *Eur J Cell Biol* 1992;**58**:291–5.

35. Matsui T, Ozeki Y, Suzuki M, Hino A, Titani K. Purification and characterization of two Ca^{2+}-dependent lectins from coelomic plasma of sea cucumber, *Stichopus japonicus*. *J Biochem* 1994;**116**:1127–33.

36. Giga Y, Ikai A, Takahashi K. The complete amino acid sequence of echinoidin, a lectin from the coelomic fluid of the sea urchin *Anthocidaris crassispina*. Homologies with mammalian and insect lectins. *J Biol Chem* 1987;**262**:6197–203.

37. Ozeki Y, Matsui T, Titani K. Cell adhesive activity of two animal lectins through different recognition mechanisms. *FEBS Lett* 1991;**289**:145–7.

38. D'Souza SE, Ginsberg MH, Plow EF. Arginyl-glycyl-aspartic acid (RGD): a cell adhesion motif. *Trends Biochem Sci* 1991;**16**:246–50.

39. Ruoslahti E. RGD and other recognition sequences for integrins. *Annu Rev Cell Dev Biol* 1996;**12**:697–715.

40. Hatakeyama T, Nagatomo H, Yamasaki N. Interaction of the hemolytic lectin Cel-III from the marine invertebrate *Cucumaria echinata* with the erythrocyte-membrane. *J Biol Chem* 1995;**270**:3560–4.

41. Sodergren E, Weinstock GM, Davidson EH, Cameron RA, Gibbs RA, Angerer RC, et al. The genome of the sea urchin *Strongylocentrotus purpuratus*. *Science* 2006;**314**:941–52.

42. Hibino T, Loza-Coll M, Messier C, Majeske AJ, Cohen AH, Terwilliger DP, et al. The immune gene repertoire encoded in the purple sea urchin genome. *Dev Biol* 2006;**300**:349–65.

43. Rast JP, Smith LC, Loza-Coll M, Hibino T, Litman GW. Genomic insights into the immune system of the sea urchin. *Science* 2006;**314**:952–6.

44. Buckley KM, Rast JP. Dynamic evolution of toll-like receptor multigene families in echinoderms. *Front Immunol* 2012;**3**:136.

45. Nair SV, Del Valle H, Gross PS, Terwilliger DP, Smith LC. Macroarray analysis of coelomocyte gene expression in response to LPS in the sea urchin. Identification of unexpected immune diversity in an invertebrate. *Physiol Genomics* 2005;**22**:33–47.

46. Terwilliger DP, Buckley KM, Mehta D, Moorjani PG, Smith LC. Unexpected diversity displayed in cDNAs expressed by the immune cells of the purple sea urchin, *Strongylocentrotus purpuratus*. *Physiol Genomics* 2006;**26**:134–44.

47. Smith LC, Clow LA, Terwilliger DP. The ancestral complement system in sea urchins. *Immunol Rev* 2001;**180**:16–34.

48. Clow LA, Gross PS, Shih CS, Smith LC. Expression of SpC3, the sea urchin complement component, in response to lipopolysaccharide. *Immunogenetics* 2000;**51**:1021–33.

49. Clow LA, Raftos DA, Gross PS, Smith LC. The sea urchin complement homologue, SpC3, functions as an opsonin. *J Exp Biol* 2004;**207**:2147–55.

50. Multerer KA, Smith LC. Two cDNAs from the purple sea urchin, *Strongylocentrotus purpuratus*, encoding mosaic proteins with domains found in factor H, factor I, and complement components C6 and C7. *Immunogenetics* 2004;**56**:89–106.

51. Ganz T. Defensins: antimicrobial peptides of innate immunity. *Nat Rev Immunol* 2003;**3**:710–20.

52. Maroti G, Kereszt A, Kondorosi E, Mergaert P. Natural roles of antimicrobial peptides in microbes, plants and animals. *Res Microbiol* 2011;**162**:363–74.

53. Brogden KA. Antimicrobial peptides: pore formers or metabolic inhibitors in bacteria? *Nat Rev Microbiol* 2005;**3**:238–50.

54. Hancock REW, Sahl HG. Antimicrobial and host-defense peptides as new anti-infective therapeutic strategies. *Nat Biotechnol* 2006;**24**:1551–7.

55. Oren Z, Shai Y. Mode of action of linear amphipathic α-helical antimicrobial peptides. *J Pept Sci* 1998;**47**:451–63.

56. Steiner H. Secondary structure of the cecropins: antibacterial peptides from the moth *Hyalophora cecropia*. *FEBS Lett* 1982;**137**:283–7.

57. Shai Y. Mechanism of the binding, insertion and destabilization of phospholipid bilayer membranes by α-helical antimicrobial and cell non-selective membrane-lytic peptides. *Biochim Biophys Acta* 1999;**1462**:55–70.

58. Mahalka AK, Kinnunen PK. Binding of amphipathic α-helical antimicrobial peptides to lipid membranes: lessons from temporins B and L. *Biochim Biophys Acta* 2009;**1788**:1600–9.

59. Matsuzaki K. Why and how are peptide-lipid interactions utilized for self-defense? Magainins and tachyplesins as archetypes. *Biochim Biophys Acta* 1999;**1462**:1–10.

60. Yeaman MR, Yount NY. Mechanisms of antimicrobial peptide action and resistance. *Pharmacol Rev* 2003;**55**:27–55.

61. Maget-Dana R, Ptak M. Penetration of the insect defensin A into phospholipid monolayers and formation of defensin A-lipid complexes. *Biophys J* 1997;**73**:2527.

62. Nguyen LT, Haney EF, Vogel HJ. The expanding scope of antimicrobial peptide structures and their modes of action. *Trends Biotechnol* 2011;**29**:464–72.

63. Selsted ME, Novotny MJ, Morris WL, Tang YQ, Smith W, Cullor JS. Indolicidin, a novel bactericidal tridecapeptide amide from neutrophils. *J Biol Chem* 1992;**267**:4292–5.

64. Frank RW, Gennaro R, Schneider K, Przybylski M, Romeo D. Amino acid sequences of two proline-rich bactenecins. Antimicrobial peptides of bovine neutrophils. *J Biol Chem* 1990;**265**:18871–4.

65. Falla TJ, Karunaratne DN, Hancock RE. Mode of action of the antimicrobial peptide indolicidin. *J Biol Chem* 1996;**271**:19298–303.

66. Subbalakshmi C, Sitaram N. Mechanism of antimicrobial action of indolicidin. *FEMS Microbiol Lett* 1998;**160**:91–6.

67. Romeo D, Skerlavaj B, Bolognesi M, Gennaro R. Structure and bactericidal activity of an antibiotic dodecapeptide purified from bovine neutrophils. *J Biol Chem* 1988;**263**:9573–5.

68. Scott MG, Gold MR, Hancock RE. Interaction of cationic peptides with lipoteichoic acid and gram-positive bacteria. *Infect Immun* 1999;**67**:6445–53.

69. Zhao H, Mattila JP, Holopainen JM, Kinnunen PK. Comparison of the membrane association of two antimicrobial peptides, magainin 2 and indolicidin. *Biophys J* 2001;**81**:2979–91.

70. Matsuzaki K, Murase O, Fujii N, Miyajima K. An antimicrobial peptide, magainin 2, induced rapid flip-flop of phospholipids coupled with pore formation and peptide translocation. *Biochemistry* 1996;**35**:11361–8.

71. Lee MT, Chen FY, Huang HW. Energetics of pore formation induced by membrane active peptides. *Biochemistry* 2004;**43**:3590–9.

72. Yang L, Harroun TA, Weiss TM, Ding L, Huang HW. Barrel-stave model or toroidal model? A case study on melittin pores. *Biophys J* 2001;**81**:1475–85.

73. Yount NY, Bayer AS, Xiong YQ, Yeaman MR. Advances in antimicrobial peptide immunobiology. *Biopolymers* 2006;**84**:435–58.

74. Brotz H, Bierbaum G, Leopold K, Reynolds PE, Sahl HG. The lantibiotic mersacidin inhibits peptidoglycan synthesis by targeting lipid II. *Antimicrob Agents Chemother* 1998;**42**:154–60.

75. Zasloff M. Antimicrobial peptides in health and disease. *N Engl J Med* 2002;**347**:1199–200.

76. Bowdish DM, Davidson DJ, Lau YE, Lee K, Scott MG, Hancock RE. Impact of LL-37 on anti-infective immunity. *J Leukoc Biol* 2005;**77**:451–9.

77. Brown KL, Hancock RE. Cationic host defense (antimicrobial) peptides. *Curr Opin Immunol* 2006;**18**:24–30.
78. Ammar B, Périanin A, Mor A, Sarfati G, Tissot M, Nicolas P, et al. Dermaseptin, a peptide antibiotic, stimulates microbicidal activities of polymorphonuclear leukocytes. *Biochem Biophys Res Commun* 1998;**247**:870–5.
79. Beauregard KA, Truong NT, Zhang H, Lin W, Beck G. The detection and isolation of a novel antimicrobial peptide from the echinoderm, *Cucumaria frondosa*. *Adv Exp Med Biol* 2001;**484**:55–62.
80. Maltseva AL, Aleshina GM, Kokryakov VN, Krasnodembsky EG. Diversity of antimicrobial peptides in acidic extracts from coelomocytes of starfish *Asterias rubens* L. *Biologiya* 2007;**1**:10.
81. Gowda NM, Goswami U, Khan MI. T-antigen binding lectin with antibacterial activity from marine invertebrate, sea cucumber (*Holothuria scabra*): possible involvement in differential recognition of bacteria. *J Invertebr Pathol* 2008;**99**:141–5.
82. Ng TB, Cheung RCF, Wong JH, Ye XJ. Antimicrobial activity of defensins and defensin-like peptides with special emphasis on those from fungi and invertebrate animals. *Curr Protein Pept Sci* 2013;**14**:515–31.
83. Hatakeyama T, Suenaga T, Eto S, Niidome T, Aoyagi H. Antibacterial activity of peptides derived from the C-terminal region of a hemolytic lectin, CEL-III, from the marine invertebrate *Cucumaria echinata*. *J Biochem* 2004;**135**:65–70.
84. Li C, Haug T, Styrvold OB, Jorgensen TO, Stensvag K. Strongylocins, novel antimicrobial peptides from the green sea urchin, *Strongylocentrotus droebachiensis*. *Dev Comp Immunol* 2008;**32**:1430–40.
85. Li C, Blencke HM, Smith LC, Karp MT, Stensvag K. Two recombinant peptides, SpStrongylocins 1 and 2, from *Strongylocentrotus purpuratus*, show antimicrobial activity against Gram-positive and Gram-negative bacteria. *Dev Comp Immunol* 2010;**34**:286–92.
86. Li C, Haug T, Moe MK, Styrvold OB, Stensvag K. Centrocins: isolation and characterization of novel dimeric antimicrobial peptides from the green sea urchin, *Strongylocentrotus droebachiensis*. *Dev Comp Immunol* 2010;**34**:959–68.
87. Haug T, Kjuul AK, Styrvold OB, Sandsdalen E, Olsen OM, Stensvag K. Antibacterial activity in *Strongylocentrotus droebachiensis* (Echinoidea), *Cucumaria frondosa* (Holothuroidea), and *Asterias rubens* (Asteroidea). *J Invertebr Pathol* 2002;**81**:94–102.
88. Schillaci D, Arizza V, Parrinello N, Di Stefano V, Fanara S, Muccilli V, et al. Antimicrobial and antistaphylococcal biofilm activity from the sea urchin *Paracentrotus lividus*. *J Appl Microbiol* 2010;**108**:17–24.
89. Schillaci D, Vitale M, Cusimano MG, Arizza V. Fragments of beta-thymosin from the sea urchin *Paracentrotus lividus* as potential antimicrobial peptides against staphylococcal biofilms. *Ann NY Acad Sci* 2012;**1270**:79–85.
90. Hisamatsu K, Tsuda N, Goda S, Hatakeyama T. Characterization of the alpha-helix region in domain 3 of the haemolytic lectin CEL-III: Implications for self-oligomerization and haemolytic processes. *J Biochem* 2008;**143**:79–86.
91. Schillaci D, Cusimano MG, Cunsolo V, Saletti R, Russo D, Vazzana M, et al. Immune mediators of sea-cucumber *Holothuria tubulosa* (Echinodermata) as source of novel antimicrobial and anti-staphylococcal biofilm agents. *AMB Express* 2013;**3**:35.
92. Tan J, Liu Z, Perfetto M, Han L, Li Q, Zhang Q, et al. Isolation and purification of the peptides from *Apostichopus japonicus* and evaluation of its antibacterial and antitumor activities. *Afr J Microbiol Res* 2012;**6**:8.
93. Hall-Stoodley L, Stoodley P. Evolving concepts in biofilm infections. *Cell Microbiol* 2009;**11**:1034–43.

94. Obst U, Schwartz T, Volkmann H. Antibiotic resistant pathogenic bacteria and their resistance genes in bacterial biofilms. *Int J Artif Organs* 2006;**29**:387–94.

95. Mah T-FC, O'Toole GA. Mechanisms of biofilm resistance to antimicrobial agents. *Trends Microbiol* 2001;**9**:34–9.

96. Van Loosdrecht M, Lyklema J, Norde W, Zehnder A. Influence of interfaces on microbial activity. *Microbiol Rev* 1990;**54**:75–87.

97. Costerton JW, Lewandowski Z, Caldwell DE, Korber DR, Lappin-Scott HM. Microbial biofilms. *Annu Rev Microbiol* 1995;**49**:711–45.

98. Schurr MJ, Martin DW, Mudd MH, Deretic V. Gene cluster controlling conversion to alginate-overproducing phenotype in *Pseudomonas aeruginosa*: functional analysis in a heterologous host and role in the instability of mucoidy. *J Bacteriol* 1994;**176**:3375–82.

99. Boyd A, Chakrabarty AM. *Pseudomonas aeruginosa* biofilms: role of the alginate exopolysaccharide. *J Ind Microbiol* 1995;**15**:162–8.

100. Post JC, Stoodley P, Hall-Stoodley L, Ehrlich GD. The role of biofilms in otolaryngologic infections. *Curr Opin Otolaryngol Head Neck Surg* 2004;**12**:185–90.

101. Stoodley P, Lewandowski Z, Boyle JD, Lappin-Scott HM. The formation of migratory ripples in a mixed species bacterial biofilm growing in turbulent flow. *Environ Microbiol* 1999;**1**:447–55.

102. Horswill AR, Stoodley P, Stewart PS, Parsek MR. The effect of the chemical, biological, and physical environment on quorum sensing in structured microbial communities. *Anal Bioanal Chem* 2007;**387**:371–80.

103. Spoering AL, Gilmore MS. Quorum sensing and DNA release in bacterial biofilms. *Curr Opin Microbiol* 2006;**9**:133–7.

104. Brogden NK, Brogden KA. Will new generations of modified antimicrobial peptides improve their potential as pharmaceuticals? *Int J Antimicrob Ag* 2011;**38**:217–25.

105. Montanaro L, Poggi A, Visai L, Ravaioli S, Campoccia D, Speziale P, et al. Extracellular DNA in biofilms. *Int J Artif Organs* 2011;**34**:824–31.

106. Barken KB, Pamp SJ, Yang L, Gjermansen M, Bertrand JJ, Klausen M, et al. Roles of type IV pili, flagellum-mediated motility and extracellular DNA in the formation of mature multicellular structures in *Pseudomonas aeruginosa* biofilms. *Environ Microbiol* 2008;**10**:2331–43.

107. Hale JD, Hancock RE. Alternative mechanisms of action of cationic antimicrobial peptides on bacteria. *Expert Rev Anti Infect Ther* 2007;**5**:951–9.

108. Chan DI, Prenner EJ, Vogel HJ. Tryptophan- and arginine-rich antimicrobial peptides: structures and mechanisms of action. *Biochim Biophys Acta* 2006;**1758**:1184–202.

109. Schillaci D, Cusimano MG, Russo D, Arizza V. Antimicrobial peptides from echinoderms as antibiofilm agents: a natural strategy to combat bacterial infections. *Ital J Zool* 2014;**81**: 312–21.

110. Schillaci D, Cusimano MG, Spinello A, Barone G, Russo D, Vitale M, et al. Paracentrin 1, a synthetic antimicrobial peptide from the sea-urchin *Paracentrotus lividus*, interferes with staphylococcal and *Pseudomonas aeruginosa* biofilm formation. *AMB Express* 2014;**4**:78.

111. Huff T, Muller CS, Otto AM, Netzker R, Hannappel E. Beta-thymosins, small acidic peptides with multiple functions. *Int J Biochem Cell Biol* 2001;**33**:205–20.

112. Tang YQ, Yeaman MR, Selsted ME. Antimicrobial peptides from human platelets. *Infect Immun* 2002;**70**:6524–33.

113. Fontana R, Mendes MA, de Souza BM, Konno K, Cesar LM, Malaspina O, et al. Jelleines: a family of antimicrobial peptides from the Royal Jelly of honeybees (*Apis mellifera*). *Peptides* 2004;**25**:919–28.

114. Mendes MA, de Souza BM, Marques MR, Palma MS. Structural and biological characterization of two novel peptides from the venom of the neotropical social wasp *Agelaia pallipes pallipes*. *Toxicon* 2004;**44**:67–74.

115. Maselli VM, Brinkworth CS, Bowie JH, Tyler MJ. Host-defence skin peptides of the Australian common froglet *Crinia signifera*: sequence determination using positive and negative ion electrospray mass spectra. *Rapid Commun Mass Spectrom* 2004;**18**:2155–61.

116. Saberwal G, Nagaraj R. Cell-lytic and antibacterial peptides that act by perturbing the barrier function of membranes - facets of their conformational features, structure-function correlations and membrane-perturbing abilities. *Biochim Biophys Acta Rev Biomembr* 1994;**1197**:109–31.

117. Tennessen JA. Molecular evolution of animal antimicrobial peptides: widespread moderate positive selection. *J Evol Biol* 2005;**18**:1387–94.

118. Viljakainen L, Pamilo P. Selection on an antimicrobial peptide defensin in ants. *J Mol Evol* 2008;**67**:643–52.

119. Fernandes JC, Tavaria FK, Fonseca SC, Ramos OS, Pintado ME, Malcata FX. Vitro screening for antimicrobial activity of chitosans and chitooligosaccharides, aiming at potential uses in functional textiles. *J Microbiol Biotechnol* 2010;**20**:311–8.

120. Arizza V. Marine biodiversity as source of new drugs. *Ital J Zool* 2013;**80**:317–8.

121. Zilberman M, Elsner JJ. Antibiotic-eluting medical devices for various applications. *J Control Release* 2008;**130**:202–15.

122. Shukla A, Fleming KE, Chuang HF, Chau TM, Loose CR, Stephanopoulos GN, et al. Controlling the release of peptide antimicrobial agents from surfaces. *Biomaterials* 2010;**31**:2348–57.

123. Glinel K, Thebault P, Humblot V, Pradier C-M, Jouenne T. Antibacterial surfaces developed from bio-inspired approaches. *Acta Biomater* 2012;**8**:1670–84.

124. Huang YB, Huang JF, Chen YX. Alpha-helical cationic antimicrobial peptides: relationships of structure and function. *Protein Cell* 2010;**1**:143–52.

Chapter 13

Inflammatory Response of the Ascidian *Ciona intestinalis*

Parrinello Nicolò[a], Cammarata Matteo[a], Parrinello Daniela[a], Vizzini Aiti[a]
University of Palermo, Palermo, Italy

INTRODUCTION

Tunicates (urochordates) are retained as the closest living relatives of vertebrates.[1,2] They share components of innate immune responses with vertebrates.[3] The sea squirt *Ciona intestinalis* is a noncolonial ascidian that lives mainly in clusters fixed in natural and artificial substrates. It is a simultaneous hermaphrodite, and the swimming small (about 2500 cells) tadpole is comprised of a notochord and dorsal neural tube. Recent reports have shown genetic divergence between populations, suggesting a species-divergence process.[4] Phylogenies inferred from mitochondrial and nuclear DNA markers accredited the existence of two cryptic species: *C. intestinalis* sp. A, genetically homogeneous, distributed in the Mediterranean Sea, Northeast Atlantic, and Pacific, and *C. intestinalis* sp. B in the North Atlantic. The recent papers by Pennati et al.[5] and Brunetti et al.,[6] based on morphological comparisons between adults and larvae of the types A and B, distinguish two species, *Ciona robusta* and *C. intestinalis*, respectively. We study the innate immune system of ascidians from the Mediterranean Sea, and it is reasonable that structures and functions of this system could be largely conserved[7,8] in microevolution. The *Ciona* whole genome has been sequenced and analyzed (about 16,000 protein-coding genes annotated), and a large number of them have single copies.[9] Further molecular analysis between immune genes from the two species and populations could disclose the divergence level of their sequences. In accordance with the previously published papers, in the present review the species nomenclature will be reported as *C. intestinalis*.

SELF/NONSELF RECOGNITION

The possibility exists that *C. intestinalis* simultaneously utilizes two types of self/nonself discrimination systems: tissue histocompatibility, indicated by

---

a. The authors have contributed equally.

Lessons in Immunity: From Single-Cell Organisms to Mammals
http://dx.doi.org/10.1016/B978-0-12-803252-7.00013-8

preliminary allograft rejection experiments,[10] and self/nonself-recognition that plays a key role in the process of interaction between sperm and the vitelline coat (VC) of the egg to block self-fertilization,[11,12] ensuring the maintenance of a high degree of polymorphism. Three highly polymorphic loci (Themis-A, Themis-B, and vCRL1) are retained and are responsible for prevention of self-fertilization.[13,14] v-Themis (a Greek goddess of divine order who prohibits incest) is a component of the VC, whereas s-Themis is expressed in the testis. The recognition of autologous v-Themis on the VC results in sperm detachment or quiescence. The highly polymorphic vCRL1 (variable complement receptor-like 1) gene encodes for a transmembrane protein that structurally resembles mammal complement receptors CD46 (membrane cofactor protein) and CD55 (decay accelerating factor), which regulates the activation of the alternative complement pathway, preventing the destruction of self cells. The vCRL1 gene is expressed in follicle cells, on all nucleated cells, including hemocytes, and serves as a "self" marker in the "missing self" strategy of innate immunity.[14] Themis loci have been identified in both *C. intestinalis* A and B, while vCRL1 has been identified only in B (North Atlantic),[15] supporting the species divergence by affecting their interfertility.

INFLAMMATORY RESPONSES

Inflammation is the body's first response for self-protection by removing harmful stimuli, including damaged cells, irritants, or pathogens, and begins the healing process. Pattern recognition receptors (PRRs) generically recognize the pathogen-associated molecular patterns (PAMPs), including lipopolysaccharides (LPS) on the surface of pathogens or parasites. In invertebrates, circulating coelomocytes or hemocytes exert phagocytosis, cytotoxicity, encapsulation, and synthesize and release inflammatory factors. Phagocytic cells and granulocytes, which synthesize and store bioactive proteins, including microbicidal agents, are common to the majority of species. Cell death appears to be inherent in immune reactivity of many invertebrates with new cells produced by mesodermal hematopoietic tissues.[16]

The *C. intestinalis* inflammatory response is mediated by hemocytes, mainly agranular/hyaline (HA) and granular amebocytes (GA), unilocular refractile granulocytes (URGs, cytoplasm occupied by a unique large granule), compartment cells (cytoplasm occupied by some large vacuoles), signet ring cells (cytoplasm occupied by a unique large vacuole), and morula cells (large granules give a morular feature).[17,18] Hematogenic nodules with hemoblasts are abundant in the pharyngeal wall and around the gut-loop.[19] Circulating lymphocyte-like cells (LLCs) can proliferate and differentiate hemocyte types[20,21]: they express a CD34-like transmembrane protein in agreement with the potential role as pluripotent cells, and a slight but significant frequency increase of CD34+ hemocytes was found after bacteria were inoculated into the body, and few LLCs underwent cell division.[21] GAs and HAs exert phagocytosis, which can be enhanced when the targets are opsonized with lectins, suggesting that a lectin recognition mechanism could also be involved.[22] In addition, GAs produce immune receptor variable regions containing chitin-binding proteins[23] and antimicrobial peptides (AMPs). Notably, these AMPs are not only found inside the tunic large granules but also within other granulocyte subtypes residing in the tunic. URGs express phenoloxidases,[24] can synthesize AMPs,[25] and can be cytotoxic cells with a mechanism that involves both soluble phospholypase A2 (blocked by specific inhibitors and sphingomyelin) and galectin-like lectins (reviewed in Refs 26,27). Infection experiments with EGFP (enhanced green fluorescent protein)-expressing *Escherichia coli* show that HAs promptly engulf bacteria, GAs degranulate, and LLCs proliferate. In addition, infected cells underwent cell death either by necrosis or apoptosis.[21] Likewise, inflammatory cells in the tunic matrix (see section Inflammatory Reaction in the Tunic), including HAs and GAs, lost their membrane integrity, broke completely, and released inner organelles, while some hemocytes underwent apoptosis stages. Finally, a cDNA/EST study identified genes expressed in the hemocytes that appeared to be related to the host defense mechanism. The transcripts have been retained to be involved in detoxification, inflammation, and apoptosis.

Inflammatory Reaction in the Tunic

The tunic is a unique tissue in metazoan, which covers and defends the ascidian soft body. It consists of a matrix containing fibrous material with cellulosic components, collagen-like proteins, elastin, and mucopolysaccharide complex; the outer layer is lined by a thin cuticle and, at the inner layer, by a monolayered epithelium connected to the pharynx by a lacunar connective containing hemocytes.[28–30] Free cells are scattered in the matrix[31]; they probably originate from hematogenetic sites in lacunar connective and migrate across the mantle epithelium into the tunic from the lacunae.[32] In addition, electron microscope observations of inflamed tissues showed proliferating figures in the mantle epithelium, releasing cells into the tunic and thus providing an increased renewal of tunical cells in restricted zones of the adult.[33]

The presence of collagens in the tunic matrix has been shown by histochemical and biochemical methods.[34] In addition, on the basis of cDNA analysis, a type IX-like collagen (with interrupted triple-helices, FACIT) with significant similarity to human and mouse 1α chain type-IX collagen[34,35] has been identified. In situ hybridization revealed the transcript in inflammatory cells in the tunic and pharynx. In the histological section, heterologous antibody showed epitopes of collagen type I-like.[34]

The epidermis consists of flattened or cuboid cells, lined by a basement membrane containing microfibrils and bordered by a basal lamina on the luminal surface. Following the inflammatory stimulus, epidermis cells release vacuolar content into the tunic matrix and, in some points, multilayered tissue suggests

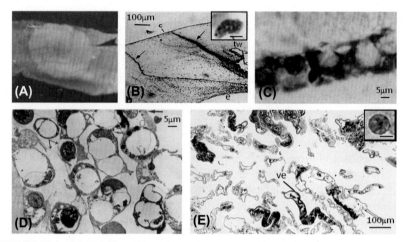

FIGURE 13.1 (A–D) Inflammatory response in the *Ciona intestinalis* tunic matrix and epidermis, at 6–7 days after erythrocyte inoculation. (A) Front view of the capsule. (B) Inflamed tunic transverse section stained with Mallory's stain; in the spot: granular amebocyte (bar: 5 μm). (C) Histological transverse section (Mallory's staining) of epidermis tissue. (D) Transmission electron microscopy. Vacuolization of inflammatory cells and cell membrane dissolution. (E) Pharynx vessels at 4 h after lipopolysaccharides inoculation; in situ hybridization with CiTNFα riboprobe of histological transverse section; in the spot: positive compartment cell (bar: 5 μm). *c*, cuticle; *e*, epidermis; *tw*, tunic wound due to foreign material inoculation; *ve*, vessel epithelium.

epithelium proliferation with consequent cell detachment.[33] The tunic inflammatory process occurs when foreign material is inoculated just below the outer cuticular layer of the tunic matrix, into the middle region of the body that lacks vessels (Fig. 13.1A–D). The inoculated particulate material is mainly maintained in the tunic matrix where the reaction occurs. Subsequent experiments with LPS (see below) revealed that the inflammatory reaction involves the underlying pharynx, which is challenged by the foreign materials or their products.

Encapsulation

An aspecific response was obtained by subcuticular inoculation of corpuscolate ($1–4 \times 10^7$ erythrocytes or their ghosts per ascidian) or soluble materials (40–50 μg bovine serum albumin and hemoglobin, *Octopus* hemocyanin, per ascidian).[36–38] The reaction time for a visible response ranged from some hours (about 24 h) to a few days, and 60–80% treated ascidians showed a whitish circular/elliptical capsule (about 1–2 cm) around the foreign material (Fig. 13.1A), visible through the transparent tunic. There is variability in the response time and deepness of the capsule, presumably dependent on the ascidian populations collected at different seasonal times and collection sites. In any case, histological observations revealed that an incipient cellular response was also present in specimens that did not reveal any visible capsule. Hemagglutination assays of the serum hemolymph with sheep or rabbit erythrocytes as a target disclosed that hemagglutinins, usually present at a low titer in the hemolymph of naïve ascidians,[39] were not found in the hemolymph of treated ascidians at any time after the erythrocyte inoculation, indicating that they could already be involved in the response.[38]

Histological sections and histochemical reactions showed several aspects of the response, as revealed by examining various specimens at different inflammatory stages following a challenge with various particulate materials/ erythrocytes. The response involves both the epidermis and the tunic hemocyte populations (Fig. 13.1B–D). The active epidermis can release granular material gathered to form clusters (histochemical reactions positive for protein and mucopolysaccharides) that contain collagen 1-like protein, as shown by an immunohistochemical reaction with a heterologous antibody.[34] Such a material, together with numerous univacuolated large "signet ring cells," forms dense bands that envelope the reaction area (Fig. 13.1D). Likewise, in the response of circulating hemocytes affected by EGFP-expressing *E. coli*, amorphous substances are released from their vacuoles through plasma membrane dissolution (Fig. 13.1C,D). Vacuolization and membrane dissolution, also shown by a transmission electron microscopy study (Fig. 13.1D), strongly characterize the cellular responses.[37,38,40–42] In several experiments, a very variable number of inoculated specimens (about 3–40%) showed a tissue injury produced independently from the inoculated material type, while amebocytes, granulocytes with small granules and "signet ring cells," were lined to form a layer under the tunic wound. The wound may be related to the severe degranulation process of granulocytes, cytoplasm vacuolization, and cell autolysis of granulocytes and vacuolated cells.[41–43] Finally, phagocytes and URGs were scattered in the inflamed tissue, and some LLCs could be found. URGs and, mainly, compartment/morula cells, contain and presumably release AMPs into the tunic matrix.[44]

In general, two main events occur: (1) autolysis (necrosis/apoptosis) of inflammatory cells that contributes to the destruction of the inflamed tunic, causing a wound, and (2) release of a substance that could contribute to building the tunic matrix. Likewise, circulating HAs and GAs from specimens infected with EGFP-*E. coli* undergo death either by necrosis or apoptosis.[21] In this respect, a granulation phase in which fibroblast-like hemocytes (compartment/morula cells) express Ci-type-IX collagen 1α-chain[45] and collagen type I-like fibers[34] could contribute to capsule composition as well as to tunic wound repair. Since the tunic matrix in the median region of the body lacks vessels, the highly dense cell populations that enriched the tunic could be due to both hemocyte migration through the mantle epithelium and cell proliferation from the underlying connective and pharynx tissues.[32,33]

The aspecificity of the reaction was also supported by priming experiments with sheep erythrocytes by a second inoculation into the body side opposite to the first one, in specimens in which the first inoculation (six dd p.i.) did not cause a visible capsule within 6 days postinoculation.[38] In any case, no significant effect of the priming procedure was found.

THE PHARYNX IS PROMPTLY INVOLVED IN THE INFLAMMATORY REACTION

Pharynx is the foremost part of the ascidian digestive tract and consists of two epithelial monolayers perforated by rows of ciliated stigmata aligned dorso-ventrally and enclosing a mesh of vessels (transversal and longitudinal bars) where hemolymph, rich in hemocytes, flows.[46,47] Epithelial host stationary cells gathered in clusters, called lymph nodules, could originate the hemocyte type from dividing hemoblasts.[19] The ciliated stigmata generate water current that serves for respiration and a supply of organic particles, including bacteria. In the floor of the pharynx, the endostyle is a groove on the bottom of the pharynx that produces mucus, a complex mucoprotein for filter feeding.[48,49] This organ is histologically divided into functional "zones" (1–9 from the groove bottom) of which the zones 2, 4, and 6 are the main secretory regions.[49]

Pharynx is considered the main ascidian immune-competent organ,[50] and during the *C. intestinalis* encapsulation process, small lymph nodules and folding of the vessel epithelium proliferate and extrude cells.[32,33]

To examine the role of the pharynx in the inflammatory response, LPS (200 μg/ascidian) was inoculated according to the above reported procedure. LPS, part of the outer membrane of gram-negative bacteria, is one of the most potent inducers of inflammation.[51] In mammals, LPS challenge occurs via CD14 and Toll-like receptors (TLRs) involving the activation of transcription factor NF-κB. In brief, LPS-binding protein binds LPS and catalyzes the transfer of individual LPS molecules to CD14 that acts as a coreceptor.[52,53] TLRs consist of an ectodomain that encompasses several tandem leucine-rich repeats (LRRs) and a cytoplasmic Toll/interleukin-1 receptor (TIR) domain. The signaling induces the production of proinflammatory cytokines responsible for a direct innate response and for triggering adaptive immune cells.

Although LPS was not an optimal irritant to induce a well-visible capsule in the tunic of *C. intestinalis*, it can reach and challenge the pharynx epithelium, hemocytes, and lymph nodules, eliciting inflammatory factors. Homologous of mammal TLRs-4-6-7 have been identified by screening the genome sequences of *C. intestinalis*,[54] and several genes involved in the TLR signaling, including MyD88, IRAK, TRAF, IκB, and NF-κB, have been annotated. Sasaki et al.[55] examined CiTLR1 and CiTLR2 putative protein sequences, which showed the typical TLR architecture with extracellular transmembrane domains and multiple extracellular LRRs. Both genes are expressed in the stomach, intestine, and in hemocytes; their products interact with multiple PAMPs and show equipotent NF-κB activation. Counterparts of *Ciona* LPS-binding protein and bactericidal/permeability-increasing protein (CiBPI) sequence cluster with oyster LBP/BPI and form a group with mammalian homologues.[56] The inclusion into the gene family was supported by further phylogenetic analysis.[57]

Apparently, *Ciona* is comprised of LPS-challenged machinery components. Cloning, real-time PCR analysis, in situ hybridization, and immunohistochemistry were performed on pharynx tissue before and after LPS inoculation (reviewed in Ref. 58). The following pharynx inflammatory factors and pathways are promptly elicited (few hours) by LPS inoculation.

C-Type Lectins

CD94

In general, lectins are carbohydrate recognition proteins characterized by a typical domain (CRD), which can be Ca^{2+}-dependent or Ca^{2+}-independent, useful for their activity, and form wide protein superfamilies present in both vertebrates and invertebrates.[59] Many members bind to proteins, rather than sugars, in a Ca^{2+}-independent manner. One such C-type protein, CD94, is part of several receptors of vertebrate innate immunity cells and interacts with MHC class I molecules expressed predominantly on the surface NK (natural killer) cells and a subset of CD8+ T-lymphocytes. A *C. intestinalis* CiCD94-1, homologue to human CD94, shares structural features with the C-type lectin-like domain (CTLD)-containing molecules that recognize proteins.[60] None of the tunic cells express CiCD94-1 mRNA, whereas immunohistochemistry analysis indicated that both tunic and hemolymph GAs contain the protein, supporting that they reach the tunic already equipped with the gene product. In this respect, following LPS inoculation, the CiCD94-1 gene transcription was upregulated in circulating granular amebocytes in which mRNA and protein were found. In vitro experiments revealed that the percentage of CiCD94-1 positive granular amebocytes increase up to 80% and can exert CiCD94-dependent phagocytosis.[60]

Lectin-Dependent Complement Pathway

Mannose-binding lectins (MBLs) are collagen-containing Ca^{2+}-dependent C-type lectins that belong to the collectin family as soluble PRRs. MBLs exert several functions, including complement activation, microbe agglutination, opsonization, and modulation of the inflammatory response.[61] A differential screening between LPS-challenged and naïve *C. intestinalis* allowed the isolation of a full-length cDNA encoding for a CiMBL that, as shown by the phylogenetic tree, forms a cluster related to the vertebrate MBL, suggesting that CiMBL evolved early as a prototype of vertebrate collectins.[62,63] The CiMBL gene transcription is strongly upregulated by LPS inoculation, and the collectin is expressed by granular amebocytes and hemocytes with large granules. In the gut epithelia, two MBL homologues have also been reported.[63] These CiMBLs colocalize with an MBL-associated serine protease (MASP), responsible for complement activation, supporting their involvement in a lectin-mediated complement pathway. In vertebrates, three pathways (antibody-mediated, lectin-mediated, and alternative) triggered by pathogens converge to the proteolysis of the C3 central complement component. In *Ciona*, two CiC3-like genes from hemocytes have been cloned.[64] The putative proteins exhibit canonical processing sites, including a typical thioester site with the His residue required for nucleophilic activation. In addition, four CiMASPs that exert trypsin-like activity and the corresponding CiCR3/CR4 receptors have been recognized in the genome, while ESTs revealed transcripts in hemocytes[65] and intestine/stomach epithelia.[63] On the whole, genome sequence analysis, EST analysis, cloning, and expression studies identified nine mannose-binding lectins (CiMBLs), nine ficolins, and four CiMBL-associated serine proteases (CiMASPs C1r/C1s-like). The pathway (CiMBLs/ficolins as PRPs) is initiated by the recognition of PAMPs and is activated by CiMASPs, leading to CiC4, CiC2, and CiC3 cleavage.[66] LPS upregulates the CiC3 gene transcription in hemocytes and activates the CiC3 proteolysis, leading to an anaphylotoxin-like proinflammatory peptide (CiC3a) that exerts a chemotactic effect on hemocytes interacting with a receptor molecule, CiC3aR, coupled with Gi protein.[67,68] In addition, the genome analysis identified 11 presumptive genes with the membrane attack complex (MAC)/perforin domain, nine of them exhibiting domain structures similar to those of late complement components, which form a cytolytic complex. Finally, the pathway may be regulated by two proteinase inhibitors similar to α2 macroglobulin.[66] Phylogenetic analysis suggests that CiC3 1, 2 genes are produced by duplication, and CiMASPs are diverged from a common ancestor of vertebrate C3/C4/C5 and MASP/C1r/C1s, respectively.

Galectins

Galectins are Ca^{2+}-independent lectins (reviewed in Ref. 69) that contain either one (mono-CRD) or two (bi-CRD) evolutionary conserved CRDs that bind β-galactosides. They are mainly cytosolic or exert extracellular functions by binding to and cross-linking glycan groups of glycoproteins and/or glycolipids on the surface of various cell types. They are involved in numerous biological processes, including immune responses. Recently, Nita-Lazar et al.[70] demonstrated both in vitro and in vivo expression and secretion of galectins (Gal1, Gal3) modulated during IAV infection. In vitro, they disclosed the galectin binding to the epithelial cell surface that modulates the expression of SOCS1 and RIG1 and activates ERK, AKT, or JAK/STAT1 signaling pathways, leading to a disregulated expression and release of proinflammatory cytokines.

The sequences of two *C. intestinalis* genes encoding bi-CRD galectins (CiLgals-a and CiLgals-b) have been deducted from ESTs and genome analysis.[71] Phylogenetic analysis showed that CiLgals resulted aligned with bi-CRD galectins from vertebrates, cephalochordates, echinoderms, and a mono-CRD galectin from the ascidian *Clavelina picta*. Previous results have shown that the LPS treatment increases the hemolymphatic level of galectin-like molecules with opsonic properties.[71] On the other hand, real-time PCR analysis and in situ hybridization have shown that CiLgals-a and CiLgals-b are inducible by LPS, which upregulates the gene transcription.[71] Both galectins are promptly expressed (in situ hybridization and immunohistochemistry) in the inflamed pharynx, localized in multivacuolar (compartment) cells, and they can be components of the vessel epithelium basal membrane. In addition, both galectins are produced by endostyle zones. CiLgals-a and CiLgals-b are constitutively expressed in zone 2 and 3, respectively, and the gene transcription is differentially upregulated by LPS[72]: both are upregulated in zone 2, whereas CiLgals-b is also upregulated in zone 3 and 4. These findings suggest that CiLgals-a and -b could have a role both in filter feeding and defense.[72]

Cytokines

Vertebrate tumor necrosis factor (TNFα) is a component of a wide TNF family. A membrane-bound form can be cleaved, and the mature cytokine may be released as a soluble form by cells of innate immunity; it regulates inflammatory reactions and recruits and activates inflammatory cells.[73] In the *C. intestinalis* genome, one CiTNF-like and three CiTNF receptor-like genes have been identified.[74] The CiTNFα has been cloned from the pharynx before and after LPS inoculation,[75] and the deduced amino acid sequence clusters at a phylogenetic position close to vertebrate TNFα. It is constitutively expressed by pharynx hemocytes and promptly enhanced by LPS. A larger cell-bound cytokine form in the hemocytes and a smaller one in the serum hemolymph suggest roles in both local and systemic responses. After LPS inoculation, in situ hybridization with CiTNFα riboprobe and immunohistochemistry with specific antibody showed an increased number of positive amebocytes with large granules, contained in the pharynx vessels, in the connective tissue lining the tunic and vessel epithelium (Fig. 13.1E) as well as in circulating hyaline amebocytes and granulocytes. The gene transcription can also be upregulated in stomach and intestine epithelia in response to CiTLR ligands.[53]

Vertebrate IL-17 is a proinflammatory cytokine that plays a key role in the clearance of extracellular bacteria promoting cell infiltration and the production of several cytokines and chemokines. In humans, six IL-17 family members (IL-17A-F) and five IL-17 receptors (IL-17RA-E) have been identified.[76] IL-17 displays proinflammatory properties, like those of TNFα, in its capacity to induce other inflammatory effectors, and it synergizes with other cytokines at the center of the inflammatory network to activate the NF-κB. Three *Ciona* IL-17 homologues (*Ci*IL17 1–3) show structure, gene organization, and phylogenetic relationships with the mammalian IL-17A and IL-17F supporting a molecular common ancestor in the chordate lineage. These cytokines are promptly expressed on induction by LPS inoculation. The gene transcription is upregulated in the pharynx and expressed by hemocytes (granulocytes and URGs) inside the pharynx vessels.[77] In addition, hemocytes express a CiIL-17 receptor gene that shows homology to the cytoplasmic region of mammalian IL-17R.

Prophenoloxidase

In invertebrates, the cascade reaction named "prophenoloxidase activating system" (proPO) is a melanogenic pathway that has been co-opted in immune reactions (reviewed in Ref. 78). This pathway also participates in ascidian tunic formation. In the tunic of *C. intestinalis*, proteases diverse from serine proteases could activate the pathway, and quinones, mainly contained in the matrix, can be the substrate. The proenzyme is also activated by LPS in a Ca^{2+}-independent pathway to produce a Cu^{2+}-dependent orthodiphenoloxidase. Following LPS inoculation, the tunic matrix is densely populated by hemocytes (among them many URGs, granulocytes with several granules and rare morula cells) that show PO activity.[79] Two POs (CiPO-1, CiPO-2) distinct in their sizes have been reported,[80] and the CiPO2 seems to be a constitutive component. The two phenoloxidases have been sequenced, and they display similarity to arthropod hemocyanins.[78] Studies on the CiPO2 showed that the gene transcription is upregulated by LPS, suggesting that the PO is inducible and highly expressed in the inflamed tissues. The transcripts were found in pharynx granulocytes, mainly in URGs.[80] There is indirect evidence that CiproPO activation products have an effect on hemocyte activity, including the uptake of bacteria by phagocytes[78] and cytotoxicity.[26,27]

Fibril-Associated Collagen With Interrupted Triple Helix-Like Collagen

Collagens are major structural components of the extracellular matrix in vertebrate and invertebrate organisms where they are also involved in defense responses, including reparative processes.[81] The nonfibril-forming collagen class includes the type IX that is "fibril-associated collagen with interrupted triple helice" (FACIT). In vertebrates, acute inflammatory reactions result in a regulated pattern of tissue repair with collagen fiber bundles increasingly organized during remodeling. A Ci-type IX-Col 1α-chain nucleotide sequence is contained in the *Ciona* genome, and the protein sequence deduced from the cDNA cloned from pharynx tissue is characterized by three short triple-helical domains interspersed with four nontriple-helical sequences and shows the structural features of fibril-associated FACIT collagen.[35] The structure appears to be formed by Gly–X–Y repeats in three short triple-helical domains interspersed with four nontriple-helical sequence domains. The structural homologies suggest that, like in mammals, it may be involved in forming a network of nonfibril-forming collagens of the tunic matrix. Real-time PCR analysis disclosed that LPS inoculation or in vitro treatment enhances the gene expression, while in situ hybridization and immunocytochemistry indicated hemocytes, mainly morula cells, as collagen-producing cells.[45] Following LPS inoculation, transcripts and proteins were also found in the epidermis and in cells associated with the epidermis. These findings suggest that a granulation tissue could participate in inflammation and wound healing.

Catabolite Activator Protein

Transcription activation is a process carried out by a combination of a complex set of gene activators. The catabolite activator protein (CAP, also known as cAMP receptor protein, CRP) is a transcriptional activator, present as homodimer in solution, each subunit including a ligand-binding domain at the N-terminus and a DNA-binding domain at the C-terminus.[82] Two cAMP molecules bind dimeric CAP and function as allosteric effectors by increasing the affinity for DNA. Components of the CAP superfamily have been linked to several biological functions, including immune defense. Many components contain a CAP domain, whereas others contain additional C-terminus extensions related to biological roles. A differential screening between LPS-treated and naïve *C. intestinalis* allowed the isolation of a full-length cDNA. Analysis of the deduced amino acid sequence showed that the protein (CiCAP) displays a modular structure with similarities to the vertebrate CAP superfamily as well as to a collagen-binding adhesin of *Streptococcus mutans*.[83] Quantitative mRNA expression, performed by real-time PCR analysis, showed that the gene transcription is promptly activated in the pharynx after LPS inoculation. Moreover, in situ hybridization assay disclosed that CiCAP mRNA is highly produced by hemocytes with large granules that are contained inside the pharynx vessels. Thus CiCAP represents a protein with novel structural domains, involved in ascidian immune responses, probably as a component of the transcription activation complex.

CONCLUSIONS

Animal evolution is the result of diverse and interactive biological processes between elements of the ecosystems on which life depends. Damaging interactions between a species and foreign materials lead to the body's self-protection to avoid host homeostasis disruption. That forms the basis of the immune responses devoted to the recognition and rejection of unrelated materials through appropriate receptors and effector cells. Since the *C. intestinalis* inflammatory response can be aspecifically challenged by several irritants, the possibility exists that it can be based on the "missing self" strategy of innate immunity.

Various innate and adaptive immune responses may have developed under pressure of various invader diversity in several environmental conditions. In *Ciona*, prodromes of higher chordate inflammation have been observed, including cell vacuolization, signet ring cells differentiation, and plasma membrane dissolution, while molecular diversification of common immune ancestral genes has been driven to fit with invader diversity. In addition preserved sequences and molecular traits of an ancestral chordate appear as building materials for the increasing complexity of the vertebrate immune systems. Similarly to vertebrates, the *C. intestinalis* inflammatory reactions also result in a pattern of tissue repair with collagen-like expression during remodeling. Conversely, the prophenoloxidase system of *Ciona* can be related to a typical response of the invertebrate immunity. Findings on *C. intestinalis* immune gene's involvement in several developmental phases[60,84,85] strengthen the concept of gene co-option during evolution. Finally, immune gene expression and functions of this nonvertebrate chordate could help to clarify how chordates originated and how vertebrate developmental innovations evolved. Further comparative analysis between *Ciona* populations could reveal the effects of reproductive isolation and diversity of their environments on inflammatory machinery and immune genes' evolution.

ACKNOWLEDGMENTS

This work was supported by a research grant from the Italian Ministry of Education (PRIN 2006 and 2010–11 to NP), co-funded by the University of Palermo.

REFERENCES

1. Delsuc F, Brinkmann H, Chourrout D, Philippe H. Tunicates and not cephalochordates are the closest living relatives of vertebrates. *Nature* 2006;**439**:965–8.
2. Delsuc F, Tsagkogeorga G, Lartillot N, Philippe H. Additional molecular support for the new chordate phylogeny. *Genesis* 2008;**46**:592–4.
3. Khalturin K, Panzer Z, Cooper MD, Bosch TC. Recognition strategies in the innate immune system of ancestral chordates. *Mol Immunol* 2004;**41**:1077–87.
4. Caputi L, Andreakis N, Mastrototaro F, Cirino P, Vassillo M, Sordino P. Cryptic speciation in a model invertebrate chordate. *PNAS* 2007;**29**:9364–9.
5. Brunetti R, et al. Morphological evidence that the molecularly determined *Ciona intestinalis* type A and type B are different species: *Ciona robusta* and *Ciona intestinalis*. *J Zool Syst Evol Res* 2015;**53**. http://dx.doi.org/10.1111jzs. 12101.
6. Pennati, et al. Morphological differences between larvae of the *Ciona intestinalis* species complex: hints for a valid taxonomic definition of distinct species. *PLoS One* 2015;**10**(5):e0122879. http://dx.doi.org/10.1371/journal.pone.0122879.
7. Dzik JM. The ancestry and cumulative evolution of immune reactions. *Acta Biochim Pol* 2010;**57**:443–6.
8. Du Pasquier L. Innate immunity in early chordates and the appearance of adaptive immunity. *CR Biol* 2004;**327**:591–601.
9. Dehal P, Satou R, Campbell J, Chapman J, Degnan B, DeTomaso A, et al. The draft genome of *Ciona intestinalis*: insights into chordate and vertebrate origins. *Science* 2002;**298**:2157–67.
10. Reddy AL, Bryan B, Hildemann H. Integumentary allograft versus autograft reactions in *Ciona intestinalis*: a protochordate species of solitary tunicate. *Immunogenetics* 1975;**1**:584–90.
11. Pinto MR, De Santis R, Marino R, Usui N. Specific induction of self-discrimination by follicle cells in *Ciona intestinalis* oocytes. *Dev Growth Differ* 1995;**37**:287–91.
12. Kürn U, Sommer F, Bosch TC, Khalturin K. In the urochordate *Ciona intestinalis* zona pellucida domain proteins vary among individuals. *Dev Comp Immunol* 2007;**31**:1242–54.
13. Harada Y, Takagaki Y, Sunagawa M, Saito T, Yamada L, Taniguchi H, et al. Mechanism of self-sterility in a hermaphroditic chordate. *Science* 2008;**2008**(320):548–50.
14. Khalturin K, Bosch TCG. Self/nonself discrimination at the basis of chordate evolution: limits on molecular conservation. *Curr Opin Immunol* 2007;**19**:4–9.

15. Sommer F, Awazu S, Anton-Erxleben F, Klimovich AV, Klimovich BV, Samailovich MP, et al. Blood system formation in the urochordate *Ciona intestinalis* requires the variable receptor vCRL1. *Mol Biol Evol* 2012;**29**:3081–93.

16. Smith V. Immunology of invertebrates: cellular. In: *LS*. Chichester: John Wiley & Sons Ltd; 2010.

17. Arizza V, Parrinello D. Inflammatory hemocytes in *Ciona intestinalis* innate immune response. *Invertebr Surv J* 2009;**6**:58–66.

18. De Leo G. Ascidian hemocytes and their involvement in defense reaction. *It J Zool* 1992;**59**: 195–214.

19. Ermak TH. The hematogeneic tissues of Tunicates. In: Wright RK, Cooper EL, editors. *Phylogeny of thymus and bone marrow bursa cells*. Amsterdam: Elsevier/North Holland; 1976. p. 45–56.

20. Cooper EL, Raftos DA. The significance of cultivating cells and hemopoietic tissue from tunicates. *Adv Exp Med Biol* 1995;**371A**:321–5.

21. Liu L, Wu C, Chen T, Zhang X, Li F, Luo W, et al. Effects of infection of EGFP-expressing *Escherichia coli* on haemocytes in *Ciona intestinalis*. *J Exp Mar Biol Ecol* 2006;**332**:121–34.

22. Parrinello N, Arizza V, Cammarata M, Giaramita FT, Pergolizzi M, Vazzana M, et al. Inducible lectins with galectin properties and human IL1α epitopes opsonize yeast during the inflammatory response of the ascidian *Ciona intestinalis*. *Cell Tissue Res* 2007;**329**:379–90.

23. Dishaw LJ, Flores-Torres JA, Mueller MG, Karrer C, Skapura DP, Melillo D, et al. A basal chordate model for studies of gut microbial immune interactions. *Front Immunol* 2012;**3**:1–10.

24. Parrinello N, Arizza V, Chinnici C, Parrinello D, Cammarata M. Phenoloxidases in ascidian hemocytes: characterization of the pro-phenoloxidase activating system. *Comp Biochem Phys* 2003;**135B**:583–91.

25. Fedders H, Leippe M. A reverse search for antimicrobial peptides in *Ciona intestinalis* identification of a gene family expressed in hemocytes and evaluation of activity. *Dev Comp Immunol* 2008;**32**:286–98.

26. Parrinello N. Cytotoxic activity of tunicate hemocytes. In: Rinkevich B, Müller WEG, editors. *Invertebr Immunol Progr Mol Subcell Biol* 1996;**15**:196–216.

27. Arizza V, Parrinello D, Cammarata M, Vazzana M, Vizzini A, Giaramita FT, et al. A lytic mechanism based on soluble phospholypases A2 (sPLA2) and β-galactoside specific lectins is exerted by *Ciona intestinalis* (ascidian) unilocular refractile hemocytes against K562 cell line and mammalian erythrocytes. *Fish Shellfish Immunol* 2011;**30**:1014–23.

28. Burighel P, Cloney RA. Urochordata: Ascidiacea. In: Harrison FW, Ruppert EE, editors. *Microscopical anatomy of invertebrates*, vol. 15. New York: Wiley-Liss; 1997. p. 221–47.

29. De Leo G, Patricolo E, D'Ancona Lunetta G. Studies on the fibrous components of the test of *Ciona intestinalis* L. I. Cellulose-like polysaccharide. *Acta Zool* 1977;**58**:135–41.

30. Patricolo E, De Leo G. Studies on the fibrous components of the test of *Ciona intestinalis* Linnaeus II. Collagen-elastin-like protein. *Acta Zool* 1979;**60**:259–69.

31. De Leo G, Patricolo E, Frittitta G. Fine structure of the tunic of *Ciona intestinalis* L. II. Tunic morphology, cell distribution and their functional importance. *Acta Zool* 1981;**62**:256–71.

32. Di Bella MA, De Leo G. Hemocyte migration during inflammatory-like reaction of *Ciona intestinalis* (Tunicata, Ascidiacea). *J Invert Pathol* 2000:105–11.

33. Di Bella MA, Carbone MC, De Leo G. Aspects of cell production in mantle tissue of *Ciona intestinalis* L. (Tunicata, Ascidiacea). *Micron* 2005;**36**:477–81.

34. Vizzini A, Arizza V, Cervello M, Chinnici C, Cammarata M, Gambino R, et al. Identification of type I and IX collagens in the ascidian *Ciona intestinalis*. In: Sawada H, Yokosawa H, Lambert CC, editors. *The Biology of ascidians*. Tokyo: Springer-Verlag; 2001. p. 402–7.

35. Vizzini A, Arizza V, Cervello M, Cammarata M, Gambino R, Parrinello N. Cloning and expression of a type IX-like collagen in tissues of the ascidian *Ciona intestinalis*. *Biochim Biophys Acta* 2002;**1577**:38–44.

36. Parrinello N. The reaction of *Ciona intestinalis* L. to subcuticular erythrocyte and protein injection. *Dev Comp Immunol* 1981;**5**:105–10.

37. Parrinello N, Patricolo E, Canicattì C. Tunicate immunobiology. 1. Tunic reaction of *Ciona intestinalis* L. to erythrocyte injection. *Boll Zool* 1977;**44**:373–81.

38. Parrinello N, Patricolo E, Canicattì C. Inflammatory-like reaction in the tunic of *Ciona intestinalis* (Tunicata). 1. Encapsulation and tissue injury. *Biol Bull* 1984;**167**:229–37.

39. Parrinello N, Patricolo E. Erythrocyte agglutinins in the blood of certain ascidians. *Experientia* 1975;**31**:1092–3.

40. Parrinello N, Patricolo E. Inflammatory-like reaction in the tunic of *Ciona intestinalis* (Tunicata). II. Capsule components. *Biol Bull* 1984;**167**:238–50.

41. De Leo G, Parrinello N, Parrinello D, Cassara G, Di Bella MA. Encapsulation response of *Ciona intestinalis* (Ascidiacea) to intratunical erythrocyte injection. I. The inner capsular architecture. *J Invertebr Pathol* 1996;**67**:205–12.

42. De Leo G, Parrinello N, Parrinello D, Cassarà G, Russo D, Di Bella MA. Encapsulation response of *Ciona intestinalis* (Ascidiacea) to intratunical erythrocyte injection: II. The outermost inflamed area. *J Invertebr Pathol* 1997;**69**:14–23.

43. Parrinello N, De Leo G, Di Bella MA. Fine structural observations of the granulocytes involved in the tunic inflammatory-like reaction of *Ciona intestinalis* (Tunicata). *J Invertebr Pathol* 1990;**56**:181–9.

44. Di Bella MA, Fedders H, De Leo G, Leippe M. Tunic localization of antimicrobial peptides in the tunic of *Ciona intestinalis* (Ascidiacea, Tunicata) and their involvement in local inflammatory-like reactions. *Res Immunol* 2011;**1**:70–5.

45. Vizzini A, Pergolizzi M, Vazzana M, Salerno G, Di Sano C, Macaluso P, et al. FACIT collagen (1a-chain) is expressed by hemocytes and epidermis during the inflammatory response of the ascidian *Ciona intestinalis*. *Dev Comp Immunol* 2008;**32**:682–92.

46. De Leo G, Parrinello N, Di Bella MA. Fine structure of blood system in *Ciona intestinalis* L. (Tunicata). Vessels and hemocytes in pharyngeal wall. *Arch Biol Bruss* 1987;**98**:35–52.

47. Pestarino M, Fiala-Medioni A, Ravera F. Ultrastructure of the branchial wall of a lower chordate: the ascidian *Ciona intestinalis*. *J Morphol* 1988;**197**:269–76.

48. Petersen JK. Ascidian suspension feeding. *J Exp Mar Biol Ecol* 2007;**342**:127–37.

49. Flood PF, Fiala-Medioni A. Ultrastructure and histochemistry of the food trapping mucous in benthic filter feeders (Ascidians). *Acta Zool Stockh* 1981;**62**:53–65.

50. Giacomelli S, Melillo D, Lambris JD, Pinto MR. Immune competence of the *Ciona intestinalis* pharynx: complement system-mediated activity. *Fish Shellfish Immunol* 2012;**33**:946–52.

51. Galanos C, Freudenberg MA. Mechanism of endotoxin shock and endotoxin hypersensitivity. *Immunobiol* 1993;**187**:346–56.

52. Satake H, Sasaki N. Comparative overview of Toll-like receptors in lower animals. *Zool Sci* 2010;**27**:154–61.

53. Coscia MR, Giacomelli S, Oreste U. Toll-like receptors: an overview from invertebrates to vertebrates. *Invert Surviv J* 2011;**8**:210–26.

54. Azumi K, De Santis R, De Tomaso A, Rigoutsos I, Yoshizaki F, Pinto MR, et al. Genomic analysis of immunity in an Urochordate and the emergence of the vertebrate immune system: "waiting for Godot". *Immunogenetics* 2003;**55**:570–81.

55. Sasaki N, Ogasawara M, Sekiguchi T, Kusumoto S, Satake H. Toll-like receptors of the ascidian *Ciona intestinalis*: prototypes with hybrid functionalities of vertebrate Toll-like receptors. *J Biol Chem* 2009;**284**:27336–43.

56. Gonzalez M, Gueguen Y, Destoumieux-Garzon D, Romestand B, Fievet J, Pugniére M, et al. Evidence of a bactericidal permeability increasing protein in an invertebrate, the *Crassostrea gigas* Cg-BPI. *PNAS* 2007;**104**:17759–64.

57. Krasity BC, Troll JV, Weiss P, McFall-Ngai MJ. LBP/BPI proteins and their relatives: conservation over evolution and roles in mutualism. *Biochem Soc Trans* 2011;**39**:1039–44.

58. Parrinello N. Focusing on *Ciona intestinalis* (Tunicata) innate immune system. Evolutionary implications. *Invert Surviv J* 2009;**6**:S46–57.

59. Zelensky AN, Gready JE. The C-type lectin-like domain superfamily. *FEBS J* 2005;**272**:6179–217.

60. Zucchetti I, Marino R, Pinto MR, Lambris JD, Du Pasquier L, De Santis R. ciCD94-1, an ascidian multipurpose C-type lectin-like receptor expressed in *Ciona intestinalis* hemocytes and larval neural structures. *Differentiation* 2008;**76**:267–82.

61. Eddie Ip WK, Takahashi K, Ezekowitz RA, Stuart LM. Mannose-binding lectin and innate immunity. *Immunol Rev* 2009;**230**:9–21.

62. Bonura A, Vizzini A, Salerno G, Parrinello N, Longo V, Colombo P. Isolation and expression of a novel MBL-like collectin cDNA enhanced by LPS injection in the body wall of the ascidian *Ciona intestinalis*. *Mol Immunol* 2009;**46**:2389–94.

63. Skjoedt MO, Palarasah Y, Rasmussen K, Vitved L, Salomonsen J, Kliem A, et al. Two mannose-binding lectin homologues and an MBL-associated serine protease are expressed in the gut epithelia of the urochordate species *Ciona intestinalis*. *Dev Comp Immunol* 2010;**34**:59–68.

64. Marino R, Kimura Y, De Santis R, Lambris JD, Pinto MR. Complement in urochordates: cloning and characterization of two C3-like genes in the ascidian *Ciona intestinalis*. *Immunogenetics* 2002;**53**:1055–64.

65. Shida K, Terajima D, Uchino R, Ikawa S, Ikeda M, Asano K, et al. Hemocytes of *Ciona intestinalis* express multiple genes involved in innate immune host defense. *Biochem Biophys Res Comm* 2003;**302**:207–18.

66. Fujita T, Endo Y, Nonaka M. Primitive complement system—recognition and activation. *Mol Immunol* 2004;**41**:103–11.

67. Pinto MR, Chinnici C, Kimura Y, Melillo D, Marino R, Spruce LA, et al. CiC3-1a-mediated chemotaxis in the deuterostome invertebrate *Ciona intestinalis* (Urochordata). *J Immunol* 2003;**171**:5521–8.

68. Melillo D, Sfyroera G, De Santis R, Graziano R, Marino R, Lambris JD, et al. First identification of a chemotactic receptor in an invertebrate species: structural and functional characterization of *Ciona intestinalis* C3a receptor. *J Immunol* 2006;**177**:4132–40.

69. Ballarin L, Cammarata M, Franchi N, Parrinello N. Routes in innate immunity evolution: galectins and rhamnose-binding lectins in ascidians. In: Kim S-K, editor. *Marine proteins and peptides. Biological activities and applications*. Singapore: John Wiley & Sons Ltd; 2013. p. 185–205.

70. Nita-Lazar M, et al. Galectins regulate the inflammatory response in airway epithelial cells exposed to microbial neuraminidase by modulating the expression of SOCS1 and RIG1. *Mol Immunol* 2015;**68**. http://dx.doi.org/10.1016/j.molimm.2015.08.005.

71. Vizzini A, Parrinello D, Sanfratello MA, Salerno G, Cammarata M, Parrinello N. Inducible galectins are expressed in the inflamed pharynx of the ascidian *Ciona intestinalis*. *Fish Shellfish Immunol* 2012;**32**:101–9.

72. Parrinello D, Sanfratello MA, Vizzini A, Parrinello N. Cammarata M *Ciona intestinalis* endostyle zones differentially express galectins (*Ci*Lgals-a and *Ci*Lgals-b) upregulated by LPS. *Fish Shellfish Immunol* 2015;**42**:171–6.

73. Akira S, Hirano T, Taga T, Kishimoto T. Biology of multifunctional cytokines: IL 6 and related molecules (IL 1 and TNF). *FASEB J* 1990;**4**:2860–7.

74. Terajima D, Shida K, Takada N, Kasuya A, Rokhsar D, Satoh N, et al. Identification of candidate genes encoding the core components of the cell death machinery in the *Ciona intestinalis* genome. *Cell Death Differ* 2003;**10**:749–53.

75. Parrinello N, Vizzini A, Arizza V, Salerno G, Parrinello D, Cammarata M, et al. Enhanced expression of a cloned and sequenced *Ciona intestinalis* TNFalpha-like (CiTNFα) gene during the LPS-induced inflammatory response. *Cell Tissue Res* 2008;**334**:305–17.

76. Hata K, Andoh A, Shimada M, Fujino S, Bamba S, Araki Y, et al. IL-17 stimulates inflammatory responses via NF-kappaB and MAP kinase pathways in human colonic myofibroblasts. *Am J Physiol Gastrointest Liver Physiol* 2002;**282**:1035–44.

77. Vizzini A, Di Falco F, Parrinello D, Sanfratello MA, Mazzarella C, Parrinello N, et al. *Ciona intestinalis* interleukin 17-like genes expression is upregulated by LPS challenge. *Dev Comp Immunol* 2015;**48**:129–37.

78. Cammarata M, Parrinello N. The ascidian prophenoloxidase activating system. *Invert Surviv J* 2009;**6**:67–76.

79. Cammarata M, Arizza V, Cianciolo C, Parrinello D, Vazzana M, Vizzini A, et al. The prophenoloxidase system is activated during the tunic inflammatory reaction of *Ciona intestinalis*. *Cell Tissue Res* 2008;**333**:481–92.

80. Vizzini A, Parrinello D, Sanfratello MA, Trapani MR, Mangano V, Parrinello N, et al. Upregulated transcription of phenoloxidase genes in the pharynx and endostyle of *Ciona intestinalis* in response to LPS. *J Invertebr Pathol* 2015;**126**:6–11.

81. Garrone R. Collagen, a common thread in extracellular matrix evolution. *Proc Indian Acad Sci Chem Sci* 1999;**111**:51–6.

82. Gibbs GM, Roelants K, O'Bryan MK. The CAP superfamily: cysteine-rich secretory proteins, antigen 5, and pathogenesis-related 1 proteins—roles in reproduction, cancer, and immune defense. *Endocr Rev* 2008;**29**:865–97.

83. Bonura A, Vizzini A, Salerno G, Parrinello D, Parrinello N, Longo V, et al. Cloning and expression of a novel component of the CAP superfamily enhanced in the inflammatory response to LPS of the ascidian *Ciona intestinalis*. *Cell Tissue Res* 2010;**342**:411–21.

84. Parrinello N, Vizzini A, Salerno G, Sanfratello MA, Cammarata M, Arizza V, et al. Inflamed adult pharynx tissues and swimming larva of *Ciona intestinalis* share CiTNFα-producing cells. *Cell Tissue Res* 2010;**341**:299–311.

85. Parrinello D, Sanfratello MA, Vizzini A, Cammarata M. The expression of an immune-related phenoloxidase gene is modulated in *Ciona intestinalis* ovary, test cells, embryos. *J Exp Zool B Mol Dev Evol* 2015;324(2).

Chapter 14

Cytotoxic Cells of Compound Ascidians

Nicola Franchi, Loriano Ballarin

University of Padova, Padova, Italy

INTRODUCTION

Tunicates or Urochordates are a subphylum of the phylum Chordata (Fig. 14.1). The realization that they represent the sister group of vertebrates[1] led to a renewed interest toward this group of organisms and stimulated a flourishing of research dealing with them. Tunicates traditionally include three classes: the benthic and sessile Ascidiacea (ascidians), the pelagic Thaliacea, and Larvacea (or Appendicularia).

Ascidians have an indirect development, with some exceptions in Molgulids,[2–4] and a free-swimming, tadpolelike larva, which metamorphoses into a saclike adult. With the exception of the carnivorous species, once considered a separate class of tunicates (Sorberacea[5]) and today included within the family Molgulidae,[4] adult ascidians are provided with two siphons, which allow water flux, and a voluminous branchial basket provided with a ventral endostyle secreting the mucous net required for filtration. Ascidians comprise two orders: Enterogona, with two suborders (Aplousobranchia and Phlebobranchia), and Pleurogona, with the order Stolidobranchia (Burighel and Cloney[5]). Thaliaceans include three orders: the colonial Pyrosomida, Doliolida, and Salpida, which alternate solitary and colonial phases in their life cycles; they have a barrel-like adult body and, with the exception of Doliolida, are devoid of larval stages.[6,7] Larvaceans or appendicularians resemble the ascidian larvae in morphology and use the tail to create the water current for filtration; filters are included in the gelatinous house secreted by the animals themselves.[6] Ascidians include about 2300 species and coloniality developed independently many times within the taxon: Aplousobranchia are all colonial, while Phlebobranchia and Stolidobranchia include both solitary and colonial species (Fig. 14.1).[8,9]

Lessons in Immunity: From Single-Cell Organisms to Mammals
http://dx.doi.org/10.1016/B978-0-12-803252-7.00014-X

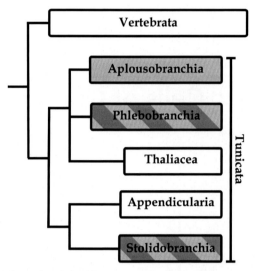

FIGURE 14.1 Phylogenetic relationships among tunicates. Ascidians, marked by *filled rectangles*, are polyphyletic. According to Delsuc et al.,[1] vertebrates represent the tunicate sister group. Light gray: solitary ascidian species; dark gray: colonial ascidian species. *From Voskoboynik A, Neff NF, Sahoo D, Newman AM, Pushkarev D, Koh W, et al. The genome sequence of the colonial chordate,* Botryllus schlosseri. *Elife 2013;2:e00569, modified according to Tsagkogeorga G, Turon X, Hopcroft RR, Tilak MK, Feldstein T, Shenkar N, et al. An updated 18S rRNA phylogeny of tunicates based on mixture and secondary structure models.* BMC Evol Biol *2009;9:187 and Tatián M, Lagger C, Demarchi M, Mattoni C. Molecular phylogeny endorses the relationship between carnivorous and filter-feeding tunicates (Tunicata, Ascidiacea).* Zool Scr *2011;40:603–12.*

ASCIDIAN CIRCULATION

Ascidians have an open circulatory system with a colorless hemolymph flowing inside blood sinuses and lacunae within the body tissues. The peristaltic waves of the tubular hearth, the direction of which reverses periodically, allow hemolymph circulation.[10,11] The hemolymph is isotonic with seawater and contains low concentrations of proteins, mainly secreted by the hemocytes and exerting important roles in humoral defense reactions.

HEMOCYTES OF COMPOUND ASCIDIANS

Many types of circulating hemocytes are commonly found in ascidians: they are involved in a variety of functions such as the storage and transport of nutrients and catabolites, asexual reproduction, tunic synthesis, allorecognition, and defense reactions (references in Ballarin et al.,[12] Cima et al.,[13] Ballarin and Cima[14]).

Various authors described the morphology of both living and fixed hemocytes of compound ascidians[13,15–20] as well as their ultrastructure.[13,19,21–26] In addition, various authors pursued the difficult task of proposing a unifying classification framework for hemolymph cells,[10,11,27] although uncertainties and doubts still exist, especially regarding hemocyte mutual relationships and differentiation pathways.

Botryllid ascidians are colonial stolidobranchs that are the subjects of most of the studies on the hemolymph of compound ascidians. In these animals, circulating cells can be grouped in at least three categories: undifferentiated cells, commonly known as hemoblasts, immunocytes (ie, cells involved in immune responses), and storage cells.[14] Immunocytes form the majority of circulating cells and are represented by phagocytes and cytotoxic cells.[13,14,20,28] Storage cells are vacuolated cells, which include trophocytes that transport nutrients, pigment cells that contain pigment crystals, and nephrocytes that store uric acid crystals.[14,20,23,24,26]

Hematopoietic sites of compound ascidians are mainly located in peripharyngeal regions. Although mitotic figures have been occasionally observed in circulating hemoblasts (Ermak[29]), stem cell niches have been recently identified in the endostyle of adult zooids of *Botryllus schlosseri* from which they colonize the aggregates of hemocytes located along the sides of the endostyle, known as cell islands. From these sites, hemocytes enter the circulation and contribute to various zooid tissues, germ line and hemolymph included.[30–32]

CYTOTOXIC CELLS

Cytotoxic cells of compound ascidians are granular cells easily recognizable with simple cytoenzymatic assays[33] for the presence of phenoloxidase (PO) inside their granules. Due to their berrylike morphology, especially evident after fixation with aldehydes, they are generally known as morula cells (MCs). Usually, they are the most abundant hemocyte type, and they represent up to 60% of the total circulating cells.[28,34]

In *B. schlosseri*, where they have been particularly studied, MCs have a mean diameter of 10–15 μm, and their cytoplasm is filled with many granules, 2 μm in diameter, which assume a yellowish color after aldehyde treatment. The granular content is acidophilic, has reducing properties, shows positivity for PO and arylsulfatase activities and for the presence of quinones, and results immunopositive to antitunichrome antibody.[14,28,34,35] Tunichromes are considered fragments of larger DOPA-containing proteins, present inside *Botryllus* MCs,[35] and they likely represent the substrates of PO, stored with the enzyme inside MC vacuoles.[36–38]

CYTOTOXICITY

In *B. schlosseri*, MCs degranulate and release their granular content upon the recognition of foreign molecules: this results in the induction of cytotoxicity. The effect is directly related to the presence, in the medium, of active PO released by MCs.[39,40] Experimental evidences indicate that cytotoxicity is related to the production of reactive oxygen species (ROS) by PO and the consequent induction of oxidative stress related to the depletion of reduced glutathione and total thiols.[41]

In agreement with this assumption, ROS scavengers (superoxide dismutase, catalase, and sorbitol) and PO inhibitors (sodium benzoate, phenylthiourea, and diethyldithiocarbamate) can significantly reduce the extent of cytotoxicity observed in vitro when hemocytes are challenged with foreign molecules, such as those in the plasma from genetically incompatible colonies, on the surface of yeast (*Saccharomyces cerevisiae*) or gram-positive bacterial (*Bacillus clausii*) cells.[40,41]

PHENOLOXIDASE

PO is a copper-containing enzyme widely distributed in invertebrates, able to convert phenol substrata to quinones, which can polymerize to form melanin. PO exerts its cytotoxic role through the production of ROS and semiquinones, which can either induce oxidative stress or react with biomolecules, altering their functionality.[39,41] Quinones and melanin are also toxic as they can contribute to the generation of oxidative stress through their reaction with thiol groups on biomolecules.[42–44]

The use of specific inhibitors in in vitro assays has clearly demonstrated the cytotoxic role of PO in ascidians, in both solitary and colonial species.[39,40,45–49]

As far as compound ascidians are concerned, *B. schlosseri* PO has been purified and partially characterized biochemically: it forms polymers starting from monomeric units of 80 kDa of molecular weight.[50] The PO transcripts of the colonial species *B. schlosseri* and *Polyandrocarpa misakiensis* were recently identified and characterized[51]: the analysis of nucleotide and deduced amino acid sequences of these POs confirmed their high similarity of ascidian POs to arthropod hemocyanins, already suggested in the study of the PO transcripts from the solitary species *Ciona intestinalis*,[52] and gave an estimated molecular weight of 86 and 74 kDa, respectively, in good agreement with available biochemical data.

As regards to the control of PO activity, there is a general consensus that the regulation of ascidian PO is analogous to that of arthropods, ie, with the enzyme stored in MC granules and released as a proenzyme subsequently cleaved by extracellular serine proteases.[53] However, evidences are emerging indicating that, in botryllid ascidians, the situation could be different. For instance, no treatment with proteases is required to reveal PO activity in cytoenzymatic assays,[14] suggesting that the enzyme is, at least in part, already active inside MCs. In addition, MCs have polyphenol and quinones (ie, products of PO activity) as ready to use cytotoxic molecules.[35,54] Furthermore, a prodomain is not present in the putative amino acid sequence of *B. schlosseri* PO.[51]

ALLORECOGNITION AND INFLAMMATION

Allorecognition, ie, the capability of intraspecific recognition of nonself, typically manifests itself in botryllid ascidians in the form of colony specificity, which occurs when colonies of different genotypes at a single, highly polymorphic histocompatibility/fusibility (HC/Fu) locus, with codominant alleles, contact each other at the level of their growing edges or are experimentally forced to contact their cut surfaces. Two different outcomes are possible: when colonies share at least one allele at the HC/Fu locus, they either fuse, forming a chimeric colony with common tunic and vasculature, or reject each other. Rejection is accomplished with the formation of a series of cytotoxic foci, called points of rejection, along the contact border,[55,56] which contain melanin deposits due to PO activity.[39,57] A typical inflammatory reaction occurs with the selective recruitment of MCs in the contact region: they cross the vessel epithelium (usually at the level of the blind termini, called ampullae, of the colonial marginal vessel) and migrate in the tunic of the contact region where they degranulate and induce cytotoxicity as a consequence of the release of their granular content, in particular the enzyme PO, its polyphenol substrata, and quinones.[39,41,54,58–65] Recent results indicate that MC degranulation is mediated by ion fluxes and is inhibited by the presence of the ionophore monensin or the anion channel-blocking agent 4-acetamido-4′-isothiocyanatostilbene-2,2′-disulfonic acid and requires the activation of both protein kinase A (PKA) and protein kinase C (PKC) as indicated by the mitogen-activated protein kinases signal transduction pathway, as indicated by its inhibition in the presence of H-89 and calphostin C, inhibitors of PKA and PKC, respectively.[35] As a consequence of the nonfusion reaction, a change in the growth direction of the contacting colonies (retreat growth) occurs.[66]

IMMUNORECOGNITION AND IMMUNOMODULATION

In *B. schlosseri*, *Botrylloides leachi*, and *Botrylloides simodensis*, MCs synthesize and release immunomodulatory molecules (cytokines), which result immunopositive to antibodies raised against mammalian IL-1α and TNFα, upon the recognition of nonself molecules.[40,64,65,67] In *B. schlosseri*, these molecules are involved in the induction of cytotoxicity during the rejection reaction[61] and exert chemotactic activity toward MCs, recruiting additional cells to the infection site. In addition, they can promote phagocytosis and the release of lectins with opsonic activity by phagocytes.[68–70] Moreover if, in the site of infection, lectin concentration reaches a certain threshold, MCs degranulate with consequent cytotoxic effects.[71]

Recently, two of the most important proteins of the complement system, C3 and B-factor (Bf), have been identified in *B. schlosseri*.[72] In particular, C3 is the main actor of the complement system while Bf is the serine protease involved in the alternative pathway of complement activation. In mammals and teleosts, C3 and Bf are mainly expressed in liver[73] and immunocytes.[74] In *B. schlosseri*, MCs are the sole source of C3 (BsC3) and Bf (BsBf). In normal and immune-stimulated conditions, the fraction of MCs involved in the expression of BsC3 remains constant, which suggests a constitutive production of such a molecule acting as a sentinel molecule in the bloodstream.[72] C3, as demonstrated in *B. schlosseri* and in other

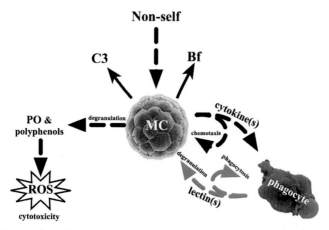

FIGURE 14.2 Schematic representation of activation of morula cell (MC) and their interaction with phagocytes. MC cytokines promote phagocytosis and induce the synthesis of lectin(s) by phagocytes. *Dashed lines*: induced events upon nonself recognition. *Full lines*: constitutive secretions. *Black lines* refer to MC events whereas *gray lines* indicate phagocyte responses.

ascidians, such as *Halocynthia roretzi*,[75] is able to influence phagocytosis similarly to vertebrate C3.[72,76] Again, MCs produce molecules with effects on phagocytes, stressing the importance of the cross talk between immunocytes and highlighting a high level of complexity of the immune system.

Collectively, all the available data suggest that, at least in *B. schlosseri*, MCs are the major sentinel cells able to sense nonself molecules. They release molecules important in the immune surveillance, as C3 are recruited in the infection sites, and, depending on the nature of the nonself, can trigger a cytotoxic response or promote phagocytosis through complement activation and/or the release of opsonic lectins (Fig. 14.2).[28]

FUTURE PERSPECTIVES: NEW ROLES FOR OLD CELLS

Until the end of the 1980s, although abundant in the circulation, ascidian MCs received little attention by scientists and were considered too differentiated to exert any important role in the organism biology. Only a few researchers paid attention to them, mainly interested in the unusual acidic content of their granules and in the ability of MCs to concentrate metals, such as iron, inside them.[23,77–79] The situation started to change after the observation that they contained PO[80] and, in botryllid ascidians, they were recruited in the course of the rejection reaction between genetically incompatible colonies[58,60]: this paved the way for studies of their role as immunocytes in inflammatory responses and immunomodulation.[34]

Today, new important roles for MCs in immune responses are emerging: they can transcribe important genes of the complement system linked to immunosurveillance and modulate, through the release of C3 and/or cytokines, the activity of phagocytes, which, in turn, can enhance the activation of MCs through the release of lectins.[28,72] In addition, evidences are accumulating denoting the ability of ascidian cytotoxic cells to face stress conditions by increasing the transcription of genes for antioxidant responses[81-84] and to trigger a rapid defense reaction upon the recognition of molecules of the microbial surface through the synthesis and release of molecules with antimicrobial activity[85-88] or by inducing an inflammatory reaction.[28,89,90] We are fully convinced that future research will shed new light on other important roles of these cells in ascidian biology.

REFERENCES

1. Delsuc F, Brinkmann H, Chourrout D, Philippe H. Tunicates and not cephalochordates are the closest living relatives of vertebrates. *Nature* 2006;**439**:965–8.
2. Jeffery WR, Swalla BJ. Anural development in ascidians: evolutionary modification and elimination of the tadpole larva. *Sem Dev Biol* 1990;**1**:253–61.
3. Jeffery WR, Swalla BJ. Evolution of alternate modes of development in ascidians. *Bioessays* 1992;**14**:219–26.
4. Tagawa K, Jeffery WR, Satoh N. The recently-described ascidian species *Molgula tectiformis* is a direct developer. *Zool Sci* 1997;**14**:297–303.
5. Burighel P, Cloney RA. Urochordata: ascidiacea. In: Harrison FW, Ruppert EE, editors. *Microscopic anatomy of invertebrates*, vol. 15. New York: Wiley-Liss; 1997. p. 221–347.
6. Tatián M, Lagger C, Demarchi M, Mattoni C. Molecular phylogeny endorses the relationship between carnivorous and filter-feeding tunicates (Tunicata, Ascidiacea). *Zool Scr* 2011;**40**:603–12.
7. Ruppert EE, Fox RS, Barnes RD. *Invertebrate zoology: a functional evolutionary approach.* 7th ed. Boston (MA): Thomson Learning Inc; 2004.
8. Satoh N. An advanced filter-feeder hypothesis for urochordate evolution. *Zool Sci* 2009;**26**:97–111.
9. Shenkar N, Swalla BJ. Global diversity of Ascidiacea. *PLoS One* 2011;**6**:e20657.
10. Goodbody I. The physiology of ascidians. *Adv Mar Biol* 1974;**12**:1–149.
11. Wright RK. Urochordates. In: Ratcliffe NA, Rowley AF, editors. *Invertebrate blood cells*, vol. 2. London: Academic Press; 1981. p. 565–626.
12. Ballarin L, Cima F, Sabbadin A. Histoenzymatic staining and characterization of the colonial ascidian *Botryllus schlosseri* hemocytes. *Boll Zool* 1993;**60**:19–24.
13. Cima F, Perin A, Burighel P, Ballarin L. Morpho-functional characterisation of haemocytes of the compound ascidian *Botrylloides leachi* (Tunicata, Ascidiacea). *Acta Zool (Stockh)* 2001;**82**:261–74.
14. Ballarin L, Cima F. Cytochemical properties of *Botryllus schlosseri* haemocytes: indications for morpho-functional characterisation. *Eur J Histochem* 2005;**49**:255–64.
15. Pérès JM. Recherches sur le sang et les organes neuraux des Tuniciers. *Ann Inst Ocean (Monaco)* 1943;**21**:229–359.
16. Sabbadin A. Studio sulle cellule del sangue di *Botryllus schlosseri* (Pallas) (Ascidiacea). *Arch Ital Anat Embriol* 1955;**60**:33–67.
17. Andrew W. Phase microscope studies of living blood-cells of the tunicates under normal and experimental conditions, with a description of a new type of motile cell appendage. *Quart J Microsc Sci* 1961;**102**:89–105.
18. Schlumpberger JM, Weissman IL, Scofield VL. Separation and labeling of specific subpopulations of *Botryllus* blood cells. *J Exp Zool* 1984;**229**:401–11.

19. Hirose E, Shirae M, Saito Y. Ultrastructures and classification of circulating hemocytes in 9 botryllid ascidians (Chordata: Ascidiacea). *Zool Sci* 2003;**20**:647–56.

20. Ballarin L, Kawamura K. The hemocytes of *Polyandrocarpa misakiensis*: morphology and immune-related activities. *Invertebr Surviv J* 2009;**6**:154–61.

21. Overton J. The fine structure of blood cells in the ascidian. *Perophora Viridis J Morphol* 1966;**119**:305–26.

22. Fujimoto H, Watanabe H. The characterization of granular amoebocytes and their possible roles in the asexual reproduction of the polystyelid ascidian, *Polyzoa vesiculiphora. J Morphol* 1976;**150**:623–38.

23. Milanesi C, Burighel P. Blood cell ultrastructure of the ascidian *Botryllus schlosseri*. I. Hemoblast, granulocytes, macrophage, morula cell and nephrocyte. *Acta Zool (Stockh)* 1978;**59**:135–47.

24. Burighel P, Milanesi C, Sabbadin A. Blood cell ultrastructure of the ascidian *Botryllus schlosseri* L. II. Pigment cells. *Acta Zool (Stockh)* 1983;**64**:15–23.

25. Hirose E, Mukai H. An ultrastructural study on the origin of glomerulocytes, a type of blood cell in a styelid ascidian, *Polyandrocarpa misakiensis. J Morphol* 1992;**211**:269–73.

26. Sugino YM, Tsuji Y, Kawamura K. An ultrastructural study of blood cells in the ascidian, *Polyandrocarpa misakiensis*: their classification and behavioral characteristics. *Mem Fac Sci Kochi Univ Ser D Biol* 1993;**14**:33–41.

27. De Leo G. Ascidian hemocytes and their involvement in defense reactions. *Boll Zool* 1992;**59**:195–213.

28. Ballarin L. Immunobiology of compound ascidians, with particular reference to *Botryllus schlosseri*: state of the art. *Invertebr Surviv J* 2008;**5**:54–74.

29. Ermak TH. The hematogenic tissues of tunicates. In: Wright RK, Cooper EL, editors. *The phylogeny of thymus and bone marrow-bursa cells*. Amsterdam: Elsevier/North Holland; 1976. p. 45–56.

30. Kawamura K, Tachibana M, Sunanaga T. Cell proliferation dynamics of somatic and germline tissues during zooidal life span in the colonial tunicate *Botryllus primigenus. Dev Dyn* 2008;**237**:1812–25.

31. Voskoboynik A, Soen Y, Rinkevich Y, Rosner A, Ueno H, Reshef R, et al. Identification of the endostyle as a stem cell niche in a colonial chordate. *Cell Stem Cell* 2008;**3**:456–64.

32. Rinkevich Y, Voskoboynik A, Rosner A, Rabinowitz C, Paz G, Oren M, et al. Repeated, long-term cycling of putative stem cells between niches in a basal chordate. *Dev Cell* 2013;**24**:76–88.

33. Ballarin L, Cammarata M, Cima F, Grimaldi A, Lorenzon S, Malagoli D, et al. Immune-neuroendocrine biology of invertebrates: a collection of methods. *Invertebr Surviv J* 2008;**5**: 192–215.

34. Ballarin L. Ascidian cytotoxic cells: state of the art and research perspectives. *Invertebr Surviv J* 2012;**9**:1–6.

35. Franchi N, Ballarin L, Cima F. Insights on cytotoxic cells of the colonial ascidian *Botryllus schlosseri. Invertebr Surviv J* 2015;**12**:109–17.

36. Bruening RC, Oltz EM, Furukawa J, Nakanishi K, Kustin K. Isolation of tunichrome B-1, a reducing blood pigment of the sea squirt, *Ascidia nigra. J Nat Prod* 1986;**49**:193–204.

37. Oltz EM, Bruening RC, Smith MJ, Kustin K, Nakanishi K. The tunichromes. A class of reducing blood pigments from sea squirts: isolation, structures, and vanadium chemistry. *J Am Chem Soc* 1988;**110**:6162–72.

38. Sugumaran M, Robinson WE. Structure, biosynthesis and possible function of tunichromes and related compounds. *Comp Biochem Physiol* 2012;**163B**:1–25.

39. Ballarin L, Cima F, Sabbadin A. Phenoloxidase and cytotoxicity in the compound ascidian *Botryllus schlosseri. Dev Comp Immunol* 1998;**22**:479–92.

40. Ballarin L, Menin A, Franchi N, Bertoloni G, Cima F. Morula cells and non-self recognition in the compound ascidian *Botryllus schlosseri. Invertebr Surviv J* 2005;**2**:1–5.

41. Ballarin L, Cima F, Floreani M, Sabbadin A. Oxidative stress induces cytotoxicity during rejection reaction in the compound ascidian *Botryllus schlosseri*. *Comp Biochem Physiol* 2002;**133C**:411–8.

42. Kato T, Ito S, Fujita K. Tyrosinase-catalyzed binding of 3,4-dihydroxyphenylalanine with proteins through the sulfhydryl group. *Biochim Biophys Acta* 1986;**881**:415–21.

43. Nappi AJ, Vass E. Melanogenesis and the generation of cytotoxic molecules during insect cellular immune reactions. *Pigment Cell Res* 1993;**6**:117–26.

44. Nappi AJ, Ottaviani E. Cytotoxicity and cytotoxic molecules in invertebrates. *Bioessays* 2000;**22**:469–80.

45. Akita N, Hoshi M. Hemocytes release phenoloxidase upon contact reaction, an allogeneic interaction, in the ascidian *Halocynthia roretzi*. *Cell Struct Funct* 1995;**20**:81–7.

46. Cammarata M, Arizza V, Parrinello N, Candore G, Caruso C. Phenoloxidase-dependent cytotoxic mechanism in ascidian (*Styela plicata*) hemocytes active against erythrocytes and K562 tumor cells. *Eur J Cell Biol* 1997;**74**:302–7.

47. Cammarata M, Arizza V, Cianciolo C, Parrinello D, Vazzana M, Vizzini A, et al. The prophenoloxidase system is activated during the tunic inflammatory reaction of *Ciona intestinalis*. *Cell Tissue Res* 2008;**333**:481–92.

48. Hata S, Azumi K, Yokosawa H. Ascidian phenoloxidase: its release from hemocytes, isolation, characterization and physiological role. *Comp Biochem Physiol* 1998;**119B**:767–76.

49. Parrinello N, Arizza V, Chinnici C, Parrinello D, Cammarata M. Phenoloxidases in ascidian hemocytes: characterization of the pro-phenoloxidase activating system. *Comp Biochem Physiol* 2003;**135B**:583–91.

50. Frizzo A, Guidolin L, Ballarin L, Sabbadin A. Purification and characterisation of phenoloxidase from the colonial ascidian *Botryllus schlosseri*. *Mar Biol* 1999;**135**:483–8.

51. Ballarin L, Franchi N, Schiavon F, Tosatto SC, Mičetić I, Kawamura K. Looking for putative phenoloxidases of compound ascidians: haemocyanin-like proteins in *Polyandrocarpa misakiensis* and *Botryllus schlosseri*. *Dev Comp Immunol* 2012;**38**:232–42.

52. Immesberger A, Burmester T. Putative phenoloxidase in the tunicate *Ciona intestinalis* and the origin of the arthropod hemocyanin superfamily. *J Comp Physiol* 2004;**174B**:169–80.

53. Cerenius L, Söderhäll K. The prophenoloxidase-activating system in invertebrates. *Immunol Rev* 2004;**198**:116–26.

54. Shirae M, Ballarin L, Frizzo A, Saito Y, Hirose E. Involvement of quinones and phenoloxidase in the allorejection reaction in a colonial ascidian, *Botrylloides simodensis*: histochemical and immunohistochemical study. *Mar Biol* 2002;**141**:659–65.

55. Sabbadin A. Le basi genetiche della capacità di fusione fra colonie in *Botryllus schlosseri* (Ascidiacea). *Rend Accad Naz Lincei* 1962;**32**:1021–35.

56. Oka H. Colony specificity in compound ascidians. The genetic control of fusibility. In: Yukawa H, editor. *Profiles of Japanese science and scientists*. Tokyo: Kodanska; 1970. p. 196–206.

57. Ballarin L, Cima F, Sabbadin A. Morula cells and histocompatibility in the colonial ascidian *Botryllus schlosseri*. *Zool Sci* 1995;**12**:757–64.

58. Hirose E, Saito Y, Watanabe H. Allogeneic rejection induced by cut surface contact in the compound ascidian, *Botrylloides simodensis*. *Invertebr Reprod Dev* 1990;**17**:159–64.

59. Hirose E, Saito Y, Watanabe H. Subcuticular rejection: an advanced mode of the allogeneic rejection in the compound ascidians *Botrylloides simodensis* and *B. fuscus*. *Biol Bull* 1997;**192**:53–61.

60. Sabbadin A, Zaniolo G, Ballarin L. Genetic and cytological aspects of histocompatibility in ascidians. *Boll Zool* 1992;**59**:167–73.

61. Cima F, Sabbadin A, Ballarin L. Cellular aspects of allorecognition in the compound ascidian *Botryllus schlosseri*. *Dev Comp Immunol* 2004;**28**:881–9.

62. Shirae M, Hirose E, Saito Y. Behavior of hemocytes in the allorejection reaction in two compound ascidians, *Botryllus scalaris* and *Symplegma reptans*. *Biol Bull* 1999;**197**:188–97.
63. Zaniolo G, Manni L, Ballarin L. Colony specificity in *Botrylloides leachi*. I. Morphological aspects. *Invertebr Surviv J* 2006;**3**:125–36.
64. Ballarin L, Zaniolo G. Colony specificity in *Botrylloides leachi*. II. Cellular aspects of the nonfusion reaction. *Invertebr Surviv J* 2007;**4**:38–44.
65. Franchi N, Hirose E, Ballarin L. Cellular aspects of allorecognition in the compound ascidian *Botrylloides simodensis*. *Invertebr Surviv J* 2014;**11**:219–23.
66. Rinkevich B, Weissman IL. Retreat growth in the ascidian *Botryllus schlosseri*: a consequence of nonself recognition. In: Grosberg RK, Hedgecock D, Nelson K, editors. *Invertebrate historecognition*. New York: Plenum Press; 1988. p. 93–109.
67. Ballarin L, Franchini A, Ottaviani E, Sabbadin A. Morula cells as the major immunomodulatory hemocytes in ascidians: evidences from the colonial species *Botryllus schlosseri*. *Biol Bull* 2001;**201**:59–64.
68. Menin A, Del Favero M, Cima F, Ballarin L. Release of phagocytosis-stimulating factor(s) by morula cells in a colonial ascidian. *Mar Biol* 2005;**148**:225–30.
69. Cima F, Sabbadin A, Zaniolo G, Ballarin L. Colony specificity and chemotaxis in the compound ascidian *Botryllus schlosseri*. *Comp Biochem Physiol* 2006;**145A**:376–82.
70. Menin A, Ballarin L. Immunomodulatory molecules in the compound ascidian *Botryllus schlosseri*: evidence from conditioned media. *J Invertebr Pathol* 2008;**99**:275–80.
71. Franchi N, Schiavon F, Carletto M, Gasparini F, Bertoloni G, Tosatto SCE, et al. Immune roles of a rhamnose-binding lectin in the colonial ascidian *Botryllus schlosseri*. *Immunobiology* 2011;**216**:725–36.
72. Franchi N, Ballarin L. Preliminary characterization of complement in a colonial tunicate: C3, Bf and inhibition of C3 opsonic activity by compstatin. *Dev Comp Immunol* 2014;**46**:430–8.
73. Zhou Z, Liu H, Liu S, Sun F, Peatman E, Kucuktas H, et al. Alternative complement pathway of channel catfish (*Ictalurus punctatus*): molecular characterization, mapping and expression analysis of factors Bf/C2 and Df. *Fish Shellfish Immunol* 2012;**32**:186–95.
74. Lambris JD. The multifunctional role of C3, the third component of complement. *Immunol Today* 1988;**9**:387–93.
75. Nonaka M, Azumi K, Ji X, Namikawa-Yamada C, Sasaki M, Saiga H, et al. Opsonic complement component C3 in the solitary ascidian, *Halocynthia roretzi*. *J Immunol* 1999;**162**:387–91.
76. Pinto MR, Chinnici CM, Kimura Y, Melillo D, Marino R, Spruce LA, et al. CiC3-1a-mediated chemotaxis in the deuterostome invertebrate *Ciona intestinalis* (Urochordata). *J Immunol* 2003;**171**:5521–8.
77. Endean R. The blood cells of the ascidian, *Phallusia mamillata*. *Quart J Microsc Sci* 1960;**101**:177–97.
78. Smith MJ. The blood cells and tunic of the ascidian *Halocynthia aurantium* (Pallas). II. The histochemistry of blood cells and tunic. *Biol Bull* 1970;**138**:379–88.
79. Pirie BJS, Bell MV. The localization of inorganic elements, particularly vanadium and sulphur, in haemolymph from the ascidians *Ascidia mentula* (Müller) and *Ascidiella aspersa* (Müller). *J Exp Mar Biol Ecol* 1984;**74**:187–94.
80. Chaga OY. Ortho-diphenoloxidase system of ascidians. *Tsitologia* 1980;**22**:619–25.
81. Ferro D, Franchi N, Ballarin L, Cammarata M, Mangano V, Rigers B, et al. Characterization and metal-induced gene transcription of two new copper zinc superoxide dismutases in the solitary ascidian *Ciona intestinalis*. *Aquat Toxicol* 2013;**140-141**:369–79.
82. Franchi N, Boldrin F, Ballarin L, Piccinni E. CiMT-1, an unusual chordate metallothionein gene in *Ciona intestinalis* genome: structure and expression studies. *J Exp Zool* 2011;**315A**:90–100.

83. Franchi N, Ferro D, Ballarin L, Santovito G. Transcription of genes involved in glutathione biosynthesis in the solitary tunicate *Ciona intestinalis* exposed to metals. *Aquat Toxicol* 2012;**114–115**:14–22.

84. Franchi N, Piccinni E, Ferro D, Basso G, Spolaore B, Santovito G, et al. Characterization and transcription studies of a phytochelatin synthase gene from the solitary tunicate *Ciona intestinalis* exposed to cadmium. *Aquat Toxicol* 2014;**152**:47–56.

85. Azumi K, Yokosawa H, Ishii S. Halocyamines: novel antimicrobial tetrapeptide-like substances isolated from the hemocytes of the solitary ascidian *Halocynthia roretzi*. *Biochemistry* 1990;**29**:159–65.

86. Lee IH, Zhao C, Cho Y, Harwig SSL, Cooper EL, Lehrer RI. Clavanins, α-helical antimicrobial peptides from tunicate hemocytes. *FEBS Lett* 1997;**400**:158–62.

87. Menzel LP, Lee IH, Sjostrand B, Lehrer RI. Immunolocalization of clavanins in *Styela clava* hemocytes. *Dev Comp Immunol* 2002;**26**:505–15.

88. Cai M, Sugumaran M, Robinson WE. The crosslinking and antimicrobial properties of tunichrome. *Comp Biochem Physiol* 2008;**151B**:110–7.

89. Cammarata M, Candore G, Arizza V, Caruso C, Parrinello N. Cytotoxic activity of *Styela plicata* hemocytes against mammalian cell targets: II. Properties of the in vitro reaction against human tumour cell lines. *Anim Biol* 1995;**4**:139–44.

90. Parrinello N, Cammarata M, Arizza V. Univacuolar refractile hemocytes from the tunicate *Ciona intestinalis* are cytotoxic for mammalian erythrocytes *in vitro*. *Biol Bull* 1996;**190**:418–25.

Chapter 15

Fish Transcriptomics

Francesco Buonocore, Giuseppe Scapigliati
University of Tuscia, Viterbo, Italy

INTRODUCTION

Transcriptomics is a branch of the -omics sciences that during the last ten years has had a great impetus, becoming more and more fundamental for studies regarding both the functional elements of the genome and aiming to discover the molecular constituents of cells and tissues. Other important aspects that are determined during transcriptome analysis are the structure of the genes and the differential expression levels of each transcript during development and under various experimental or environmental conditions. The technologies that have been developed for unraveling the transcriptome are based on hybridization or sequence approaches, and they have been continuously improved. The most known hybridization technique is the microarray, which typically is based on the interactions between a fluorescently labeled cDNA with custom-made or high-density short probes of nucleotide sequences fixed on a solid surface.[1] The limitations of the microarray technology are mainly related to the need for an extensive knowledge about the genome sequence, to the possible saturation of the signal for high-abundance transcripts, and to the background noise that could be quite disturbing in the case of nonspecific hybridization.[2] The sequence-based approaches aim to determine the nucleotide sequence of each transcript present in the explored transcriptome. At the beginning, these technologies provide the sequencing of cDNA or expressed sequence tag libraries,[3] but they suffer some limitations due to the relatively low output, the quite high cost, and the lack of any quantitative analysis. Successively, other methods—based on the addition of a tag to the RNA molecules prior to cloning and sequencing—have been developed,[4–8] but they are mostly based on the expensive Sanger sequence technology, and to annotate the tags they need the whole genome available.[9] More recently, a new method, termed RNA-sequencing (RNA-seq), has been produced, and it immediately showed clear advantages compared to existing approaches. It is expected to change the way transcriptomes will be analyzed in the future.[10] This methodology uses deep-sequencing technologies[11] that are usually called next-generation sequencing, like Illumina

Lessons in Immunity: From Single-Cell Organisms to Mammals
http://dx.doi.org/10.1016/B978-0-12-803252-7.00015-1

205

IG, Applied Biosystems SOLiD, and Roche 454 Life Science. After sequencing, the reads have to be aligned to a reference genome or transcriptome or assembled de novo to produce a transcription map if no genome is available; another output of the methodology is the level of expression of each gene.[12] The major advantages compared to existing technologies are the absence of limitations if a reference genomic sequence is not present, the precise location of transcription boundaries and single-nucleotide polymorphisms are not known, and the absence of any background signal.[10]

TRANSCRIPTOMICS ANALYSIS OF FISH LEUKOCYTES

RNA-seq technology has been widely used in the last ten years to study fish transcriptomes[13,14] with the aim of gaining new information on the biology, physiology, and evolution of fish, sometimes taking into account the analysis of tissues known to be involved in immune responses and therefore containing leukocytes. Table 15.1 summarizes some of the research performed on this last topic from a database search (using the PubMed website).

Physiological Processes

Different physiological processes involving fish leukocytes have been analyzed by RNA-seq. In *Salmo trutta* (brown trout), the toxicity in water of the glyphosate, the active ingredient of the herbicide Roundup, was studied.[15] This environmental contaminant should induce a broad range of negative biological effects, and the authors focused on the study of the oxidative stress. RNA-seq was performed on liver samples, and 1020 differentially regulated transcripts were evidenced after the various performed treatments. These changes seem to be consistent with the presence of an oxidative stress and with the successive induction of compensatory cellular stress response pathways. Significant alterations were observed even at the lowest tested concentrations and, for this reason, there are high concerns for the potential toxicity of this herbicide to fish populations inhabiting contaminated rivers.[15] Moreover, differentially expressed transcripts have been studied in brown trout specimens exposed to a waterborne mixture of metals (the River Hayle in South West England), compared to brown trout from a relatively uncontaminated river.[27] RNA-seq analyses from different tissues (gill, liver, and head kidney) evidenced 998 transcripts, most of them linked to metal- and ion-homeostasis pathways, which therefore should be the most important mechanisms contributing to the fish metal tolerance. In medaka (*Oryzias latipes*), the transcripts linked to hyperosmotic stress have been investigated by RNA-seq in the fish intestine and, among the about 50 identified upregulated transcription factors, five were confirmed by real-time PCR to be specific for the studied physiological process.[18] In the Antarctic notothenioid fish *Pagothenia borchgrevinki*,[21] researchers have studied the gene expression changes in the liver in response to elevated body temperature.

TABLE 15.1 Analysis of Fish Transcriptomes by RNA-Sequencing

Main Application	Fish Species	Examined Tissues	References
Physiological processes	*Salmo trutta*	Liver, spleen, head kidney, gill, gut	15,27
	Oryzias latipes	Intestine	18
	Pagothenia borchgrevinki	Liver	21
	Megalobrama amblycephala	Liver	25
	Lates calcarifer	Intestine	28
	Melanotaenia duboulayi	Liver	29
	Ictalurus punctatus	Gill and liver	30
	Fundulus grandis	Liver	31
Parasite response	*Scophthalmus maximus*	Head kidney, spleen, pyloric caeca	16
Transcripts in specific tissues	*Trematomus bernacchii*	Head kidney, liver, gill, brain	17,39
	Basilichthys microlepidotus	Liver	19
	Oncorhynchus mykiss	Spleen	20
	Dicentrarchus labrax	Liver, brain, gill	23,37
	Takifugu rubripes	Gill, swim bladder	24
Bacterial infection	*I. punctatus*	Intestine, gill	34,35
	Oreochromis niloticus	Spleen, head kidney	26
	Danio rerio	Liver	32
	D. labrax	Hind gut and head kidney	33
	Lateolabrax japonicus	Head kidney and spleen	36
Virus infection	*Ctenopharyngodon idella*	Gill, intestine, liver, spleen	22
Evolution biology	*Latimeria menadoensis*	Liver, testis	38

Starting from a large number of annotated transcripts, hundreds of significantly differentially expressed genes were identified after 2 and 4 days of 4°C exposure (that was 5°C more than the naïve water temperature). As an example, all classes of molecular chaperones and most genes involved in cellular proliferation were downregulated after 2 days, whereas for molecules participating in protein biosynthesis the same phenomenon happens after 4 days.

In *Megalobrama amblycephala*,[25] the transcripts linked to nitrite toxicity in liver have been investigated. Gene expression analysis identified a total of 357 differentially expressed molecules that were mainly related to oxidative stress, apoptotic pathway, oxygen transport, immune responses, and metabolism of proteins and fats. Different stressors and modulators of immune responses (lipopolysaccharide, infection with *Vibrio harveyi*, high salinity, and fasting) were applied to Asian sea bass (*Lates calcarifer*).[28] The differentially expressed genes were observed in the intestine leading to the identification of about 200 regulated pathways for each stressor. In *Melanotaenia duboulayi*, RNA-seq technology was used to study its plasticity to a temperature stress.[29] The aim was to identify genes that could be of high interest due to the changing environment that fish need to be faced with. The investigated species was selected as it was predicted to be negatively impacted by the ongoing climatic change. Two fish groups were maintained at different temperatures, and 614 upregulated and 349 downregulated transcripts were annotated. The differentially expressed genes correspond to metabolic pathways shown to be linked to temperature tolerance in other fish species. In catfish (*Ictalurus punctatus*) a heat stress was also performed to study the molecular mechanism that is involved in tolerance to temperature fluctuations.[30] RNA-seq analyses identified more than 2000 differentially expressed transcripts with a cutoff of twofold change, and real-time PCR was used to validate these results. Genes related to oxygen transport, protein folding and degradation, and metabolic processes were upregulated, while general protein synthesis was highly downregulated in response to temperature stress. The environmental impact of an ecological disaster, the release of oil resulting from the blowout of the Deepwater Horizon drilling platform, was investigated studying its effects on the genetic response of the *Fundulus grandis*.[31] RNA-seq was applied on fish exposed and not exposed to the oil release and, after the use of a statistical framework, 1070 downregulated and 1251 upregulated transcripts were selected. Some of the identified genes were correlated with an aryl hydrocarbon receptor and cytochrome-mediated responses.

Parasite Response

In *Scophthalmus maximus*,[16] the immune response against the presence of the intestinal myxozoan parasite *Enteromyxum scophthalmi* has been studied by RNA-seq. Different organs (head kidney, spleen, and pyloric caeca) of severely infected fish have been investigated in order to better elucidate the pathogenetic mechanisms of the parasite. More than 4000 differentially expressed transcripts were identified, and associated functions were related mainly to immune and defense responses; apoptosis and cell proliferation; iron metabolism and erythropoiesis; cytoskeleton and extracellular matrix; and metabolism and digestive functions.

Transcripts in Specific Tissues

The transcripts in the head kidney, liver, brain, and gill of the Antarctic fish *Trematomus bernacchii* (Teleostea, Notothenioidea) have been investigated in two different papers.[17,39] Two different methodologies were used to obtain the sequences: the 454 Roche pyrosequencing[39] and the Illumina platform[16] (see Table 15.2).

The Illumina approach gave a rather high sequencing throughput, and only about 28% of the sequences coming out from the study performed with Illumina were found in the previous one made by 454 sequencing, while the rest of the annotated gene models were completely new. In *Basilichthys microlepidotus*, the liver transcriptome[19] was investigated to obtain information on this fish that is considered a vulnerable species due to the effects of the anthropic activity on the rivers where it lives. The information could be useful in developing an appropriate conservation strategy for this freshwater species. In *Oncorhynchus mykiss*, the RNA-seq technology was applied to identify immune-related genes from the spleen.[20] KEGG annotation revealed about 900 sequences related to the immune system, and some of them were completely unknown before. The transcripts in the liver, brain, and gill of *Dicentrarchus labrax* were studied by two research groups.[23,37] Both analyses were made by using the Illumina platform and generated a high number of unique genes that will be useful for the final annotation of the genome[40,41] of this important aquacultured fish species. In *Takifugu rubripes*, gill and swim bladder transcripts were examined in order to gain information in one case on immune-related genes linked to mucosal immunity and, in the other, on the function of this poorly studied organ and its relationship with lungs.

TABLE 15.2 Sequencing and De Novo Assembly Statistics

	454 Roche	Illumina
Number of paired-end reads	738,379	70,525,666
Total sequencing output	412 Mbases	7 Gbases
Number of assembled contigs	468,721	96,641
Average contig length (bp)	605	1209
N50	671	2485

Bacterial Infection

Various studies have been performed on *I. punctatus* using RNA-seq to define the genes that are up- or downregulated after a bacterial challenge. In one paper, the investigated pathogen was the *Flavobacterium columnare*, which is an important aquaculture pathogen, and the target organs were the gills.[34] Differential expression analyses of the transcripts evidenced an upregulation of a rhamnose-binding lectin, suppression of NF-κB signaling, and strong induction of IFN-inducible responses after a challenge. In the other research, the infection was made with *Edwardsiella ictaluri*, and the role of the intestinal epithelial barrier was investigated.[35] Transcripts related to genes involved in actin cytoskeletal polymerization/remodeling, junctional regulation in pathogen entry, and inflammatory responses were differentially expressed after a challenge. In *Oreochromis niloticus*, the effects of an infection with the *Streptococcus agalactiae* were investigated.[26] A total of 774 significantly upregulated and 625 significantly downregulated genes were identified, including 17 immune-related pathways. Six genes in the Toll-like receptor signaling pathway were involved, and their regulation was confirmed using real-time PCR. RNA-seq analysis was used in *Danio rerio* to investigate the effects of an immunization with an *Edwardsiella tarda* live attenuated vaccine.[32] It was demonstrated that different pathways involved in acute phase response, complement activation, immune/defense response, and antigen processing and presentation were affected at the early stage of the immunization. Real-time PCR analysis confirmed that the genes encoding the factors involved in the major histocompatibility complex (MHC)-I processing pathway were upregulated, while those involved in the MHC-II pathway were downregulated. In *D. labrax*, the efficacy of an oral vaccine against the bacterium pathogen *Vibrio anguillarum* was tested.[33] Differential transcripts were analyzed both in hind gut and head kidney, and a set of genes upregulated or downregulated were evidenced. Finally, the transcriptome profiling of *Lateolabrax japonicus* challenged with the pathogen *V. harveyi* was studied. The analysis of the up- or downregulated transcripts revealed the presence of genes involved in both innate and adaptive immune responses.

Virus Infection

The effects of the hemorrhagic disease of the grass carp, *Ctenopharyngodon idella*, caused by a reovirus (grass carp reovirus), were analyzed by RNA-seq in different tissues (gill, intestine, liver, and spleen) and at various time points before and after the challenge with the virus. The results showed that all tissues were involved in the immune response against the pathogen and that the expression of genes involved in lipid and carbohydrate metabolism, complement system, and cellular immunity was altered.

Evolution Biology

RNA-seq was used to study the transcriptome from the liver and testis of *Latimeria menadoensis*,[38] a coelacanth species identified for the first time in

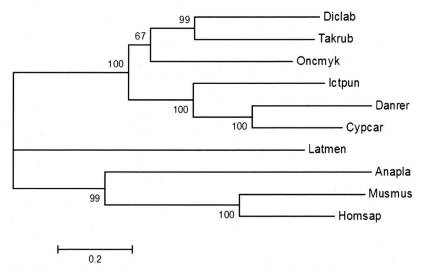

FIGURE 15.1 Phylogenetic tree showing the relationship between the CD4 amino acid sequence from *Latimeria menadoensis* with other known CD4 molecules. The tree was constructed by the "neighbor-joining" method using the bootstrap test with 10,000 replications. 0.2 indicates the genetic distance. Accession numbers: *Dicentrarchus labrax* AM849811; *Takifugu rubripes* NM_001078623; *Oncorhynchus mykiss* AY973030; *Ictalurus punctatus* DQ435305; *Danio rerio* HE983359; *Cyprinus carpio* DQ400124; *L. menadoensis* KC677707; *Anas platyrhynchos* AY738732; *Mus musculus* NM_013488; *Homo sapiens* X87579.

1997 from Indonesia. About 14 GB of sequence data were obtained that generated 66,308 contigs after a de novo assembling strategy using Trinity and CLC softwares. The results were fundamental for the annotation of the sequenced genome of the African congener *Latimeria chalumnae*.[42] Substantial differences in the expression profiles coming from the two examined tissues were evidenced and, moreover, the analysis of the immune-related gene sequences revealed that they more closely resemble orthologous genes in tetrapods than those in teleost fish (Fig. 15.1), consistent with current phylogenomic interpretations.[43,44]

CONCLUSION

The knowledge about the molecular immunology of fish has received a great speedup by RNA-seq technology. The number of newly discovered immune-related sequences has increased a lot. Moreover, the possibility to study the quantitative expression of all genes in one step has improved our data on the plasticity and dynamicity of fish biological processes linked to the immune system. This last feature will help to have information on the possible function of the different genes identified from the transcriptome analysis. With no doubt, RNA-seq technology will continue to evolve, and its cost will decrease in the future. Therefore it will become more widely used in the field of fish immunology, leading to the improvement of our understanding on the evolution of the vertebrate immune system.

REFERENCES

1. Schena M, Shalon D, Davis RW, Brown PO. Quantitative monitoring of gene expression patterns with a complementary DNA microarray. *Science* 1995;**270**:467–70.
2. Okoniewski MJ, Miller CJ. Hybridization interactions between probesets in short oligo microarrays lead to spurious correlations. *BMC Bioinformatics* 2006;**7**:276.
3. Boguski MS, Tolstoshev CM, Bassett Jr DE. Gene discovery in dbEST. *Science* 1994;**265**: 1993–4.
4. Velculescu VE, Zhang L, Vogelstein B, Kinzler KW. Serial analysis of gene expression. *Science* 1995;**270**:484–7.
5. Harbers M, Carninci P. Tag-based approaches for transcriptome research and genome annotation. *Nat Methods* 2005;**2**:495–502.
6. Kodzius R, Kojima M, Nishiyori H, Nakamura M, Fukuda S, Tagami M, et al. CAGE: cap analysis of gene expression. *Nat Methods* 2006;**3**:211–22.
7. Shiraki T, Kondo S, Katayama S, Waki K, Kasukawa T, Kawaji H, et al. Cap analysis gene expression for high-throughput analysis of transcriptional starting point and identification of promoter usage. *Proc Natl Acad Sci USA* 2003;**100**:15776–81.
8. Brenner S, Johnson M, Bridgham J, Golda G, Lloyd DH, Johnson D, et al. Gene expression analysis by massively parallel signature sequencing (MPSS) on microbead arrays. *Nat Biotechnol* 2000;**18**:630–4.
9. Costa V, Angelini C, De Feis I, Ciccodicola A. Uncovering the complexity of the transcriptomes with RNA-seq. *J Biomed Biotechnol* 2010;**2010**:853916.
10. Wang Z, Gerstein M, Snyder M. RNA-seq: a revolutionary tool for transcriptomics. *Nat Rev Genet* 2009;**10**:57–63.
11. Holt RA, Jones SJ. The new paradigm of flow cell sequencing. *Genome Res* 2008;**18**: 839–46.
12. Mortazavi A, Williams BA, McCue K, Schaeffer L, Wold B. Mapping and quantifying mammalian transcriptomes by RNA-Seq. *Nat Methods* 2008;**5**:621–8.
13. Qian X, Ba Y, Zhuang Q, Zhong G. RNA-seq technology and its application in fish transcriptomics. *OMICS* 2014;**18**:98–110.
14. Collins JE, White S, Searle SM, Stemple DL. Incorporating RNA-seq data into the zebrafish Ensembl gene-build. *Genome Res* 2012;**22**:2067–78.
15. Uren Webster TM, Santos EM. Global transcriptomic profiling demonstrates induction of oxidative stress and of compensatory cellular stress responses in brown trout exposed to glyphosate and Roundup. *BMC Genomics* 2015;**16**:32.
16. Robledo D, Ronza P, Harrison PW, Losada AP, Bermúdez R, Pardo BG, et al. RNA-seq analysis reveals significant transcriptome changes in turbot (*Scophthalmus maximus*) suffering severe enteromyxosis. *BMC Genomics* 2014;**15**:1149.
17. Gerdol M, Buonocore F, Scapigliati G, Pallavicini A. Analysis and characterization of the head kidney transcriptome from the Antarctic fish *Trematomus bernacchii* (Teleostea, Notothenioidea): a source for immune relevant genes. *Mar Genomics* 2015;**20**:13–5.
18. Wong MK, Ozaki H, Suzuki Y, Iwasaki W, Takei Y. Discovery of osmotic sensitive transcription factors in fish intestine via a transcriptomic approach. *BMC Genomics* 2014;**15**:1134.
19. Vega-Retter C, Véliz D. Liver transcriptome characterization of the endangered freshwater silverside *Basilichthys microlepidotus* (Teleostei: Atherinopsidae) using next generation sequencing. *Mar Genomics* 2014;**18PB**:147–50.
20. Ali A, Rexroad CE, Thorgaard GH, Yao J, Salem M. Characterization of the rainbow trout spleen transcriptome and identification of immune-related genes. *Front Genet* 2014;**5**:348.

21. Bilyk KT, Cheng CH. RNA-seq analyses of cellular responses to elevated body temperature in the high Antarctic cryopelagic notothenioid fish *Pagothenia borchgrevinki*. *Mar Genomics* 2014;**18PB**:163–71.

22. Shi M, Huang R, Du F, Pei Y, Liao L, Zhu Z, et al. RNA-seq profiles from grass carp tissues after reovirus (GCRV) infection based on singular and modular enrichment analyses. *Mol Immunol* 2014;**61**:44–53.

23. Magnanou E, Klopp C, Noirot C, Besseau L, Falcón J. Generation and characterization of the sea bass *Dicentrarchus labrax* brain and liver transcriptomes. *Gene* 2014;**544**:56–66.

24. Cui J, Liu S, Zhang B, Wang H, Sun H, Song S, et al. Transcriptome analysis of the gill and swimbladder of *Takifugu rubripes* by RNA-Seq. *PLoS One* 2014;**9**:e85505.

25. Sun S, Ge X, Xuan F, Zhu J, Yu N. Nitrite-induced hepatotoxicity in Bluntsnout bream (*Megalobrama amblycephala*): the mechanistic insight from transcriptome to physiology analysis. *Environ Toxicol Pharmacol* 2014;**37**:55–65.

26. Zhang R, Zhang LL, Ye X, Tian YY, Sun CF, Lu MX, et al. Transcriptome profiling and digital gene expression analysis of Nile tilapia (*Oreochromis niloticus*) infected by *Streptococcus agalactiae*. *Mol Biol Rep* 2013;**40**:5657–68.

27. Uren Webster TM, Bury N, van Aerle R, Santos EM. Global transcriptome profiling reveals molecular mechanisms of metal tolerance in a chronically exposed wild population of brown trout. *Environ Sci Technol* 2013;**47**:8869–77.

28. Xia JH, Liu P, Liu F, Lin G, Sun F, Tu R, et al. Analysis of stress-responsive transcriptome in the intestine of Asian seabass (*Lates calcarifer*) using RNA-seq. *DNA Res* 2013;**20**:449–60.

29. Smith S, Bernatchez L, Beheregaray LB. RNA-seq analysis reveals extensive transcriptional plasticity to temperature stress in a freshwater fish species. *BMC Genomics* 2013;**14**:375.

30. Liu S, Wang X, Sun F, Zhang J, Feng J, Liu H, et al. RNA-Seq reveals expression signatures of genes involved in oxygen transport, protein synthesis, folding, and degradation in response to heat stress in catfish. *Physiol Genomics* 2013;**45**:462–76.

31. Garcia TI, Shen Y, Crawford D, Oleksiak MF, Whitehead A, Walter RB. RNA-Seq reveals complex genetic response to Deepwater Horizon oil release in *Fundulus grandis*. *BMC Genomics* 2012;**13**:474.

32. Yang D, Liu Q, Yang M, Wu H, Wang Q, Xiao J, et al. RNA-seq liver transcriptome analysis reveals an activated MHC-I pathway and an inhibited MHC-II pathway at the early stage of vaccine immunization in zebrafish. *BMC Genomics* 2012;**13**:319.

33. Sarropoulou E, Galindo-Villegas J, García-Alcázar A, Kasapidis P, Mulero V. Characterization of European sea bass transcripts by RNA SEQ after oral vaccine against *V. anguillarum*. *Mar Biotechnol (NY)* 2012;**14**:634–42.

34. Sun F, Peatman E, Li C, Liu S, Jiang Y, Zhou Z, et al. Transcriptomic signatures of attachment, NF-κB suppression and IFN stimulation in the catfish gill following columnaris bacterial infection. *Dev Comp Immunol* 2012;**38**:169–80.

35. Li C, Zhang Y, Wang R, Lu J, Nandi S, Mohanty S, et al. RNA-seq analysis of mucosal immune responses reveals signatures of intestinal barrier disruption and pathogen entry following *Edwardsiella ictaluri* infection in channel catfish, *Ictalurus punctatus*. *Fish Shellfish Immunol* 2012;**32**:816–27.

36. Xiang LX, He D, Dong WR, Zhang YW, Shao JZ. Deep sequencing-based transcriptome profiling analysis of bacteria-challenged *Lateolabrax japonicus* reveals insight into the immune-relevant genes in marine fish. *BMC Genomics* 2010;**11**:472.

37. Nunez Ortiz N, Gerdol M, Stocchi V, Marozzi C, Randelli E, Bernini C, et al. T cell transcripts and T cell activities in the gills of the teleost fish sea bass (*Dicentrarchus labrax*). *Dev Comp Immunol* 2014;**47**:309–18.

38. Pallavicini A, Canapa A, Barucca M, Alfoldi J, Biscotti MA, Buonocore F, et al. Analysis of the transcriptome of the Indonesian coelacanth *Latimeria menadoensis*. *BMC Genomics* 2013;**14**:538.

39. Huth TJ, Place SP. De novo assembly and characterization of tissue specific transcriptomes in the emerald notothen, *Trematomus bernacchii*. *BMC Genomics* 2013;**14**:805.

40. Kuhl H, Beck A, Wozniak G, Canario AV, Volckaert FA, Reinhardt R. The European sea bass *Dicentrarchus labrax* genome puzzle: comparative BAC-mapping and low coverage shotgun sequencing. *BMC Genomics* 2010;**11**:68.

41. Tine M, Kuhl H, Gagnaire PA, Louro B, Desmarais E, Martins RS, et al. European sea bass genome and its variation provide insights into adaptation to euryhalinity and speciation. *Nat Commun* 2014;**5**:5770.

42. Amemiya CT, Alföldi J, Lee AP, Fan S, Philippe H, Maccallum I, et al. The African coelacanth genome provides insights into tetrapod evolution. *Nature* 2013;**496**:311–6.

43. Boudinot P, Zou J, Ota T, Buonocore F, Scapigliati G, Canapa A, et al. A tetrapod-like repertoire of innate immune receptors and effectors for coelacanths. *J Exp Zool B Mol Dev Evol* 2014;**322**:415–37.

44. Saha NR, Ota T, Litman GW, Hansen J, Parra Z, Hsu E, et al. Genome complexity in the coelacanth is reflected in its adaptive immune system. *J Exp Zool B Mol Dev Evol* 2014;**322**:438–63.

Chapter 16

Developmental Biology of Teleost Lymphocytes

Luigi Abelli
University of Ferrara, Ferrara, Italy

List of Abbreviations
AID Activation-induced cytidine deaminase
BSAP B cell-specific activator protein
CLP Common lymphoid progenitor
EBF-1 Early B cell factor 1
ICM Intermediate cell mass
MALT Mucosa-associated lymphoid tissue
NCC Nonspecific cytotoxic cells
NITR Novel immune-type receptors
NK Natural killer
Pf Postfertilization
Ph Posthatch
RAG Recombination-activating gene
TECs Thymic epithelial cells.

INTRODUCTION

Teleost bony fish (as cartilaginous fish) possess the basic components of the adaptive immune system of gnathostome vertebrates, such as specialized primary lymphoid organs, B and T lymphocytes with antigen receptors that undergo V(D)J recombination, major histocompatibility complex (MHC) molecules, antigen-presenting cells, cytokines and interferon pathway, together with peculiar features. The analysis of developmental pathways of teleost leukocytes has also been gathering considerable information.

The embryos of most teleost species hatch in the water, becoming free-living at an early vital stage, and therefore must defend against a variety of potential pathogens when adaptive immunity is not yet functional.[1] Innate immunity thus develops early to exert defense mechanisms,[2,3] in part relying on a maternally derived supply of effector molecules, such as complement components, lysozyme, lectins, protein inhibitors, and Ig, already present in the eggs.[4]

Lessons in Immunity: From Single-Cell Organisms to Mammals
http://dx.doi.org/10.1016/B978-0-12-803252-7.00016-3
215

It can be suggested that environmental factors, such as feeding, microbes, and pathogens, could also affect the maternal transfer of immunity.[5] Furthermore, it is well established that, at least in some species, the expression of complement and acute phase protein genes and embryonic formation of blood cells begin before hatching[2] to provide the embryo with precocious humoral and cellular defense systems.

Much work has been performed on the ontogeny of the zebra fish (*Danio rerio*), a model teleost species extensively used for embryological studies, due to powerful genetics, which can be applied for the generation of mutant and transgenic individuals, and the huge availability of molecular markers. However, significant differences can be observed regarding early development and organogenesis among the teleost species. At least three modalities of early hematopoiesis have been described in teleosts.[1] The process can start (1) in the blood islands of the extraembryonic yolk sac, as in angelfish, (2) in the embryonic intermediate cell mass (ICM), as in zebra fish, or (3) in the yolk sac for a short time before continuing in the ICM, as in rainbow trout.

Developmental studies in zebra fish and carp (*Cypinus carpio*) described an "embryonic" hematopoiesis producing myeloid precursors that migrate in the yolk sac and differentiate into primitive macrophages and neutrophils already at 22–33 h postfertilization (pf), thus just before and soon after hatching. Thereafter the multilineage hematopoiesis begins in the posterior blood island that becomes the main site of production of erythroid and myeloid precursors that migrate and start colonizing the "definitive" hematopoietic tissues (3–4 days pf).

The first lymphocytes can be detected in the thymus and intestine.[6] B cells can be first detected only 1–2 weeks later in lymphoid organs, such as the kidney and the spleen of carp,[6] and in the pancreas of zebra fish,[7] while several more weeks are needed before typical B cells appear in the intestine and gills of carp or sea bass (*Dicentrarchus labrax*).[8] Otherwise, cells with innate activity (eg, neutrophils) can be observed in the intestine of developing teleosts from the start of exogenous feeding. In gnotobiotic zebra fish, a neutrophil influx was observed in response to microbiome, indicating that commensals, like pathogenic microbes, could stimulate the activity of immune cells at very early developmental stages. The fundamental role played by the innate response in teleosts was strikingly shown by the possibility of rearing *rag1*$^{-/-}$ zebra fish in sterile conditions, when instead *rag1* knockout mammals undergo severe immunodeficiency and death. The integrity of epithelial barriers is, however, indispensable for fish survival.[9]

In general, the previously mentioned developmental studies indicate that teleost lymphoid cell populations differentiate in a progressive way. This idea is supported by functional proofs about a progressive establishment throughout the development of allograft responses, anamnestic responses,[10] and the later onset of adaptive responses against T-dependent antigens compared with antibody production against T-independent antigens.[11] Even the possibility for tolerance induction in young fish, still missing a complete adaptive system, should be taken into account, especially for the vaccination procedure at an early age. At any rate, full immunocompetence is, in general, achieved slowly, depending on the maturation of the lymphocyte function rather than the morphological appearance of lymphoid organs or the identification of lymphoid cells and varying among teleost species according to the general growth rate.

The major lymphoid organs of teleosts are thymus, kidney (pronephros and mesonephros), and spleen. In most species, the hematopoietic tissue of the kidney develops first, followed by the spleen (mainly erythropoietic in larval fish), and finally by the thymus. The anatomy of the lymphoid system of teleosts shows some notable differences compared with mammals, for instance the lack of a bone marrow. In adults, the hematopoietic activity resides in the intertubular tissue inside the kidneys, also named as kidney marrow. The occurrence there of definitive hematopoietic lineage cells has been demonstrated by long-term reconstitution experiments.[12] As the mammalian bone marrow, the teleost kidneys produce all the leukocyte types, except the naïve T lymphocytes that are generated in the thymus.

The secondary lymphoid tissues are less developed than in mammals. Fish drain efficiently the superficial tissues of the body by lymphatic vessels but lack lymph nodes. The spleen, simply organized, filters the blood and is the site where the different steps of immune responses against circulating antigens develop. Such a secondary role is played by the kidneys, being together with the spleen the main sites of production of circulating antibodies and the localization of antigen-specific T lymphocytes. However, both tissues do not contain any germinal centers (sites of B lymphocytes proliferation where class switch and somatic hypermutation of Ig occur in endothermic vertebrates). Mucosa-associated lymphoid tissues (MALT) are well developed, especially housing numerous leukocytes in the epithelia (intestine, skin, gills), but are less organized than in mammals, eg, in the intestine there are no equivalents of Peyer's patches. Such organization apparently depicts compartments where efficient local responses can occur, but their dependence on central compartments is still disputed. The peculiar adaptations of fish to the aquatic environment provide them with a special reinforcement of epithelial barriers against pathogen penetration; therefore an abundant production of mucus enriched by antimicrobial molecules frequently occurs.

The main categories of immune cells of teleost fish resemble, for morphology and function, the equivalents described in more developed vertebrates, such as monocytes/macrophages, granulocytes, natural killer (NK) cells, and T and B lymphocytes. The macrophages are the main phagocytic population, which play a role in the elimination of cell debris as well as pathogens, already acquired at a very early embryonic development. Other phagocytic populations are represented by granulocytes that are recruited very quickly at inflammatory sites. It is worth mentioning that some teleost granulocytes could play roles usually ascribed to tissue resident macrophages, as those undergoing recirculation in most organs even in the absence of inflammation,[13] or acidophilic granulocytes able to phagocyte live bacteria that could play a role for antigen presentation, underlined by their MHC II expression.[14] Otherwise, the occurrence of cells specialized for interferon secretion or typical dendritic cells specialized for antigen presentation is still debated, even if some evidences are accumulating.[15,16]

The occurrence of NK equivalents is proposed, although their relationship with nonspecific cytotoxic cells is not yet clarified. A number of potential receptors have been identified, most convincingly falling into the novel immune-type receptors superfamily.

Teleost lymphocytes, as those of all gnathostome vertebrates, recombine the *V(D)J* genes by means of the enzymes recombination-activating gene (RAG) 1 and 2. Their absence, as in *rag1* zebra fish mutants,[17] does not allow the rearrangement of genes encoding for the lymphocyte antigen receptors (TCR and Ig). T cell subpopulations are still incompletely characterized, even if a distinction between helper and cytotoxic cells is presumed, according to distinctive patterns of expression of genes coding for MHC class I and class II molecules and CD4 and CD8 coreceptors. The occurrence of four types of TCR chains implies the presence of at least two main populations of T cells, alternatively expressing TCRαβ or TCRγδ, thus called Tαβ and Tγδ. The main subpopulation of B lymphocytes expresses both IgM and IgD, while another expresses another isotype, named IgT or IgZ, according to the species (trout and zebra fish) where discovered.[18,19]

T CELL DEVELOPMENT

The adaptive immune system of gnathostome vertebrates is distinguished by the occurrence of the thymus as the primary lymphoid organ for the maturation and selection of T lymphocytes, self-MHC restricted and tolerant. Thymopoiesis is a highly organized process that involves the development of neural crest cells and their migration in the pharyngeal region, where epithelial–mesenchymal interactions govern the proliferation and differentiation of thymic epithelial cells (TECs) to allow colonization of the epithelial organ anlagen by lymphoid progenitor cells, their commitment to the T cell lineage, and subsequent differentiation, including tolerance induction.

In bony fish, the thymus usually develops involving pharyngeal pouches II–IV. Fundamental studies in zebra fish have defined basic molecular principles of thymopoiesis.[9,20,21] The developmental process involves neural crest cells that migrate from the neuroectoderm of the sixth rhombomere into the pharyngeal pouches III and IV, where they interact with the pharyngeal endoderm and mesoderm and with the ectoderm (all three germ layers). The proliferation and differentiation of epithelial cells is induced, then an intrathymic net is established, the capsule and trabeculae. Critically important are *Hoxa3* genes, specifically involved in primordium formation, then *Foxn1* for the differentiation of epithelial progenitor cells and to attract (via chemokines) lymphoid progenitors, whose source is thought to be the head kidney.[22] Finally, *Notch-1* signaling determines the T cell specification contrasting the B fate of lymphocytes. Many factors (eg, Bmp, Shh, Wnt, Foxn1, Dll, Ccl25, Hoxa, Pax1/9, Aire) implicated in the genetic networks of TECs occur in teleost fish and are remarkably conserved throughout vertebrate evolution.

Although morphological studies aimed at characterizing the stromal cell subpopulations in teleost thymus, their cellular interactions with thymocytes remain an important issue for future research. Evidence about the establishment of different thymic compartments, with specific roles in differentiation pathways, has been derived mainly from studies in a few species (sea bass, carp, Atlantic halibut) that provided preliminary insights into the mechanisms of thymocyte selection. T cells rely on a functional zonation of the thymus in cortical, corticomedullary, and medullary regions that constitute throughout organogenesis. In sea bass, the thymus progressively develops from 25 to 51 days posthatch (ph) a cortex filled by small thymocytes, followed by the appearance of a medulla. At this latter stage, the first expression of the T cell coreceptors CD4 and CD8-α was recorded,[23] and *MHC II-β* transcripts significantly increased compared with earlier stages.[24] The successful generation of a mature and self-tolerant T cell repertoire requires that developing thymocytes pass at least two checkpoints: positive and negative selection. The sea bass thymocytes residing in the cortex (site of *TCR* genes rearrangement in zebra fish and carp) possibly archived positive selection mediated by interactions with cortical TECs. In addition, MHC II+ cells in the medulla (*RAG1⁻* in zebra fish and carp), and notably at the corticomedullary border, could exert a key control of thymocyte negative selection.[24] Apoptotic thymocytes significantly increase in number, notably concentrated at the corticomedullary border, only at 74 days ph,[25] which is almost the time showing the appearance of specialized nonepithelial medullary stromal cells.

The thymus houses lymphocytes and thymic microenvironments specialized to support various differentiation steps that can ultimately lead to the maturation of naïve T cells, as indicated by reports that in a one-year-old sea bass nearly all cortical thymocytes expressed both CD4 and CD8 (double positive), while the medullary ones had a coreceptor (single positive).[23] Mature naïve T cells migrate from the thymus to secondary lymphoid organs (kidney, spleen), mucosal tissues, peritoneal cavity, and blood. Early data about the origin of T cells in the thymus, later localized in the head kidney and spleen, are derived from studies with monoclonal antibodies in sea bass.[26] However, the full comprehension of developmental pathways of T-cytotoxic and T-helper cells (and their subsets) is still a matter of investigation. In addition, it is worth mentioning that in some species, cells expressing thymocyte antigenic determinants (putative T cells or their precursors) have been detected in early developing intestine,[27] even indicated as a possible site of extrathymic T lymphopoiesis. These cells, mainly intraepithelial Tγδ endowed with innate and/or regulatory functions, apparently expand in the intestine at the onset of exogenous feeding of the larvae; however, their origin is not yet clarified.

B CELL DEVELOPMENT

B cell developmental pathways in teleost fish are still poorly understood.[28] Differences were found among different species at early developmental stages; however, there is a general agreement that B cell lymphopoiesis appears and occurs mainly in the kidney. The hematopoietic tissue is already present in the larval pronephros that later becomes the head (cephalic) kidney, where endocrine roles are also exerted by the adrenal homologue (steroidogenic and chromaffin cells). Developmental studies have shown a role of teleost head kidney as the primary lymphoid organ for the B lymphocytes.

In zebra fish, the first VHDHJH rearrangements were detected around 4 days pf,[7] while the pronephros was the earliest extrathymic site of RAG expression, observed at 8 days pf in *RAG2-Gfp* transgenic fish.[29] The pancreas was proposed as the site of origin of B cells,[7] but indeed the same authors later suggested that the rearrangement likely corresponds to Igζ instead of Igμ.[18] The first cells expressing IgM are found between the dorsal aorta and posterior cardinal veins and in the kidney around 3 weeks pf, suggesting a rather slow process of B cell differentiation,[30] as it is observed in most teleosts. In general, Ig-producing cells first appear in the kidney, later in the spleen, and last in the MALTs. The kidney then becomes a secondary lymphoid organ, with a prominent role in the induction and elaboration of immune responses. The parenchyma becomes structured in a wide system of sinusoids and is supported by the reticular-endothelial stroma that also plays an important role in innate immunity. The endothelium of sinusoids and macrophages (MHC II⁺) participate to the uptake and trapping of particles and molecules from the circulating blood. The head kidney is the major organ that produces antibodies, can maintain the antigens for a long time after vaccination, and has an undisputed role in immunological memory. The teleost spleen slowly (months) acquires the ability to capture and trap antigens and develops a scant regionalization compared with more evolved vertebrates. Poorly developed areas of white pulp (more evident after immunization) can house more lymphoid elements than the red pulp, while a marginal zone is lacking.

The rainbow trout B lymphopoiesis could be analyzed in depth studying transcription factors (Ikaros, E2A, EBF, Pax5, Blimp-1, and Xbp-1) conserved throughout gnathostome evolution and differentially expressed during development.[31] *Ikaros* genes are highly expressed during the earliest immune cell development and in common lymphoid progenitor (CLP), pro-B, and pre-B cells within the B cell lineage. E2A drives early B cell development and regulates the expression of genes essential for Ig rearrangement. Early B cell factor 1 (EBF-1), like E2A, also drives B lineage commitment and B cell determination. In the rainbow trout head kidney, EBF-1 is expressed (often with RAG1) in μchain-negative lymphoid cells.[32] EBF-1 and Pax5 cross-regulate their expression during B cell development. Late developing B cells express Pax5 and membrane IgM, while lacking EBF and RAG1. During B cell activation, suppression of

Pax-5 is necessary to complete terminal differentiation into a plasma cell, and this is done through the transcriptional repressor Blimp-1 (directly repressed by Pax5). Blimp-1 not only directly represses Pax5 but also regulates in activated B cells the shift from membrane to secreted forms of Ig RNA. In addition, Pax5 directly represses Xbp-1 in resting, mature B cells, thereby blocking terminal differentiation until the B cell is induced through engagement with the antigen. Xbp1-S levels increase during terminal differentiation to regulate plasma cell survival.[33]

Based on the expression patterns recorded in trout, B cell progenitors are dominant in the head kidney, from where mature naïve B cells enter circulation to reach the spleen and posterior kidney, where they encounter antigen and differentiate into short-lived plasma blasts and plasma cells.[31,34] A small subset may migrate back to the head kidney where they might subsist in particular niches as long-lived plasma cells.[34]

In addition, Pax5 isoforms with paired domain deletions (lacking exon 2) are expressed in early B cell progenitors (CLP/pro-B) in trout head kidney, and even in a few cells in the blood and spleen,[35] where they could be stored for need or simply transported to secondary sites. The homeodomain type transcription factor B cell-specific activator protein encoded by *Pax5* gene binds to DNA as a monomer, acting on numerous potential target genes. Both the activation and repressor domains at the C-terminus of the protein are common targets for alternative splicing that could maximize functional specificity. Seven alternatively spliced Pax5 isoforms were reported in rainbow trout,[35] and their analysis appears to be a very promising tool for future discoveries on B lymphopoiesis.

Ikaros forms homo- and heterodimers with its family members, leading to highly diverse functions. In trout, Ikaros has been detected in both primary and secondary lymphoid organs. In zebra fish, Ikaros expression is seen during embryogenesis in the ventral side of the dorsal aorta and near the developing thymus and is maintained mainly in adult primary lymphoid organs. A zebra fish mutant for an Ikaros protein, lacking the two C-terminal zinc-fingers and thus unable to dimerize with other Ikaros proteins, lacked IgT-expressing cells, while low levels of IgM$^+$ B cells (oligoclonal, formed later, and with a lower frequency of productive heavy chain rearrangements) were detected in the head kidney.[36] Hence, proper dimerization of Ikaros appears to be required for IgT-rearrangement and facilitates IgM-rearrangement. This important finding indicated that the development of IgM$^+$IgD$^+$ B cells and IgT$^+$ B cells involves two different pathways. Indeed, the structure of the trout and zebra fish *IgH* loci already predicted that the expression of IgT/IgZ cannot occur in IgM/IgD-expressing cells.[18,19,37] These subpopulations also have different localization in some species (IgM$^+$IgD$^+$ as the main components in spleen, kidney, and blood, while IgT$^+$ in mucosal tissues) and, notably, functional properties.[38] In most species, IgD is coexpressed with IgM through alternative splicing of the same pre-mRNA; however, a distinct population of IgM$^-$IgD$^+$ B cells has been identified in the channel catfish, which preferentially expresses σ Ig light chain.[39] Furthermore, novel splicing mechanisms were discovered that produce secretory IgD.[40] Other studies are needed to establish the functional meaning and developmental processes.

Teleost IgM is, by far, the most abundant antibody in serum and is thought to play the prevalent role in systemic immunity. Booster immunization can produce a significant increase of serum IgM; however, heterogeneity of antibodies is limited, as is anamnestic response, with little increase in IgM affinity. Among the activation-induced cytidine deaminase-mediated mechanisms that could modify the initial receptor repertoire generated by RAG, only somatic hypermutation is operative in teleosts. However, teleost IgM typically associate into larger polymers, varying the number of disulfide bridges that bind monomers and subunities, to produce heterogeneous mixtures that can raise the antibody affinity.[41] Rather abundant natural antibodies might compensate for the lack of high-affinity antibodies, such as in Atlantic cod lacking CD4 and MHC II molecules, thus typical T helper cells.[42]

PERSPECTIVES

The impressive mass of information gathered on teleost immunology certainly will allow further progress, which is expected to define the much in-depth phenotype/function of leukocytes, their specific/coordinated roles in the response against microbes and parasites, and boost basic and applied research. On the other hand, knowledge about leukocyte developmental pathways is rising more slowly, often referring to seminal findings from a few outstanding research groups. It can advise a much more widespread focus on Devo, which appears to be crucial for ontogenetic and cell lineage studies, providing a meaningful scientific basis for the selection/rearing of species that can have a higheconomical value.

REFERENCES

1. Zapata A, Diez B, Cejalvo T, Gutierrez-de Frias C, Cortes A. Ontogeny of the immune system of fish. *Fish Shellfish Immunol* 2006;**20**:126–36.
2. Huttenhuis HBT, Grou CPO, Taverne-Thiele AJ, Taverne N, Rombout JHWM. Carp (*Cyprinus carpio* L.) innate immune factors are present before hatching. *Fish Shellfish Immunol* 2006;**20**: 586–96.
3. Huttenhuis HBT, Taverne-Thiele AJ, Grou CPO, Bergsma J, Saeij JPJ, Nakayasu C, et al. Ontogeny of the common carp (*Cyprinus carpio* L.) innate immune system. *Dev Comp Immunol* 2006;**30**:557–74.
4. Magnadóttir B. Innate immunity of fish (overview). *Fish Shellfish Immunol* 2006;**20**:137–51.
5. Zhang S, Wang Z, Wang H. Maternal immunity in fish. *Dev Comp Immunol* 2013;**39**:72–8.
6. Huttenhuis HBT, Huising MO, Van der Meulen T, Van Oosterhoud CN, Sanchez NA, Taverne-Thiele AJ, et al. Rag expression identifies B and T cell lymphopoietic tissues during the development of common carp (*Cyprinus carpio* L.). *Dev Comp Immunol* 2005;**29**:1033–47.
7. Danilova N, Steiner LA. B cells develop in the zebrafish pancreas. *Proc Natl Acad Sci USA* 2002;**99**:13711–6.

8. Picchietti S, Terribili FR, Mastrolia L, Scapigliati G, Abelli L. Expression of lymphocyte antigenic determinants in developing gut-associated lymphoid tissue of the sea bass *Dicentrarchus labrax* (L.). *Anat Embryol* 1997;**196**:457–63.

9. Lieschke GJ, Trede NS. Fish immunology. *Curr Biol* 2009;**19**:678–82.

10. Botham JW, Grace MF, Manning MJ. Ontogeny of first set and second set alloimmune reactivity in fishes. In: Manning MJ, editor. *Phylogeny of immunological memory*. Amsterdam: Elsevier/North-Holland; 1980. p. 83–92.

11. Tatner MF. The ontogeny of humoral immunity in rainbow trout, *Salmo gairdneri*. *Vet Immunol Immunopathol* 1986;**12**:93–105.

12. Kobayashi I, Kuniyoshi S, Saito K, Moritomo T, Takahashi T, Nakanishi T. Long-term hematopoietic reconstitution by transplantation of kidney hematopoietic stem cells in lethally irradiated clonal gibuna crucian carp (*Carassius auratus langsdorfii*). *Dev Comp Immunol* 2008;**32**:957–65.

13. Le Guyader D, Redd MJ, Colucci-Guyon E, Murayama E, Kissa K, Briolat V, et al. Origins and unconventional behavior of neutrophils in developing zebrafish. *Blood* 2008;**111**:132–41.

14. Cuesta A, Esteban MA, Meseguer J. Cloning, distribution and upregulation of the teleost fish MHC class II alpha suggests a role for granulocytes as antigen-presenting cells. *Mol Immunol* 2006;**43**:1275–85.

15. Lugo-Villarino G, Balla KM, Stachura DL, Bañuelos K, Werneck MBF, Traver D. Identification of dendritic antigen-presenting cells in the zebrafish. *Proc Natl Acad Sci USA* 2010;**107**: 15850–5.

16. Bassity E, Clark TG. Functional identification of dendritic cells in the teleost model, rainbow trout (*Oncorhynchus mykiss*). *PLoS One* 2012;**7**:e33196.

17. Wienholds E, Schulte-Merker S, Walderich B, Plasterk RH. Target-selected inactivation of the zebrafish rag1 gene. *Science* 2002;**297**:99–102.

18. Danilova N, Bussmann J, Jekosch K, Steiner LA. The immunoglobulin heavy-chain locus in zebrafish: identification and expression of a previously unknown isotype, immunoglobulin Z. *Nat Immunol* 2005;**6**:295–302.

19. Hansen JD, Landis ED, Phillips RB. Discovery of a unique Ig heavy-chain isotype (IgT) in rainbow trout: implications for a distinctive B cell developmental pathway in teleost fish. *Proc Natl Acad Sci USA* 2005;**102**:6919–24.

20. Trede NS, Ota T, Kawasaki H, Paw BH, Katz T, Demarest B, et al. Zebrafish mutants with disrupted early T cell and thymus development identified in early pressure screen. *Dev Dyn* 2008;**237**:2575–84.

21. Bajoghli B, Aghaallaei N, Hess I, Rode I, Netuschil N, Tay BH, et al. Evolution of genetic networks underlying the emergence of thymopoiesis in vertebrates. *Cell* 2009;**138**:186–97.

22. Langenau DM, Ferrando AA, Traver D, Kutok JL, Hezel J-P, Kanki JP, et al. In vivo tracking of T cell development, ablation, and engraftment in transgenic zebrafish. *Proc Natl Acad Sci USA* 2004;**101**:7369–74.

23. Picchietti S, Guerra L, Buonocore F, Randelli E, Fausto AM, Abelli L. Lymphocyte differentiation in sea bass thymus: CD4 and CD8-α gene expression studies. *Fish Shellfish Immunol* 2009;**27**:50–6.

24. Picchietti S, Abelli L, Guerra L, Randelli E, Proietti Serafini F, Belardinelli MC, et al. *MHC II-β chain* gene expression studies define the regional organization of the thymus in the developing bony fish *Dicentrarchus labrax* (L.). *Fish Shellfish Immunol* 2015;**42**:483–93.

25. Abelli L, Baldassini MR, Meschini R, Mastrolia L. Apoptosis of thymocytes in developing sea bass *Dicentrarchus labrax* (L.). *Fish Shellfish Immunol* 1998;**8**:13–24.

26. Abelli L, Picchietti S, Romano N, Mastrolia L, Scapigliati G. Immunocytochemical detection of thymocyte antigenic determinants in developing lymphoid organs of sea bass *Dicentrarchus labrax* (L.). *Fish Shellfish Immunol* 1996;**6**:493–505.

27. Rombout JHMW, Abelli L, Picchietti S, Scapigliati G, Kiron V. Teleost intestinal immunology. *Fish Shellfish Immunol* 2011;**31**:616–26.

28. Fillatreau S, Six A, Magadan S, Castro R, Sunyer JO, Boudinot P. The astonishing diversity of Ig classes and B cell repertoires in teleost fish. *Front Immunol* 2013;**4**:1–13.

29. Trede NS, Langenau DM, Traver D, Look AT, Zon LI. The use of zebrafish to understand immunity. *Immunity* 2004;**20**:367–79.

30. Page DM, Wittamer V, Bertrand JY, Lewis KL, Pratt DN, Delgado N, et al. An evolutionarily conserved program of B-cell development and activation in zebrafish. *Blood* 2013;**122**:1–11.

31. Zwollo P. Dissecting teleost B cell differentiation using transcription factors. *Dev Comp Immunol* 2011;**35**:898–905.

32. Zwollo P, Mott K, Barr M. Comparative analyses of B cell populations in trout kidney and mouse bone marrow: establishing "B cell signatures". *Dev Comp Immunol* 2010;**34**:1291–9.

33. Barr M, Mott K, Zwollo P. Defining terminally differentiating B cell populations in rainbow trout immune tissues using the transcription factor XbpI. *Fish Shellfish Immunol* 2011;**31**: 727–35.

34. Bromage ES, Kaattari IM, Zwollo P, Kaattari SL. Plasmablast and plasma cell production and distribution in trout immune tissues. *J Immunol* 2004;**173**:7317–23.

35. MacMurray E, Barr M, Bruce A, Epp L, Zwollo P. Alternative splicing of the trout Pax5 gene and identification of novel B cell populations using Pax5 signatures. *Dev Comp Immunol* 2013;**41**:270–81.

36. Schorpp M, Bialecki M, Diekhoff D, Walderich B, Odenthal J, Maischein HM, et al. Conserved functions of Ikaros in vertebrate lymphocyte development: genetic evidence for distinct larval and adult phases of T cell development and two lineages of B cells in zebrafish. *J Immunol* 2006;**177**:2463–76.

37. Parra D, Takizawa F, Sunyer OJ. Evolution of B cell immunity. *Annu Rev Anim Biosci* 2013;**1**:65–97.

38. Zhang YA, Salinas I, Li J, Parra D, Bjork S, Xu Z, et al. IgT, a primitive immunoglobulin class specialized in mucosal immunity. *Nat Immunol* 2010;**11**:827–35.

39. Edholm ES, Bengten E, Wilson M. Insights into the function of IgD. *Dev Comp Immunol* 2011;**35**:1309–16.

40. Ramirez-Gomez F, Greene W, Rego K, Hansen JD, Costa G, Kataria P, et al. Discovery and characterization of secretory IgD in rainbow trout: secretory IgD is produced through a novel splicing mechanism. *J Immunol* 2012;**188**:1341–9.

41. Kaattari S, Evans D, Klemer J. Varied redox forms of teleost IgM: an alternative to isotypic diversity? *Immunol Rev* 1998;**166**:133–42.

42. Star B, Nederbragt AJ, Jentoft S, Grimholt U, Malmstrøm M, Gregers TF, et al. The genome sequence of Atlantic cod reveals a unique immune system. *Nature* 2011;**477**:207–10.

Chapter 17

Cathelicidins: An Ancient Family of Fish Antimicrobial Peptides

Marco Scocchi, Michela Furlan
University of Trieste, Trieste, Italy

Paola Venier
University of Padova, Padova, Italy

Alberto Pallavicini
University of Trieste, Trieste, Italy

Fish live in aquatic environments, which are ideal for microorganisms' growth, in comparison to terrestrial habitats. For this reason, they have to cope with high loads of microbes, which circulate through and reach every mucosal epithelial barrier of the body.[1] A danger signal at a mucosal barrier can be detected and triggers an innate defensive response, which directs release of multiple immune effectors.[2] It is well known that fish mucosal secretions, including gut, skin, and the gills, carry a wide variety of molecules involved in the innate immunity, including complement proteins, lysozyme, proteases, esterases, and antimicrobial peptides (AMPs).[1]

The study of AMPs represents one of the fastest growing fields in innate immunity. AMPs are a broad category of different families of highly conserved host-protective peptides, widely found in nature and commonly exhibiting broad-spectrum antimicrobial activity in vitro.[3] Similar to mammals, fish produce many different AMPs displaying antibacterial, antiviral, and antifungal activities, which are detectable in mucosal secretions and tissues as skin, intestine, gills, and hematopoietic tissues.[4]

While the discovery of vertebrate AMPs in amphibians, humans, and rabbits started in the mid-1980s, reports on an increasing number of teleost AMPs, based on their antibacterial activity or identified by genomic analysis, are more recent.[3,5–8] Different groups of AMPs coexist in the same fish. Some of them, such as defensins and cathelicidins, have a counterpart in other classes of vertebrates (eg, mammals),[7,9,10] whereas others, such as piscidins, have been specifically recognized only in teleosts.[11] Whereas a detailed description of the main class of AMPs of fish has been reported in excellent reviews,[34] this chapter is focused

Lessons in Immunity: From Single-Cell Organisms to Mammals
http://dx.doi.org/10.1016/B978-0-12-803252-7.00017-5

on fish cathelicidins, their main features, and activities. Until now, only scattered and incomplete information has been available. Experimental data show that fish cathelicidins share several common characteristics but also have distinguished features in respect to their mammal counterpart, and their emerging functions underlie their importance within the innate immunity of fish. Cathelicidins were originally identified in mammalian neutrophils[12] and later were characterized in tissues of other classes of vertebrates, including birds,[13,14] fish,[15] reptiles,[16,17] and amphibians.[18] Although members of this AMP family have a highly divergent C-terminal antimicrobial sequences, both intraspecies and across species, cat-helicidins share a typical N-terminal proregion of ≈100 amino acids named the cathelin-like domain[10] (Fig. 17.1). Cathelicidins are produced as a pre-proprotein, with an N-terminal signal sequence, the cathelin-like domain, and a variable antimicrobial domain in the C-terminal region.[19] After the cleavage of the signal sequence, the proprotein may be further removed by proteases, thus releasing an AMP, which can vary greatly in sequence and size.

The highly conserved cathelin domain has been used to search for novel members of this family in other species. In 2005, Chang and collaborators revealed the presence of a first cathelicidin gene, *cath-1*, in rainbow trout *Oncorhynchus mykiss*[15] and a second cathelicidin gene, *cath-2*, was reported one year later, both in rainbow trout with homologs in Atlantic salmon *Salmo salar*.[20] Homologs of one or both types of cathelicidins have been subsequently identified in other Sal-monidae, including brown trout *Salmo trutta fario*,[21,22] grayling *Thymallus thy-mallus*,[22] brook trout *Salvelinus fontinalis*,[21,22] Chinook salmon *Oncorhynchus tshawytscha*,[23] Arctic charr *Salvelinus alpinus*,[21] and in the ancient salmonid lenox *Brachymystax lenok*.[24] In addition to the previous findings, two more cathe-licidin genes and multiple transcripts were recently identified in rainbow trout,[25] suggesting that a more complex family of cathelicidins could exist in salmonids.

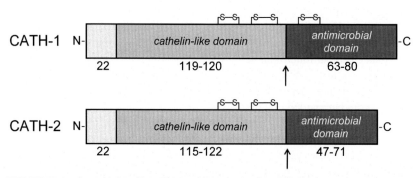

FIGURE 17.1 **Organization of the fish cathelicidins of type I (CATH-1) and type II (CATH-2) characterized in salmonids.** The signal peptides (light gray), cathelin-like proregion, and C-terminal antimicrobial domain are shown in the gray color of different intensity. Conserved cys-teines and putative disulfide bridges are shown. A minimum and maximum number of amino acid residues of known cathelicidins and putative cleavage sites for the release of the C-terminal antimi-crobial peptide (*arrow*) are also indicated.

Homologs have also been identified in other fish, such as the Osmeridae *Plecoglossus altivelis*[26] and the rainbow smelt *Osmerus mordax*,[22] while three almost identical members have been discovered in Atlantic cod *Gadus morhua*, the unique one found in a fish not belonging to Protacanthopterygii.[21,27]

THE PRESENCE OF CATHELICIDIN IN BONY FISH GENOMES

The first cathelicidins identified in marine animals, previously only found in mammals, were initially isolated as AMPs from the Atlantic hagfish, *Myxine glutinosa*.[28] The cathelin domain was then used as a probe to mine large-scale cDNA sequencing data and, in a couple of years, cathelicidin transcripts were described from salmonids and cods,[15,20–22,24] as reported in the introduction.

Few new cathelicidin transcripts were described in bony fish from these initial reports, despite growing knowledge of the biological activity of this group of molecules in fish. To date, besides salmonids and cods, only six nonredundant cathelicidins are annotated in the nucleotide public database. One putative sequence is codified in the guppy genome (GB:XP_008426081), a model organism for ecology and evolution studies in Cypriniformes, obtained as an output of a whole-genome shotgun project and annotated by automated computational analysis using gene prediction methods. Similarly to the guppy sequence, another putative sequence annotated as cathelicidin resulted from the whole-genome sequence project of the croaker *Larimichthys crocea* (GB:XP_010742358). Irrespective of their annotation, we are doubtful about the goodness of this automatic analysis. Two probably genuine cathelicidin transcripts from the Japanese eel (GB:AFP72291, AFP72292) were submitted to the public database 3 years ago, unfortunately not related to any scientific report. Another undoubted sequence publicly available is from the ayu *P. altivelis*, a relative of the smelts placed in the order Osmeriformes.

The presence of two distinctive cathelicidins in the Elopomorpha, a basal superorder lineage of Teleostei likely diverged about 250 million years ago, reinforces the hypothesis of a cathelicidin ancestor gene at least in the basal bony fish, if not in the whole Actinopterygii class. The lack of genetic information about this important immunity gene in almost all bony fish families could have both technical and biological reasons. Technically speaking, the still incomplete genome sequences of many bony fish make the automatic annotation of variable and noncanonical transcripts, such as those of AMPs, more difficult. As an example of the presence of several false negatives for cathelicidin genes in the public sequence database, we could consider a sequence from the assembled transcriptome of the flat fish *Scophthalmus maximus* (GB:JU354606) strikingly similar to the eel cathelicidin 1. Taking into consideration the sequence variability of cathelicidins between salmonids and cods, the similarity of these two sequences deserves further study. More interesting is a protein sequence automatically predicted in the genome of the spotted gar *Lepisosteus oculatus* (UNIPROT:W5MSD0) showing a high similarity to the eel cathelicidin 2.

The structure of these two transcripts is identical and their organization absolutely comparable to that described in Fig. 17.1 but with a putative active peptide of only 14 amino acids. Because of the ancestral characteristics of the orders Lepisosteiformes and Elopomorpha, we can assume these sequences as the most primitive among the bony fish. Starting from this initial information, we have mined the genomic data of all the ancestral fish species available, and we could identify this ancestral cathelicidin form also in the Chondrosteans. Fig. 17.2 depicts the presence or absence of cathelicidins in all vertebrate lineages. The biological explanation of the absence of annotated cathelicidins in most of the Euteleost may be linked to the genome duplication and the huge evolutive radiation of bony fish. Ohno[29] proposed that the increased complexity and genome size of vertebrates have resulted from two rounds of whole-genome duplication in early vertebrate evolution (2R), which provided raw materials for the evolutionary diversification of vertebrates. Genomic sequence data provide substantial evidence for the abundance of duplicated genes in many organisms. Extensive comparative analyses have demonstrated that teleost fish experienced another round of genome duplication, the so-called fish-specific genome duplication.[30–32] This event, which occurred about 350 million years ago, has accelerated the radiation and diversification of bony fish by losing genes or by gaining new features, as paradigmatically reported for the Hox genes.[33] Cathelicidin genes, appearing and disappearing in the fish phylogeny, can be just another target of this phenomenom. We can argue that the most ancestral cathelicidin gene (indicated with a square in Fig. 17.2) was lost during the Euteleosteomorpha radiation, and the duplicated cathelicidin gene (the circle in Fig. 17.2) extended the sequence codified by the fourth exon, acquiring the amino acid profile rich in GlyArgSer repeats that we can find in salmonids and cods. Fig. 17.3

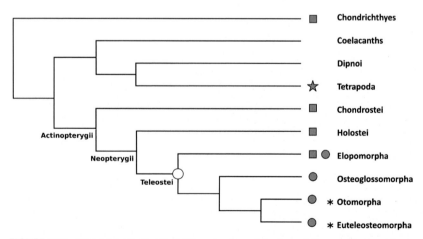

FIGURE 17.2 **The presence of cathelicidin genes in vertebrate evolutionary lineages.** A *star* indicates the cathelicidins from tetrapods, a *square* is used to show where we have identified an ancestral sequence, and, finally, the *circle* is placed on the fish superorders in which the cathelicidin was previously studied. An *empty circle* indicates the fish-specific genome duplication. *Probably only in very few orders.

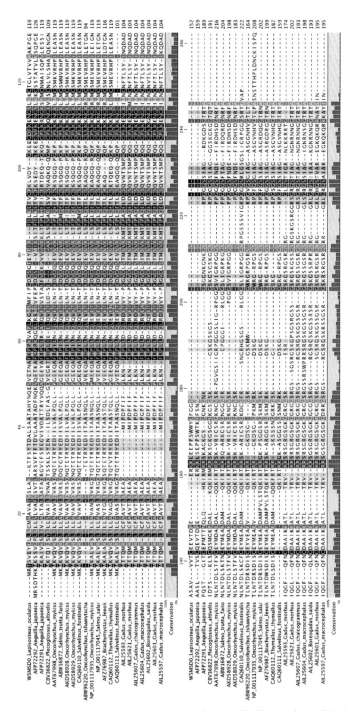

FIGURE 17.3 Multiple sequence alignment of the fish cathelicidin proteins. All the bony fish cathelidins retrievable from the public database are shown with their accession numbers. The sequence variants with a similarity greater than 97% are collapsed with CD-Hit software (http://cd-hit.org). Amino acid residues with at least 50% of conservation are indicated with a gray to black background.

shows the alignment of fish cathelicidins, including those of eel and spotted gar. The first two aligned proteins are those supposed to be the ancestral gene. In other Euteleosteomorpha lineages, such as in Percomorpha, a genome reduction event likely caused the loss of the second cathelicidin. A study in yeast demonstrated that speciation of polyploid yeasts may be associated with reciprocal gene loss at duplicated loci.[34] Thus speciation accompanied by differential retention and loss of duplicated genes after genome duplication may be a powerful lineage-splitting force.[35] Fig. 17.2 reflects our speculation, a hypothesis to be verified with comparative genomic studies.

STRUCTURE OF CATHELICIDIN GENE AND TRANSCRIPTS

Fish cathelicidins share several characteristics with their mammalian counterparts, such as four-exon organization of their genes and a conserved proregion with four-clustered cysteines. The lowest sequence similarity of exon 1 with mammalian sequences suggests a substantially different signal peptide in fish species.[15] A multiple sequence alignment of fish cathelicidins (Fig. 17.3) displayed the high-amino acid conservation across species of the N-terminal region, composed by the signal peptide sequence and the cathelin-like domain and encompassing the exons 1, 2, and 3. Compared with mammals, fish have a shorter signal peptide, with about 22–26 residues versus 29–30, and a longer cathelin-like domain, with 115–127 residues versus 94–114.[15,20]

Different from mammalian cathelicidins, in which exon 4 codes for peptides of 12–45 amino acids endowed with antimicrobial activity, the fish cathelicidin exon 4 codes for long and highly divergent peptides of 47–80 amino acids.[22] Despite the sequence variability, all these C-terminal peptides are invariably highly cationic with a net positive charge over +10, with the unusually high number of Gly (25–30%) and Ser (8–21%) representing a hallmark for this class of AMPs.[22]

Based on sequence analysis, salmonid cathelicidins can be divided into two groups (identified with the Arabic numbers 1 and 2) (Fig. 17.1). The CATH-1 group is characterized by the presence of two cysteine residues, which probably lead to the formation of a disulfide bond, which are absent in CATH-2.[21] In *O. mykiss* and *S. fontinalis* the two cysteines are separated by five residues, whereas in *S. salar* and *S. trutta fario* the dividing sequence is longer, with 9–12 residues. Furthermore, the central region of the mature peptide is characterized by the six amino acid repeat RPGGGS. In particular, up to eight copies of this motif are present in CATH-1 sequences, whereas there are almost one or two copies in CATH-2 members and in phylogenetically distant *Osmerus* and *Thymallus* CATH-1. This motif can also be comprised in another longer repeat R(L/P)GGGSLIG, detected in the CATH-1 group. Recently, Zhang and colleagues described two more cathelicidin genes in rainbow trout, CATH-1d and CATH-2b, and multiple alternative splicing sites.[25] They also reported an energy-saving form of cathelicidins with the deletion of the characteristic cathelin-like domain, a deletion also reported for *S. fontinalis*.[22] Concerning the two Atlantic cod cathelicidin genes, a slightly different motif GSRGG(S/K) is present in 2–3 copies.

An overview of this situation outlines the presence of a genetically unstable region, predisposed to duplication, which could denote a common mechanism responsible for cathelicidin gene diversification (Scocchi et al.[22]). Recently, a third gene was reported in cod.[36] Most genome-wide studies show high-frequency polymorphisms in genes related to immunity, in particular AMPs.[37] The investigation of cathelicidin genes throughout a wide distributional range of individuals in the Atlantic cod, as well as in closely related species, highlighted a highly variable polymorphism in the antimicrobial domain, with a transspecies variation level that suggests maintenance by some form of balancing selection.[36]

Cathelicidin Gene Expression

Most of the data elucidating the cathelicidin role in vivo come from expression studies. Cathelicidin genes are expressed in several tissues of healthy rainbow trout, including gill, head kidney, intestine, skin, and spleen.[15,20,22] This is similar to the expression patterns observed in cod where cathelicidin transcripts have been detected in spleen and kidney and to a lesser extent in gills, pyloric caeca, and intestine.[21] Transcripts of the only cathelicidin gene of the thick-lipped lenok, *B. lenok*, were principally detected in gill and, at lower levels, in the gut and muscle. In the Atlantic cod, cathelicidin mRNA was also present at low levels in newly hatched larvae, and its expression varied over the 68 days examined, thus suggesting an active defense role also in very early developmental stages.[27]

Several studies highlighted the cathelicidin induction in cell lines or live organisms following stimulation. In responsive cells of the Atlantic salmon, as*cath-1* can be induced by inflammatory cytokines such as TNF-α,[38] whereas trout IL-6 induced rt*cath-2* but not rt*cath-1* expression in the monocyte/macrophage-like RTS-11 cells.[39] Both bacteria and bacterial DNA induced cathelicidin expression in a cultured embryonic salmon cell line, thus confirming the antibacterial role of fish homologs.[23] Surprisingly, purified lipopolysaccharide (LPS) (that is, treated with DNase I) could not induce the cathelicidin expression. Assays with poly I:C, LPS, and flagellin demonstrated a wide variability in the response of the Chinook salmon embryonic cell line.[40] Further clue of the participation of these proteins in the immune response derived from in vitro and in vivo studies with different pathogens.[40] During yersiniosis of Atlantic salmon, triggered by bath exposure to *Yersinia ruckeri*, both the cathelicidin genes, especially as*cath-2*, were differentially expressed in the gills and spleen with expression peaks at 96 h postinfection.[41] Similar results were obtained in the ayu *P. altivelis* following intraperitoneal injection of *Vibrio anguillarum*. However, in this case, *cath-2* induction was observable in multiple tissues very early, already after 6 h postinoculum, and further increased at 24 h.[26] Interestingly, the rt*cath-2* gene was also found upregulated, even if at a low extent, after exposing rainbow trout fry and larvae to *Y. ruckeri*[42] and the skin parasite *Ichthyophthirius mul-tifiliis*,[43] respectively. Overall, these results indicate that cathelicidins are early expressed during ontogenesis and are highly inducible in adult fish.

Despite several gene expression studies, few data are available on the cellular location of cathelicidin expression. Using specific antibodies raised in trout, CATH-1a and CATH-2a peptides could be detected by immunofluorescence in the head kidney: the immunoreactive signals were observed in circulating lymphoid cells around sinusoids and in the gut, with intense immunopositivity, at the mucosal layer, especially in the columnar epithelial cells of the villus, and in some lymphoid cells in the lamina propria.[25] Overall, these results indicate that, similar to their mammalian orthologs, fish cathelicidins form the first line of host defense.

Protein Processing and Expression

The conserved N-terminal QKIRTRR sequence encoded by exon 4 has been suggested to contain a cleavage site for a processing enzyme between the Thr and Arg residues.[20,24,26] Like in mammals, this would lead to a mature peptide in which elastase and proteinase 3 cleave cathelicidin precursors into functional C-terminal domains.[44] Actually, some recombinant fish cathelicidins subjected to the action of human elastase resulted in the generation of peptides of the expected size. At the moment, no elastase homolog has been identified in salmonids[45] and, thereby, the substrate specificity of a hypothetical elastase-like enzyme is unknown (the true-processing site and the protease involved remain unknown). The only mature peptide so far purified from fish tissues, a 67 amino acid peptide isolated from cod, has a predicted cleavage site different from that of salmonid cathelicidins. On the other hand, the starting sequence of the purified peptide, SRSG (Ser-Arg-Ser-Gly), suggests that the precursor has been cleaved between the fifth and sixth amino acid (Arg-Ser) specified by exon 4.[27]

Surprisingly, data on the mature peptide forms and their differential expression in different tissues are scarce. Western blot analysis is available only for cod CATH in infected fish. A band of 7 kDa, consistent with the presence of a mature peptide, was detected, and its intensity was more pronounced in the kidney than in the spleen of infected fish.[27] The presence of the cathelicidin peptide at a low level in infected tissues is apparently in contrast with the very high level of their transcripts induced in cod and in different salmonids after infection with bacterial pathogens (mentioned previously).

Biological Activity of the C-Terminal Peptides

In other vertebrates, the C-terminal mature peptides exert antimicrobial activity. In most cases, in fish, antibacterial assays have been carried out using peptide fragments representing different portions of the deduced amino acid sequences. In a few cases, the full-length peptides[25] or purified natural peptide[27] has been employed.

The variability of the C-terminal region of the analyzed peptides and differences in the applied experimental protocols make a precise comparison of the resulting antibacterial data difficult. It is quite clear that both rtCATH-1 and rtCATH-2 possess bacteriostatic more than bactericidal activity not only against the gram-negative fish pathogens *Aeromonas salmonicida*, *Photobacterium damselae*, and *Y. ruckeri* but also against the gram-positive stains of *Lactococcus garvieae*.[15,20] Growth inhibition assays have been used to evidence the antibacterial properties of trout CATHs and of their truncated variants against *Edwardsiella ictaluri*, *Vibrio fluvialis*, *Aeromonas hydrophila*, and *Streptococcus dysgalactiae* (Zhang et al.[25]). Recombinant asCATH-1 and asCATH-2 from Atlantic salmon showed direct microbicidal activity against *Vibrio anguillarum* and *Escherichia coli* but little or no bactericidal activity against *Y. ruckeri*,[41] and these findings suggest that specificity of the same cathelicidin may vary in different species.

Interestingly, all the different methods used to detect antimicrobial activity of cathelicidin peptides have been carried out testing them in diluted media, such as 0.25× Mueller-Hinton broth[15,20] or even a more diluted media.[46] A decrease of function has been shown for rtCATH-1(R151-V186) against *A. salmonicida* MT004 by supplementing the medium with calcium or magnesium ions.[15] This aspect is consistent with a sensitivity for this type of AMPs to high concentrations of salts, a feature already observed for other AMPs such as the mammal defensins.[47]

Data on antibacterial properties toward various pathogens using synthetic fragments have been collected for the salmonid lenok[24] and for aCATH-m of ayu.[26] Both peptides exhibited strong activity against several bacteria strains although in both cases it is unclear if low salt or diluted media have been used.[26] Radial diffusion assays in low ionic strength conditions were also used to determine the activity of synthetic codCATH against different pathogens. It is highly active against gram-negative species, the gram-positive strain *Bacillus megaterium* Bm11, and against the fungus *Candida albicans*.[46] The 67-residue natural peptide of cod was found to be quite active against the strain Bm11 in the same assay conditions.[27]

Overall, the sequence diversity of the mature peptides, suggestive of positive diversifying selection in response to various and quickly evolving pathogens, appears to direct the specificity of the antimicrobial activities.[3] However, these results do not definitely demonstrate that the biological function of the C-terminal peptides is a direct antibacterial activity. It is also possible that the antimicrobial activity is exerted in particular and unknown conditions or those cathelicidin peptides have to assume particular structures. In this respect, few data exist on the structures of C-terminal polypeptides. Some insights were inferred by CD spectroscopy carried out in different solvent environments.[25] In phosphate buffer, rtCATHs and their truncated variants showed mostly a random-coiled conformation, while in TFE solvent, mimicking the bacterial cell membrane environment, the CD spectra of CATH-1 peptides changed accordingly to the presence in the peptides of a certain degree of α-helical and β-sheet conformations.[25]

A remarkable feature that distinguishes fish cathelicidin from most AMPs is the low toxicity against eukaryotic cells. Neither hemolytic nor a very modest effect has been detected for Atlantic salmon CATHs[41]; nor has cytotoxicity toward the rainbow trout gonadal 2 cells been revealed by trout CATHs.[15,25] In contrast, human cathelicidin LL-37 exhibited strong hemolytic and cytotoxic activities against all cells tested.[25] No cytotoxicity was observed up to a concentration of $40\,\mu M$ for cod in fish cells, and its cell selectivity has been confirmed by using bacterial and mammalian membrane mimetics.[46] The thick-lipped lenok also does not show toxic activity even at 10-fold the bactericidal concentration.[24]

In mammals, cathelicidins have been demonstrated to exhibit multiple activities, both immune and nonimmune, and antimicrobial activity far beyond the levels has been observed in vitro.[48] In fish, research has not reached this point. However, recent studies demonstrated that the two cathelicidins of Atlantic salmon induced the rapid and transient expression of IL-8 in peripheral blood leukocytes.[41] Trout cathelicidins could also bind LPS in a dose-dependent manner and, using different fragments, it was clear that the N-terminal binding site has a higher affinity for LPS than does the central one.[25] Very recent data indicate that rtCATH-2, produced by an intestinal epithelial cell line in response to β-glucans, induced the production of IL-1β in RTgutGC cells and displayed a synergic effect with zymosan in the IL-1β upregulation. Importantly, the colocalization of both rtCATH-2 and IL-1β was detected in the intestinal epithelial cells of rainbow trout fed with a zymosan-supplemented diet.[49] These preliminary data indicate that some of the immunomodulatory activities of mammalian cathelicidins may be shared by their fish counterparts, and thus they probably are an evolutionarily conserved mechanism of innate immune regulation.

CONCLUSIONS

In the last few years, extensive studies on fish cathelicidins have provided a detailed initial characterization of this important AMP family on structural, genetic, and functional levels. This has led to a better understanding of the role of these peptides in the innate host defense of fish. Furthermore, studies on the similarities and differences of cathelicidins from other species have contributed to our understanding of the evolutionary relationships of innate host defense mechanisms among vertebrates.

One of the main reasons for studying AMPs is the possibility to design novel therapeutic agents against microbial infections. The cathelicidins described in this chapter have shown to have activity against fish pathogens and the capacity to stimulate the innate immune responses of fish. For these reasons, a comprehensive knowledge of their functions could find potential applications in aquaculture where there is a constant risk of large-scale microbial infection that can lead to significant economic losses and which demands new strategies to prevent or treat these pathogens.

ACKNOWLEDGMENTS

MF is supported by grants from the project "InnovH$_2$O" Italy–Slovenia cross-border cooperation 2007–13 financed by the European Regional Development Fund for Territorial Cooperation and cofinancing of national public funds.

REFERENCES

1. Salinas I. The mucosal immune system of teleost fish. *Biology (Basel)* 2015;**4**:525–39.
2. Gomez D, Sunyer JO, Salinas I. The mucosal immune system of fish: the evolution of tolerating commensals while fighting pathogens. *Fish Shellfish Immunol* 2013;**35**:1729–39.
3. Masso-Silva JA, Diamond G. Antimicrobial peptides from fish. *Pharmaceuticals (Basel)* 2014;**7**:265–310.
4. Rajanbabu V, Chen JY. Applications of antimicrobial peptides from fish and perspectives for the future. *Peptides* 2011;**32**:415–20.
5. Noga EJ, Ullal AJ, Corrales J, Fernandes JM. Application of antimicrobial polypeptide host defenses to aquaculture: exploitation of downregulation and upregulation responses. *Comp Biochem Physiol Part D Genomics Proteom* 2011;**6**:44–54.
6. Lazarovici P, Primor N, Loew LM. Purification and pore-forming activity of two hydrophobic polypeptides from the secretion of the Red Sea Moses sole (*Pardachirus marmoratus*). *J Biol Chem* 1986;**261**:16704–13.
7. Zou J, Mercier C, Koussounadis A, Secombes C. Discovery of multiple beta-defensin like homologues in teleost fish. *Mol Immunol* 2007;**44**:638–47.
8. Oren Z, Shai Y. A class of highly potent antibacterial peptides derived from pardaxin, a pore-forming peptide isolated from Moses sole fish *Pardachirus marmoratus. Eur J Biochem* 1996;**237**:303–10.
9. Lai Y, Gallo RL. AMPed up immunity: how antimicrobial peptides have multiple roles in immune defense. *Trends Immunol* 2009;**30**:131–41.
10. Zanetti M. Cathelicidins, multifunctional peptides of the innate immunity. *J Leukoc Biol* 2004;**75**:39–48.
11. Noga EJ, Silphaduang U. Piscidins: a novel family of peptide antibiotics from fish. *Drug News Perspect* 2003;**16**:87–92.
12. Zanetti M, Del Sal G, Storici P, Schneider C, Romeo D. The cDNA of the neutrophil antibiotic Bac5 predicts a pro-sequence homologous to a cysteine proteinase inhibitor that is common to other neutrophil antibiotics. *J Biol Chem* 1993;**268**:522–6.
13. Lynn DJ, Higgs R, Gaines S, Tierney J, James T, Lloyd AT, et al. Bioinformatic discovery and initial characterisation of nine novel antimicrobial peptide genes in the chicken. *Immunogenetics* 2004;**56**:170–7.
14. van Dijk A, Veldhuizen EJ, van Asten AJ, Haagsman HP. CMAP27, a novel chicken cathelicidin-like antimicrobial protein. *Vet Immunol Immunopathol* 2005;**106**:321–7.
15. Chang CI, Pleguezuelos O, Zhang YA, Zou J, Secombes CJ. Identification of a novel cathelicidin gene in the rainbow trout, *Oncorhynchus mykiss. Infect Immun* 2005;**73**:5053–64.
16. Wang Y, Hong J, Liu X, Yang H, Liu R, Wu J, et al. Snake cathelicidin from *Bungarus fasciatus* is a potent peptide antibiotics. *PLoS One* 2008;**3**:e3217.
17. Zhao H, Gan TX, Liu XD, Jin Y, Lee WH, Shen JH, et al. Identification and characterization of novel reptile cathelicidins from elapid snakes. *Peptides* 2008;**29**:1685–91.
18. Hao X, Yang H, Wei L, Yang S, Zhu W, Ma D, et al. Amphibian cathelicidin fills the evolutionary gap of cathelicidin in vertebrate. *Amino Acids* 2012;**43**:677–85.

19. Tomasinsig L, Zanetti M. The cathelicidins–structure, function and evolution. *Curr Protein Pept Sci* 2005;**6**:23–34.
20. Chang CI, Zhang YA, Zou J, Nie P, Secombes CJ. Two cathelicidin genes are present in both rainbow trout (*Oncorhynchus mykiss*) and Atlantic salmon (*Salmo salar*). *Antimicrob Agents Chemother* 2006;**50**:185–95.
21. Maier VH, Dorn KV, Gudmundsdottir BK, Gudmundsson GH. Characterisation of cathelicidin gene family members in divergent fish species. *Mol Immunol* 2008;**45**:3723–30.
22. Scocchi M, Pallavicini A, Salgaro R, Bociek K, Gennaro R. The salmonid cathelicidins: a gene family with highly varied C-terminal antimicrobial domains. *Comp Biochem Physiol B Biochem Mol Biol* 2009;**152**:376–81.
23. Maier VH, Schmitt CN, Gudmundsdottir S, Gudmundsson GH. Bacterial DNA indicated as an important inducer of fish cathelicidins. *Mol Immunol* 2008;**45**:2352–8.
24. Li Z, Zhang S, Gao J, Guang H, Tian Y, Zhao Z, et al. Structural and functional characterization of CATH_BRALE, the defense molecule in the ancient salmonoid, *Brachymystax lenok*. *Fish Shellfish Immunol* 2013;**34**:1–7.
25. Zhang XJ, Zhang XY, Zhang N, Guo X, Peng KS, Wu H, et al. Distinctive structural hallmarks and biological activities of the multiple cathelicidin antimicrobial peptides in a primitive teleost fish. *J Immunol* 2015;**194**:4974–87.
26. Lu XJ, Chen J, Huang ZA, Shi YH, Lv JN. Identification and characterization of a novel cathelicidin from ayu, *Plecoglossus altivelis*. *Fish Shellfish Immunol* 2011;**31**:52–7.
27. Broekman DC, Frei DM, Gylfason GA, Steinarsson A, Jornvall H, Agerberth B, et al. Cod cathelicidin: isolation of the mature peptide, cleavage site characterisation and developmental expression. *Dev Comp Immunol* 2011;**35**:296–303.
28. Uzzell T, Stolzenberg ED, Shinnar AE, Zasloff M. Hagfish intestinal antimicrobial peptides are ancient cathelicidins. *Peptides* 2003;**24**:1655–67.
29. Ohno S. Duplication for the sake of producing more of the same. In: Ohno S, editor. *Evolution by gene duplication*. Heidelberg: Springer-Verlag Berlin Heidelberg; 1970. p. 59–65.
30. Amores A, Force A, Yan YL, Joly L, Amemiya C, Fritz A, et al. Zebrafish hox clusters and vertebrate genome evolution. *Science* 1998;**282**:1711–4.
31. Taylor JS, Braasch I, Frickey T, Meyer A, Van de Peer Y. Genome duplication, a trait shared by 22000 species of ray-finned fish. *Genome Res* 2003;**13**:382–90.
32. Meyer A, Van de Peer Y. From 2R to 3R: evidence for a fish-specific genome duplication (FSGD). *Bioessays* 2005;**27**:937–45.
33. Hoegg S, Boore JL, Kuehl JV, Meyer A. Comparative phylogenomic analyses of teleost fish Hox gene clusters: lessons from the cichlid fish *Astatotilapia burtoni*. *BMC Genomics* 2007;**8**:317.
34. Scannell DR, Byrne KP, Gordon JL, Wong S, Wolfe KH. Multiple rounds of speciation associated with reciprocal gene loss in polyploid yeasts. *Nature* 2006;**440**:341–5.
35. Lynch M, Conery JS. The evolutionary fate and consequences of duplicate genes. *Science* 2000;**290**:1151–5.
36. Halldorsdottir K, Arnason E. Trans-species polymorphism at antimicrobial innate immunity cathelicidin genes of Atlantic cod and related species. *PeerJ* 2015;**3**:e976.
37. Rosani U, Domeneghetti S, Pallavicini A, Venier P. Target capture and massive sequencing of genes transcribed in *Mytilus galloprovincialis*. *Biomed Res Int* 2014;**2014**. 538549.
38. Hong S, Li R, Xu Q, Secombes CJ, Wang T. Two types of TNF-alpha exist in teleost fish: phylogeny, expression, and bioactivity analysis of type-II TNF-alpha3 in rainbow trout *Oncorhynchus mykiss*. *J Immunol* 2013;**191**:5959–72.

39. Costa MM, Maehr T, Diaz-Rosales P, Secombes CJ, Wang T. Bioactivity studies of rainbow trout (*Oncorhynchus mykiss*) interleukin-6: effects on macrophage growth and antimicrobial peptide gene expression. *Mol Immunol* 2011;**48**:1903–16.
40. Broekman DC, Guethmundsson GH, Maier VH. Differential regulation of cathelicidin in salmon and cod. *Fish Shellfish Immunol* 2013;**35**:532–8.
41. Bridle A, Nosworthy E, Polinski M, Nowak B. Evidence of an antimicrobial-immunomodulatory role of Atlantic salmon cathelicidins during infection with *Yersinia ruckeri*. *PLoS One* 2011;**6**:e23417.
42. Chettri JK, Raida MK, Kania PW, Buchmann K. Differential immune response of rainbow trout (*Oncorhynchus mykiss*) at early developmental stages (larvae and fry) against the bacterial pathogen *Yersinia ruckeri*. *Dev Comp Immunol* 2012;**36**:463–74.
43. Heinecke RD, Buchmann K. Inflammatory response of rainbow trout *Oncorhynchus mykiss* (Walbaum, 1792) larvae against *Ichthyophthirius multifiliis*. *Fish Shellfish Immunol* 2013;**34**:521–8.
44. Scocchi M, Skerlavaj B, Romeo D, Gennaro R. Proteolytic cleavage by neutrophil elastase converts inactive storage proforms to antibacterial bactenecins. *Eur J Biochem* 1992;**209**:589–95.
45. Wernersson S, Reimer JM, Poorafshar M, Karlson U, Wermenstam N, Bengten E, et al. Granzyme-like sequences in bony fish shed light on the emergence of hematopoietic serine proteases during vertebrate evolution. *Dev Comp Immunol* 2006;**30**:901–18.
46. Broekman DC, Zenz A, Gudmundsdottir BK, Lohner K, Maier VH, Gudmundsson GH. Functional characterization of codCath, the mature cathelicidin antimicrobial peptide from Atlantic cod (*Gadus morhua*). *Peptides* 2011;**32**:2044–51.
47. Singh PK, Jia HP, Wiles K, Hesselberth J, Liu L, Conway BA, et al. Production of beta-defensins by human airway epithelia. *Proc Natl Acad Sci USA* 1998;**95**:14961–6.
48. Hilchie AL, Wuerth K, Hancock RE. Immune modulation by multifaceted cationic host defense (antimicrobial) peptides. *Nat Chem Biol* 2013;**9**:761–8.
49. Schmitt P, Wacyk J, Morales-Lange B, Rojas V, Guzman F, Dixon B, et al. Immunomodulatory effect of cathelicidins in response to a beta-glucan in intestinal epithelial cells from rainbow trout. *Dev Comp Immunol* 2015;**51**:160–9.

Chapter 18

Evolution and Immune Function of Fish Lectins

Matteo Cammarata, Maria G. Parisi
University of Palermo, Palermo, Italy

Gerardo R. Vasta
University of Maryland School of Medicine, Baltimore, MD, United States

INTRODUCTION

The term "lectin" is commonly used to encompass a wide variety of carbohydrate-binding proteins, widely distributed in viruses, prokaryotes, and eukaryotes.[1] The first invertebrate lectins were described in the early 1900s in the snail *Helix pomatia*,[2] the horseshoe crab *Limulus polyphemus*,[3] and the lobster *Homarus americanus*.[3] Among the vertebrates, Watkins and Morgan[4] first described an L-fucose-specific lectin in the European eel *Anguilla anguilla*, which led to the discovery of the carbohydrate nature of the H blood substance.

Animal lectins are grouped into various molecular families, differing in carbohydrate recognition domain (CRD) structure and organization.[1,5–7] Based on their CRD sequence motifs and cation requirements, animal lectins can be categorized in several families, such as C-type lectins (CTLs), galectins (formerly S-type lectins), rhamnose-binding lectins (RBLs), F-type lectins (FTLs), X-type lectins (XTLs), I-type lectins, P-type lectins, and pentraxins.[1,5–7]

Lectins are involved in a variety of key biological processes, ranging from development to immune responses.[1,7–11] The roles of lectin-carbohydrate interactions in self/nonself recognition in early development and innate immunity of vertebrates have been well documented.[1,7–11] In some ("chimeric" or "mosaic") lectins, the combination of one or multiple CRDs with distinct functional domains enable additional effector functions, including opsonization and phagocytosis, and activation of the complement pathway.[12]

It is now well established that protein–carbohydrate interactions constitute the basis of mechanisms mediating signaling functions, cell communication, and self/nonself recognition that are critical in the establishment and maintenance of highly specific mutualistic associations in organism–microbe complexes.[1,13,14] In this respect, mutual benefit (symbiosis or commensalism)

Lessons in Immunity: From Single-Cell Organisms to Mammals
http://dx.doi.org/10.1016/B978-0-12-803252-7.00018-7

239

depends on the maintenance of a tightly regulated balance, whereas colonization of tissues beneficial to the microbe could lead to a loss of host fitness
(pathogenesis) unless host defense responses are able to eliminate the foreign-
ness pentraxins.[1,13,14] Microheterogeneity, originating from multiple lectin gene
copies, allelic variation, or posttranslational modifications of the gene products,
expands the molecular diversity and recognition capabilities.[7,15,16]

FISH LECTINS

In fish, CTLs, FTLs, galectins, and pentraxins have been identified in both cartilaginous and bony fish.[17] In addition, selectins and other lectin genes have been
found in the currently available fish genomes. Members of most lectin families
described in mammals, including CTLs, XTLs, and galectins, have been isolated from fish serum, skin mucus, and other tissues.[17–20] Furthermore, some
lectin families unique to fish, such as the RBLs, have been identified in eggs
and embryos[21] but are also present in the serum.[22] Lectins can exert opsonic
activity[7,9,23] or enhance respiratory burst and bactericidal activity of phagocytic
cells.[19,24,25]

Considerable heterogeneity has been identified in the FTL of the Japanese
eel[15] that exists in various isoforms. The presence of isoforms has also been
shown in C-reactive proteins from the serum of the Indian major carp, *Labeo
rohita*, in which a shift in expression from normal to diverse structural isoforms
has been demonstrated.[26]

Several fish species have proved to be useful model organisms for gaining
insight into structural, functional, and evolutionary aspects of lectin immunobiology.[17,27] For example, based on the identification of a novel CRD sequence
motif[20] and a unique structural fold,[28] the FTL family was identified both in
prokaryotes and in fluids and tissues of invertebrates and vertebrates.[29–34]

THE LECTIN REPERTOIRES IN FISH: GENOMIC, STRUCTURAL, AND FUNCTIONAL DIVERSITY

Most components of the mammalian innate and adaptive immune response are
present in elasmobranchs and teleost fish. However, it is currently accepted that
their innate immune responses carry a substantial burden of the defense functions
against infectious diseases.[17] Evidence of the presence of lectins in teleost fish,
particularly in plasma and eggs, was obtained by serological approaches. More
recently, however, the implementation of biochemical, molecular, genomic, and
structural approaches has contributed to the comprehensive genomic, structural,
and functional characterization of the fish lectin repertoires.[17]

The determination of the lectin structures by crystallization or homology
modeling using as templates lectin structures from other species has provided
detailed information on the amino acid residues that interact with the ligands.[28,29]
Like mammals, recent information suggests that the lectin repertoires are

diversified among teleost fish, including representatives from most of the known lectin families.[17] In addition, recent studies on teleost fish have identified novel families of lectins, some of them with members present in other vertebrate and invertebrate taxa.[1,17] This lectin diversity is greatly amplified by the presence of isoforms with differences in sugar specificity and recognition ability.[15-17] The available genomes of tetraodontid pufferfish (*Takifugu rubripes* and *T. nigroviridis*) (www.genoscope.com), zebrafish (*Danio rerio*) (www.sanger.ac.uk), and medaka (*Oryzias latipes*) (www.ensamble.org) are expanding this view even further.[17,20]

RHAMNOSE-BINDING LECTINS

More than 20 years ago,[35] a lectin with specificity for D-galactosides was identified in eggs of the sea urchin *Anthocidaris crassispina*. It was designated SUEL (sea urchin egg lectin), and it is now recognized as the first described member of a new family of animal lectins, the RBL family.[1] RBLs are Ca^{2+}-independent lectins with specificity for rhamnose and galactosides, particularly abundant in teleosts and aquatic invertebrate species, such as annelids, bivalves, and ascidians.[36,37] RBLs share the presence of one or multiple CRDs with a unique β/β fold, about 100 amino acids in length, with 8 highly conserved cysteine residues engaged in 4 disulfide bridges with characteristic topology.[22,38,39] In addition, conserved motifs (YGR, DPC, and KYL) are also found.[38]

RHAMNOSE-BINDING LECTINS IN FISH: BIOCHEMICAL AND MOLECULAR FEATURES

RBLs purified from fish eggs exhibited two or three tandemly repeated structures of CRD.[35,38,40-42] Three RBLs, named STL1, STL2, and STL3, were isolated from eggs of steelhead trout (*Oncorhynchus mykiss*),[41,42] and three RBLs, CSL1, CSL2, and CSL3, with a high degree of sequence identity with *O. mykiss*, were isolated from chum salmon (*Oncorhynchus keta*)[43] (Table 18.1). Only one RBL (SAL) and two RBLs (WCL1 and WCL3) were isolated from catfish (*Silurus asotus*) and whitespotted charr (*Salvelinus leucomaenis*) eggs, respectively[44,45] (Table 18.1). Fish RBLs increase their expression in response to inflammatory stimuli, enhance phagocytosis acting as opsonins, and induce the synthesis and release of proinflammatory cytokines.[21,36,40,46]

   The ability to recognize and bind lipopolysaccharides, lipoteichoic acid, and agglutinate, both gram-positive and gram-negative bacteria, has been described in trout RBLs, suggesting an antibacterial activity.[22,35,44,47] In addition, RBLs have also been found in the cortex of teleost eggs as well as in the skin mucus and serum, further confirming their protective role. The ligand of fish RBL is the glycosphingolipid globotriaosylceramide, which is abundant in membrane lipid rafts.[17,21,36] The RBL CRD appeared early in metazoan evolution, and it is found in a variety of proteins, with different domain architecture, from

TABLE 18.1 Classification of Rhamnose-Binding Lectin Family Lectins Isolated From Teleostean Fish Species

Species	Order	RBL	Type—CRD Composition (Ogawa et al.[36]; Thongda et al.[93])	Type—Sugar Specificity (Nitta et al.[96])	CRD	No. of CRD	References
Ictalurus punctatus	Siluriformes	IpRBL1a	Ia	I		3	90
		IpRBL1b	Ia	I			
		IpRBL1c	Ia	I			
		IpRBL3a	IIIg	III		2	
		IpRBL3b	IIIg	III			
		IpRBL1c	Va	–		1	
Silurus asotus		SAL	Ia	I		3	39
I. punctatus		IfRBL	Ia	I			91
Oncorhyncus keta	Salmoniformes	CSL1	II	II		3	38
Oncorhyncus mykiss		STL1	II	II			37
Savelinus leucomaenis		WCL1	II	II			32

O. keta	CLS3	IIIa		III	2	38
O. mykiss	STL3	IIIa				37
S. leucomaenis	WCL3	IIIa				32
Dicentrarchus labrax	DIRBL	IIIa				2
O. keta	CSL2	IIIb		III	2	38
O. mykiss	STL2	IIIb				37

RBLs have been classified into five groups (types I to V) based on their domain structures and the hemagglutination activity against human erythrocytes and sugar specificity against lactose.

Type I is composed of three tandemly repeated domains, while type II has two tandem-repeated domains with an extra domain. Types III and IV have two tandem-repeated domains, but they have different hemagglutination activity and sugar specificity. Type V has only one RBL domain and exists in a homodimer with a disulfide linkage between subunits.

As proposed by Thongda et al.[90] and Nitta et al.,[96] RBLs are classified into subgroups based on their structural features of RBL-CRD compositions.

Thus RBL genes containing three domains (in an N–C orientation) were classified as type Ia and type II; genes composed of two domains were classified as a different type named IIIa, IIIb. The RBL containing only one domain was termed type Va.

CRD, carbohydrate recognition domain; RBL, rhamnose-binding lectin.

mammals (eg, polycystic kidney disease 1-like, axon guidance receptor EVA-1, and latrophilin) to cnidarian (rhamnospondins). RBLs together with these proteins constitute the RBL superfamily containing RBL CRDs.[48–50]

Recently, we have purified, and characterized, both biochemically and functionally, a novel RBL from sea bass, *Dicentrarchus labrax*, serum (DlRBL).[22] The purified DlRBL had electrophoretic mobility corresponding to 24 and 100 kDa under reducing and nonreducing conditions, respectively, suggesting that in plasma, the DlRBL is present as a physiological homotetramer. DlRBL subunit transcripts revealed an open reading frame encoding 212 amino acid residues that included two tandemly arrayed CRD and an 18-residue signal sequence at the N-terminus. The deduced size of 24.1 kDa for the mature protein was in good agreement with the subunit size of the isolated lectin. The Ca^{2+}-independent agglutinating activity of DlRBL toward rabbit erythrocytes can be inhibited in the presence of rhamnose or galactose. DlRBL agglutinated gram-positive and gram-negative bacteria, and exposure of formalin-killed *Escherichia coli* to DlRBL enhanced their phagocytosis by *D. labrax* peritoneal macrophages. These results suggest that plasma DlRBL may play a role in immune recognition of microbial pathogens and facilitate their clearance by phagocytosis.[22]

RHAMNOSE-BINDING LECTIN—MOLECULAR STRUCTURE, PHYLOGENY, AND EVOLUTION

As previously described, RBLs contain variable numbers of CRDs and therefore can vary significantly in length. STL1, CSL1, WCL1, and SAL have three tandemly repeated CRDs, of about 95 amino acid residues; STL2, STL3, CSL2, CSL3, WCL3, and DlRBL contain two repeated CRDs (Table 18.1).

Comparison of the amino acid sequences among CSLs shows 42–52% identity, while CSLs show 94–97% sequence identity when compared with the corresponding three RBLs from the steelhead trout eggs, STL1, STL2, and STL3. Moreover, CSL1, CSL2, and CSL3 are formed by 4, 18, and 2 subunits, respectively, interacting via noncovalent binding. The crystal structure of CSL3 revealed that it is a homodimer of two 20 kDa subunits and forms a pseudotetrameric structure[51]; a tetrameric conformation has also been described in *D. labrax*.[22] The detailed phylogenetic analysis of the CRDs in RBLs showed highly conserved sequences in their N-CRDs or C-CRDs, indicating a probably ancient CRDs duplication. In contrast, the N and C-CRD from the echinoderm *Strongylocentrotus purpuratus* and the urochordate *Ciona intestinalis* clustered together, indicating a closer similarity between their C- and N-CRDs and a more recent origin of this duplication. The homology model of DlRBL based on the *O. mykiss* CSL3 RBL structure (40.31%, of identity E value 0.00e-1) showed substantial structural overlap.[22]

The gene organization of the fish RBL suggests that the RBL ancestral gene may have diverged and evolved by exon shuffling and gene duplication, producing functionally diversified forms in different organisms. According to Ogawa et al.,[36] animal RBL CRDs were clustered into seven groups. The composite CRD structure of RBLs allowed the identification of 13 types of RBL genes. The seven CRDs were used to classify each channel catfish RBL constituent CRD. As shown in Table 18.1, three RBL genes containing three CRDs (CRD5-3-3, in an N–C orientation) were classified as type Ia. Two RBL genes composed of two CRDs (CRD5-3) were a new type named IIIg. The RBL containing only one CRD3 domain was termed type Va.

FUCOSE-BINDING LECTINS

FTLs constitute the most recently identified lectin family, characterized by a unique amino acid sequence motif and structural fold and a nominal specificity for L-Fucose.[20] Unlike CTLs, Ca^{2+} is required for structural stabilization, rather than participating in direct cation–saccharide interactions.[28] FTLs (Table 18.2) have been identified in the serum from fish.[20] While the European eel (*A. anguilla*) agglutinin (AAA)[20,28] possesses a single CRD, those from the striped bass (*Morone saxatilis*), MsFBP32,[20] the sea bass (*D. labrax*), DlFBL,[23,30] and the sea bream (*Sparus aurata*), SauFBL,[31] exhibit two tandemly arrayed (N- and C-terminal) CRDs. The structure of MsFBP32 in complex with L-fucose revealed a trimeric organization with two globular opposite halves containing, respectively, the N-CRDs and the C-CRDs.[28] We proposed that fish F-lectins mediate immune defense responses both in the bloodstream[20,28,29] and the intestinal mucus.[20,23,30,31] They are expressed in larval and juvenile tissues and are also stored in eggs.[33]

The scarcity of bacteria possessing FTL CRDs suggests that it may have been acquired through horizontal transfer from metazoans.[20] The absence of the FTL CRDs in higher vertebrates is an evolutionary enigma that coincides with land colonization after cleidoic egg appearance.[20]

FISH FTLs: BIOCHEMICAL AND MOLECULAR FEATURES

In fish FTLs, the F-type CRD can be present either as a single CRD or as tandemly arranged F-type CRD repeats.[20] In most teleosts, FTLs contain either duplicate or quadruplicate (steelhead trout) tandemly arrayed F-type CRDs yielding subunits of variable sizes, even within a single fish species.[20] The multiple duplicate tandem homologues present in modern teleost orders appear to be the product of independent duplications.[20]

Previously, we reported the purification of sea bass (DlFBL) and gilt head bream (SauFBL) serum fucose-binding lectins,[23,30,31] and we also demonstrated that SauFBL displays epitopes recognized by anti-DlFBL–specific antibodies. Furthermore, based on the DlFBL cDNA sequence, we showed that it is a bona fide FTL, as it shares carbohydrate specificity and biochemical properties with other well-characterized FTLs.[23] FTLs have also been described in the shark

TABLE 18.2 Classification of F-Type Lectin Family Lectins Isolated From Teleostean Fish Species

Species	Order	F-Type Lectin	F-Type CRD	Recognition Specificity	Structure	No. of CRD	References
Anguilla japonica	Anguilliformes	Eel fucolectin			Two disulfide-linked dimers		17
Anguilla anguilla	Anguilliformes	AAA		L-Fucose; D-galactose; H and Lewis[a] antigens	Homotrimer	1	23
Morone saxatalis	Perciformes	MsaFBP32		Fucosilated oligosaccharides	Cylindrical trimer	2	16
D. labrax	Perciformes	DlFBL		L-Fucose; galactose; melibiose; lactulose	Cylindrical trimer	2	41,20
Sparus aurata	Perciformes	SauFBP32		L-Fucose; galactose; melibiose; lactulose	Cylindrical trimer	2	44
Oreochromis niloticus	Perciformes	TFBP		Fucose	–	2	48
Lateolabrax japonicus	Perciformes	JspFL		Fucose	–	2	95
Aristichthys nobilis	Cypriniformes	GANL		Fucose	Homomultimeric	2	47
Danio rerio						2	16

CRD, carbohydrate recognition domain.

Scylorhinus canicula,[34] and other fucose-binding lectins have been identified in bighead carp (*Aristichthys nobilis*),[52] Nile tilapia (*Oreochromis niloticus* L.),[53] and the Antarctic fish (*Trematomus bernacchii* and *Chiionotraco hamatus*) (unpublished data) although the lack of full sequence information in these two species has prevented their identification as members of the FTL family.

The crystal structures of the single-CRD FTL from *A. anguilla* (AAA) and the binary CRD FTL from *M. saxatilis* (MsFBP32) have revealed that the FTL fold consists of a jellyroll β-barrel topology.[28,29] In MsFBP32, although the overall structure of the N-CRD is highly similar to that of the C-CRD, significant differences in the topology of the N- and C-CRDs were identified, particularly in those features corresponding to the extended binding site that surrounds the primary recognition site where L-fucose binds.[29] These differences strongly suggest that the N-CRD recognizes more complex fucosylated oligosaccharides and with a relatively higher avidity than the C-CRD.[29,16] These results have suggested that the individual CRDs of *Ms*FBP32 and other binary CRD F-lectins can bind to ligands on the microbial or host cell surface, supporting the role of FTLs as opsonins. As the single-CRD AAA can form dimers, it is also possible that recognition of topologically similar ligands on the microbial and host cell surfaces can also lead to opsonization.[16] Exposure of bacteria to the FTLs, DlFBL and SauFBL, enhanced phagocytosis[23,31] and supports the notion that these lectins mediate innate immune functions as opsonins by cross-linking microbial pathogens to phagocytic host cells.[16,29] Variability of critical residues in the binding pocket and surrounding loops in the multiple isoforms[28] expressed in the Japanese eel FTL[15] suggests that alternative interactions with terminal and subterminal sugars may expand the range of diverse oligosaccharides recognized by the lectin isoform repertoire.[16,28,29]

F-TYPE LECTINS—PHYLOGENY AND EVOLUTION

Similarity searches in genomic databases revealed that the FTL sequence motif is phylogenetically broadly distributed, being present in both lophotrochozoan (ie, molluscs and planaria) and ecdysozoan protostomes, in echinoderm, in a cartilaginous vertebrate, and in both early branching clades of vertebrates, lobe-finned and ray-finned fish.[20] A large number of FTLs with diverse domain topologies were identified in a variety of taxa from prokaryotes and invertebrates to amphibians, such as the *Streptococcus pneumoniae TIGR4*, the "furrowed receptor" and CG9095 of *Drosophila melanogaster*, the *Xenopus laevis* pentraxin 1 fusion protein, *Microbulbifer degradans* ZP 00065873.1, and yeast allantoicases.[20] Further, Bianchet et al.[28] described that the FTL fold is widely distributed in other proteins even with lower sequence similarities, for example, C1 and C2 repeats of blood coagulation factor V, C-terminal domain of sialidase, N-terminal domain of galactose oxidase, APC10/DOC1 ubiquitin ligase, and XRCC1. Interestingly, in modern teleosts (ie, striped bass, zebrafish, steelhead trout, stickleback, pufferfish, and sea bass), the predominant arrangement is either duplicate or quadruplicate tandem F-type domains. Clearly, the F-type fold favors the formation of concatenated CRD topologies in numbers that appear to be lineage related.[20] It is noteworthy, however, that the FTL CRD sequence motif has not yet been identified in genomes of higher vertebrates such as reptiles, birds, and mammals.[20]

GALECTIN STRUCTURE AND EVOLUTION

Galectins, the most conserved and ubiquitous lectin family detected from protists to mammals, are characterized by their specificity for β-galactosides (such as lactose and N-acetyllactosamine), a lack of Ca^{+2} requirement for ligand binding, and the presence of a conserved sequence motif in the CRD.[54] From the structural standpoint, galectins are defined by a β-sandwich structure formed by six (S) and five (F) strand sheets, with the S4–S6 strands containing the carbohydrate-binding amino acid residues.[54] The first galectin was identified and characterized from the electric organs of the electric eel *Electrophorus electricus*,[55] and since then members of the galectin family have been found in mammals, birds, amphibians, fish, nematodes, sponges, and some fungi.[1,56,57]

Based on their domain organization, mammalian galectins have been classified into three types: "proto," "chimera," and "tandem-repeat."[1] Prototype galectins contain one CRD per subunit and are usually homodimers of noncovalently linked subunits.[1] The homodimer is necessary for binding and signaling on the cell surface.[57–59] The chimera-type galectins have a C-terminal similar to the prototype and a non-CRD N-terminal domain rich in proline and glycine. The N-terminal domain with collagen-like sequences in the presence of multivalent carbohydrate ligands could result in oligomerization.[60] Garner and Baum[61] proposed a model in which cell function may be "fine-tuned" by galectin binding. Tandem repeat galectins, in which two CRDs are joined by a linker peptide, are monomeric with a constitutive bivalency.[59]

Although the number of genes is different in various species, the galectin structures are well conserved among invertebrates and vertebrates.[57,62,63] They play important roles in morphogenesis, cell proliferation, cell death, tumor functions, and numerous pathological processes.[1,62–67]

A substantial number of galectins from the three different types have been identified and characterized in various tissues, plasma, and mucus of elasmobranch and teleost fish, which show structural and binding specificity conservation with mammalian counterparts.[17,27,68–70].

Although initially shown to be involved in the early development of vertebrates, galectins were later shown to participate in the regulation of immune homeostasis.[67] More recently, galectins have been demonstrated to participate in the recognition of microbial pathogens.[14] Extracellular galectins exhibit various degrees of affinity interactions with glycans and form complexes with glycoprotein receptors[61] that can induce cellular responses such as proliferation, cell adhesion, migration, cell motility, and apoptosis.[71,72] Intracellular galectins can participate in biological responses, including cell differentiation, and are inflammatory mediators as cytokines.[73]

Duplication and divergence events can explain the evolution of the various chordate galectins[56,62] while multiple lectin gene copies, allelic variation, or posttranslational modifications of the gene products expand the molecular diversity and recognition capabilities.[57]

C-TYPE LECTINS

The CTLs are characterized by Ca^{2+} requirement, diverse carbohydrate specificity, and multiple structural domains, sometimes forming chimeric structures.[1,12] CTLs have been classified into groups comprising collectins, proteoglycan core proteins, selectins, endocytic receptors, and the mannose-macrophage receptor, some of them directly or indirectly involved in immune function.[1,12] The collectins include the MBLs and conglutinin from serum and saliva and the pulmonary surfactant, with critical roles in innate immunity against viruses and bacteria. Some NK cell and macrophage receptors and selectins are also CTL-related.[1,12] MBL consists of multimers of an identical polypeptide chain of 32 kDa and comprises four distinct regions: a cysteine-rich N-terminal region; a collagenous domain; a neck region, a short α-helical coiled-coil domain, and a CRD at C-terminal.[12]

MBL binds terminal D-mannose, L-fucose, and N-acetyl-D-glucosamine but does not interact with D-galactose and sialic acid. Selectivity concerns the presence of conserved amino acid residues within their CRDs. The hydroxyl groups are on C3 and C4 orientated in the equatorial plane of the pyranose ring.[12,74] The CRD is approximately 120 amino acids long along with a distinctive double loop stabilized by two conserved disulfide bridges, conserved polar and hydrophobic interaction. There are four Ca^{2+} binding sites recognized in CRDs from various species, and the Ca^{2+} binding site is important for carbohydrate-binding activity.[1,12,74]

MANNOSE-BINDING LECTINS IN FISH

MBL is an important component of innate immunity capable of activating the lectin pathway of the complement system by coopting MASPs, MBL-associated serine proteases. It acts as an opsonin, promoting phagocytosis of foreign material.[1,12,74] MBL is known as an acute phase protein produced by hepatocytes and modulated by infection or during an inflammatory response. In the presence of Ca^{2+}, MBLs initiate a broad range of biological processes such as adhesion, endocytosis, complement activation, and pathogen neutralization.[1,12,18,74]

MBLs have been reported in several fish species (reviewed in Vasta et al.[17]). The first lectin was isolated from the serum of the Atlantic salmon (*Salmo salar*) by mannose-affinity chromatography; its structure and immune functions were also characterized.[75] It exhibited antibacterial activity and could enhance macrophage activity.[25,75]MBLs were also purified from rohu (*L. rohita*), rainbow trout (*O. mykiss*), sea lamprey (*Petromyzon marinus*), common carp (*Cyprinus carpio*), fugu (*T. rubripes*), and turbot (*Scophthalmus maximus*).[76–80] Moreover, the MBL gene from channel catfish (*Ictalurus punctatus*) was upregulated following exposure to gram-negative pathogens.[80] In the African catfish, *Clarias gariespinus*, MBL exhibited antimicrobial activity, and in tilapia (*O. niloticus*), it induced cytochine production.[81]

In the Japanese flounder (*Paralichthys olivaceus*), CTLs are expressed in the liver,[82] whereas in other fish species, the presence of lectins in ski and gut mucus is particularly intriguing with regard to their potential biological role(s) in the external defense against microbial pathogens. CTLs (MBL-like CTLs) are present in skin mucus of the Japanese eel (*Anguilla japonica*)[83] and in the conger eel (*Conger myriaster*).[84] In the latter, conCTL-s is expressed in club cells of external and internal mucosal tissues.[84]

In healthy fish, MBL is expressed almost exclusively in the liver. In *O. mykiss* and *C. carpio*, MBLs are expressed in the liver and spleen.[85–88] In *T. rubripes*, the mannose-specific lectin pufflectin gene is transcribed in the gills, oral cavity wall, esophagus, and skin. Only an isoform was detected in the intestine.[89]

MANNOSE-BINDING LECTIN PHYLOGENY AND EVOLUTION

MBLs are highly diversified and widely distributed in the animal kingdom, including fish as unique structural motifs and functional domains, regardless of whether they possess sugar-binding properties.[12] Bony fish MBL shows the same carbohydrate specificity of human MBL. A similar MBL molecule associated with MASP-A has been identified in the lamprey, involved in C3 system activation.[90]

It is likely that the MBLs had evolved before the emergence of agnathans, and they have been conserved as a recognition molecule of the lectin pathway throughout vertebrate evolution. MBL homologues should be present in species evolved from the common ancestor of both jawed and jawless fish.[91]

Moreover, the two forms of the mammalian MBL, MBL-A and MBL-C, must have diverged after the common ancestor of tetrapods separated from bony fish. The MBL-A/MBL-C duplication was probably an independent event in the mammalian lineage.[77] The three identified and partially characterized rainbow trout MBL homologues represent structural homologues of mammalian MBLs and are expressed in various tissues, including the anterior intestine, the liver, and spleen. A rainbow trout MASP-3 homologue was also expressed in partially overlapping tissues.[92]

The polymorphic nature of MBL genes in humans is well described. Similarly, recent research demonstrated that there are multiple copies of the MBL gene in zebrafish and that the polymorphism and copy number variation of MBL can significantly affect resistance to pathogen infection.[76] Multiple homologues of MBL also exist in rainbow trout and common carp.[73,77] In catfish, only a single copy gene in the genome is present.[94]

ACKNOWLEDGMENTS

The authors' research reviewed herein was supported by grants from the RITMARE project (CNR and CONISMA) to MC, and IOS-0822257 and IOS-1063729 from the National Science Foundation and grant 5R01 GM070589-06 from the National Institutes of Health to GRV.

REFERENCES

1. Vasta GR, Ahmed H. *Animal lectins: a functional view*. CRC Press; 2008.
2. Camus M. Recherches experimentales sur une agglutinine produite par la glande de l'albumen chez l' *Helix pomatia. CR Acad Sci* 1899:129–233.
3. Noguchi H. On the multiplicity of the serum haemagglutinins of cold-blooded animals. *Zentralbl Bakteriol Abt l Orig* 1903;**34**:286.
4. Watkins WM, Morgan WT. Neutralization of the anti-H agglutinin in eel serum by simple sugars. *Nature* 1952;**169**:825–6.
5. Kilpatrick CD. Animal lectins: a historical introduction and overview. *Biochim Biophys Acta* 2002;**1572**:187–97.
6. Loris R. Principles of structures of animal and plant lectins. *Biochim Biophys Acta* 2002;**1572**:198–208.
7. Vasta GR, Ahmed H, Odom EW. Structural and functional diversity of lectin repertoires in invertebrates, protochordates and ectothermic vertebrates. *Curr Opin Struct Biol* 2004;**14**: 617–30.
8. Kaltner H, Stierstorfer B. Animal lectins as cell adhesion molecules. *Acta Anat* 1998;**161**:162–79.
9. Arason GJ. Lectins as defense molecules in vertebrates and invertebrates. *Fish Shellfish Immunol* 1996;**6**:277–89.
10. Sharon N, Lis H. Carbohydrates in cell recognition. *Sci Am* 1993;**268**:82–9.
11. Sharon N, Lis H. History of lectins: from hemagglutinins to biological recognition molecules. *Glycobiology* 2004;**14**:53–62.
12. Zelensky AN1, Gready JE. The C-type lectin-like domain superfamily. *FEBS J* December 2005;**272**(24):6179–217.
13. Casadevall A, Pirofski L. Host-pathogen interactions: basic concepts of microbial commensalism, colonization, infection, and disease. *Infect Immun* 2000;**68**:6511–8.
14. Vasta GR. Roles of galectins in infection. *Nat Rev Microbiol* 2009;**7**:424–38.
15. Honda S, Kashiwagi M, Miyamoto K, Takei Y, Hirose S. Multiplicity, structures, and endocrine and exocrine natures of eel fucose-binding lectins. *J Biol Chem* 2000;**275**(42):33151–7.
16. Vasta GR, Ahmed H, Bianchet MA, Fernández-Robledo JA, Amzel LM. Diversity in recognition of glycans by F-type lectins and galectins: molecular, structural, and biophysical aspects. *Ann NY Acad Sci* 2012;**1253**(1):14–26.
17. Vasta GR, Nita-Lazar M, Giomarelli B, Ahmed H, Du S, Cammarata M, et al. Structural and functional diversity of the lectin repertoire in teleost fish: relevance to innate and adaptive immunity. *Dev Comp Immunol* 2011;**35**:1388–99.
18. Fujita T. Evolution of the lectin-complement pathway and its role in innate immunity. *Nat Rev Immunol* 2002;**2**(5):346–53.
19. Russel S, Lumsden JS. Function and heterogeneity of fish lectins. *Vet Immunol Immunopathol* 2005;**108**:111–20.

20. Odom EW, Vasta GR. Characterization of a binary tandem domain F-type lectin from striped bass (*Morone saxatilis*). *J Biol Chem* 2006;**281**(3):1698–713.

21. Watanabe Y, Tateno H, Nakamura-Tsuruta S, Kominami J, Hirabayashi J, Nakamura O, et al. The function of rhamnose-binding lectin in innate immunity by restricted binding to Gb3. *Dev Comp Immunol* 2009;**33**:187–97.

22. Cammarata M, Parisi MG, Benenati G, Vasta G, Parrinello N. A rhamnose-binding lectin from sea bass (*Dicentrarchus labrax*) plasma agglutinates and opsonizes pathogenic bacteria. *Dev Comp Immunol* 2014;**44**:332–40.

23. Salerno G, Parisi MG, Parrinello D, Benenati G, Vizzini A, Vazzana M, et al. F-type lectin from the sea bass (*Dicentrarchus labrax*): purification, cDNA cloning, tissue expression and localization, and opsonic activity. *Fish Shellfish Immunol* 2009;**27**:143–53.

24. Yano T. The nonspecific immune system: humoral defense. In: Iwama G, Nakanishi T, editors. *The fish immune system: organism, pathogen, and environment*. San Diego (USA): Academic Press; 2006. p. 105–53.

25. Ottinger C, Johnson S, Ewart K, Brown L, Ross N. Enhancement of anti-*Aeromonas salmonicida* activity in Atlantic salmon (*Salmo salar*) macrophages by a mannose-binding lectin. *Comp Biochem Physiol* 1999;**123C**:53–9.

26. Mitra S, Das H. A novel mannose-binding lectin from plasma of *Labeo rohita*. *Fish Physiol Biochem* 2001;**25**:121–9.

27. Vasta GR. Galectins in teleost fish: zebrafish (*Danio rerio*) as a model species to address their biological roles in development and innate immunity. *Glycoconj J* 2004;**21**:503–21.

28. Bianchet MA, Odom EW, Vasta GR, Amzel LM. A novel fucose recognition fold involved in innate immunity. *Nat Struct Biol* 2002;**9**:628–34.

29. Bianchet M, Odom E, Vasta G, Amzel L. Structure and specificity of a binary tandem domain F-Lectin from striped bass (*Morone saxatilis*). *J Mol Biol* 2010;**401**:239–52.

30. Cammarata M, Vazzana M, Chinnici C, Parrinello N. A serum fucolectin isolated and characterized from sea bass *Dicentrarchus labrax*. *Biochim Biophys Acta* 2001;**1528**:196–202.

31. Cammarata M, Salerno G, Parisi MG, Benenati G, Vizzini A, Vasta G, et al. Primary structure and opsonic activity of an F-lectin from serum of the gilt head bream *Sparus aurata* (Pisces, Sparidae). *Ital J Zool* 2012;**79**:34–43.

32. Cammarata M, Benenati G, Odom E, Salerno G, Vizzini A, Vasta G, et al. Isolation and characterization of a fish F-type lectin from gilt head bream (*Sparus aurata*) serum. *Biochim Biophys Acta* 2006;**1770**:150–5.

33. Parisi MG, Cammarata M, Benenati G, Salerno G, Mangano V, Vizzini A, et al. A serum fucose-binding lectin (D1FBL) from adult *Dicentrarchus labrax* is expressed in larva and juvenile tissue and contained in eggs. *Cell Tissue Res* 2010;**341**:279–88.

34. Cammarata M, Mangano V, Parisi MG, Benenati G, Parrinello N. Purification and characterization of an F-type lectin from small-spotted catshark (*Scyliorhinus canicula*) serum. *Biol Mar Mediterr* 2010;**17**:242–3.

35. Ozeki Y, Matsui T, Suzuki M, Titani K. Amino acid sequence and molecular characterization of a D-galactoside-specific lectin purified from sea urchin (*Anthocidaris crassispina*) eggs. *Biochemistry* 1991;**30**:2391–4.

36. Ogawa T, Watanabe M, Naganuma T, Muramoto K. Diversified carbohydrate-binding lectins from marine resources. *J Amino Acids* 2011:838914.

37. Ballarin L, Cammarata M, Franchi N, Parrinello N. Routes in innate immunity evolution: galectins and rhamnose-binding lectins in ascidians. In: Kim S-W, editor. *Marine proteins and peptides: biological activities and applications*. Singapore: John Wiley & Sons; 2013. p. 185–205.

38. Terada T, Watanabe Y, Tateno H, Naganuma T, Ogawa T, Muramoto K. Structural characterization of a rhamnose-binding glycoprotein (lectin) from Spanish mackerel (*Scomberomorous niphonius*) eggs. *Biochim Biophys Acta* 2007;**1770**:617–29.

39. Jimbo M, Usui R, Sakai R, Muramoto KH. Purification, cloning and characterization of egg lectins from the teleost *Tribolodon brandti*. *Comp Biochem Physiol* 2007;**147B**:164–71.

40. Lam YW, Ng TB. Purification and characterization of a rhamnose-binding lectin with immune enhancing activity from grass carp (*Ctenopharyngodon idellus*) ovaries. *Protein Expr Purif* 2002;**26**:378–85.

41. Tateno H, Saneyoshi A, Ogawa T, Muramoto K, Kamiya H, Saneyoshi M. Isolation and characterization of rhamnose-binding lectins from eggs of steelhead trout (*Onchorynchus mykiss*) homologous to low density lipoprotein receptor superfamily. *J Biol Chem* 1998;**273**:19190–7.

42. Tateno H, Ogawa T, Muramoto K, Kamiya H, Hirai T, Saneyoshi M. A novel rhamnose-binding lectin family from eggs of steelhead trout (*Oncorhynchus mykiss*) with different structures and tissue distribution. *Biosci Biotechnol Biochem* 2001;**65**:1328–38.

43. Shiina N, Tateno H, Ogawa T, Muramoto K, Saneyoshi M, Kamiya H. Isolation and characterization of L-rhamnose-binding lectins from chum salmon (*Oncorhychus keta*) eggs. *Fish Sci* 2002;**68**:1352–66.

44. Tateno H, Ogawa T, Muramoto K, Kamiya H, Saneyoshi M. Distribution and molecular evolution of rhamnose-binding lectins in Salmonidae: isolation and characterization of two lectins from white-spotted Charr (*Salvelinus leucomaenis*) eggs. *Biosci Biotechnol Biochem* 2002a;**66**:1356–65.

45. Hosono M, Ishikawa K, Mineki R, Murayama K, Numata C, Ogawa Y, et al. Tandem repeat structure of rhamnose-binding lectin from catfish (*Silurus asotus*) eggs. *Biochim Biophys Acta* 1999;**1472**:668–75.

46. Jia H, Liu Y, Yan W, Jia J. PP4 and PP2A regulate Hedgehog signaling by controlling Smo and Ci phosphorylation. *Development* 2009;**136**:307–16.

47. Matsui T, Ozeki Y, Suzuki M, Hino A, Titani K. Purification and characterization of two Ca^{2+}dependent lectins from coelomic plasma of sea cucumber, *Stychopus japonicus*. *J Biochem* 2004;**116**:1127–33.

48. Schwarz RS, Hodes-Villamar L, Fitzpatrick KA, Fain MG, Hughes AL, Cadavid LF. A gene family of putative immune recognition molecules in the hydroid *Hydractinia*. *Immunogenetics* 2007;**59**:233–46.

49. Vakonakis I, Langhenhan T, Promel S, Russ A, Campbell I. Solution structure and sugar-binding mechanism of mouse latrophilin-1 RBL: a 7TM receptor-attached lectin-like domain. *Structure* 2008;**16**:944–53.

50. Lopez JA, Fain MG, Cadavid LF. The evolution of the immune-type gene family rhamnospondin in cnidarians. *Gene* 2011;**473**:119–24.

51. Shirai T, Watanabe Y, Lee MS, Ogawa T, Muramoto K. Structure of rhamnose binding lectin CSL3: unique pseudo-tetrameric architecture of a pattern recognition protein. *J Mol Biol* 2009;**391**:390–440.

52. Pan S, Tang J, Gu X. Isolation and characterization of a novel fucose binding lectin from the gill of bighead carp (*Aristichthys nobilis*). *Vet Immunol Immunopathol* 2010;**133**:154–64.

53. Argayosa AM, Lee YC. Identification of (l)-Fucose-binding proteins from the *Nile tilapia* (*Oreochromis niloticus* L.) serum. *Fish Shellfish Immunol* 2009;**27**:478–85.

54. Liao D-I, Kapadia G, Ahmed H, Vasta GR, Herzberg O. Structure of S-lectin, a developmentally regulated vertebrate b-galactoside-binding protein. *Proc Natl Acad Sci USA* 1994;**91**:1428–32.

55. Teichberg VI, Silman I, Beitsch DD, Resheff G. A beta-D-galactoside binding protein from electric organ tissue of *Electrophorus electricus*. *Proc Natl Acad Sci USA* 1975;**72**(4):1383–7.

56. Houzelstein D, Goncalves IR, Fadden AJ, Sidhu SS, Cooper DNW, Drickamer K, et al. Phylogenetic analysis of the vertebrate galectin family. *Mol Biol Evol* 2004;**21**:1177–87.

57. Vasta GR, Ahmed H, Nita-Lazar M, Banerjee A, Pasek M, et al. Galectins as self/non-self recognition receptors in innate and adaptive immunity: an unresolved paradox. *Front Immunol* 2012;**3**:199.

58. Levroney EL, Aguilar HC, Fulcher JA, Kohatsu L, Pace KE, Pang M, et al. Novel innate immune functions for galectin-1: galectin-1 inhibits cell fusion by Nipah virus envelope glycoproteins and augments dendritic cell secretion of proinflammatory cytokines. *J Immunol* 2005;**175**:413–20.

59. Earl LA, Bi S, Baum LG. Galectin multimerization and lattice formation are regulated by linker region structure. *Glycobiology* 2011;**21**:6–12.

60. Ahmad N, Gabius H, Andre S, Kaltner H, Sabesan S, Roy R, et al. Galectin-3 precipitates as a pentamer with synthetic multivalent carbohydrates and forms heterogeneous cross-linked complexes. *J Biol Chem* 2004;**279**:10841–7.

61. Garner OB, Baum LG. Galectin-glycan lattices regulate cell-surface glycoprotein organization and signalling. *Biochem Soc Trans* 2008;**36**:1472–7.

62. Cooper D. Galectinomics: finding themes in complexity. *Biochim Biophys Acta* 2002;**1572**:209–31.

63. Ahmed H, Vasta GR. Galectins: conservation of functionally and structurally relevant amino acid residues defines two types of carbohydrate recognition domains. *Glycobiology* 1994;**4**:545–8.

64. Brewer CF. Binding and cross-linking properties of galectins. *Biochim Biophys Acta* 2002;**1572**:255–62.

65. Paulson JC, Blixt O, Collins BE. Sweet spots in functional glycomics. *Nat Chem Biol* 2006;**2**:238–48.

66. Gabius H, Wu AM. Galectins as regulators for tumor growth and invasion by targeting distinct cell surface glycans and implications for drug design. In: Klyosov AA, Witczak ZJ, Platt D, editors. *Galectins*. Hoboken (NJ): John Wiley & Sons; 2008. p. 71–86.

67. Sato S, Rabinovich GA. Galectins as danger signals in host-pathogen and host-tumor interactions: new members of the growing group of 'alarmins'?. In: Klyosov AA, Witczak ZJ, Platt D, editors. *Galectins*. Hoboken (NJ): John Wiley & Sons; 2008. p. 115–45.

68. Muramoto K, Kagawa D, Sato T, Ogawa T, Nishida Y, Kamiya H. Functional and structural characterization of multiple galectins from the skin mucus of conger eel, *Conger myriaster*. *Comp Biochem Physiol* 1999;**123B**:33–45.

69. Inagawa H, Kuroda A, Nishizawa T, Honda T, Ototake M, Yokomizo U, et al. Cloning and characterisation of tandem-repeat type galectin in rainbow trout (*Oncorhynchus mykiss*). *Fish Shellfish Immunol* 2001;**11**:217–31.

70. Ahmed H, Du S, O'Leary N, Vasta G. Biochemical and molecular characterization of galectins from zebrafish (*Danio rerio*): notochord-specific expression of a prototype galectin during early embryogenesis. *Glycobiology* 2004;**14**:219–32.

71. Hernandez JD, Baum LG. Ah, sweet mystery of death! Galectins and control of cell fate. *Glycobiology* 2002;**12**:127–36.

72. Rabinovich GA, Toscano MA. Turning 'sweet' on immunity: galectin-glycan interactions in immune tolerance and inflammation. *Nat Rev Immunol* 2009;**9**:338–52.

73. Liu FT, Yang RY, Hsu DK. Galectins in acute and chronic inflammation. *Ann NY Acad Sci* 2012b;**1253**:80–91.

74. Turner MW. Mannose-binding lectin: the pluripotent molecule of the innate immune system. *Immunol Today* 1996;**17**:532–40.

75. Ewart KV, Johnson SC, Ross NW. Identification of a pathogen-binding lectin in salmon serum. *Comp Biochem Physiol* 1999;**123C**:9–15.

76. Jackson AN, McLure CA, Dawkins RL, Keating PJ. Mannose binding lectin (MBL) copy number polymorphism in Zebrafish (*D. rerio*) and identification of haplotypes resistant to *L. anguillarum*. *Immunogenetics* 2007;**59**:861–72.

77. Nakao M, Kajiya T, Sato Y, Somamoto T, Kato-Unoki Y, Matsushita M, et al. Lectin pathway of bony fish complement: identification of two homologs of the mannose binding lectin associated with MASP2 in the common carp (*Cyprinus carpio*. *J Immunol* 2006;**177**:5471–9.

78. Ourth DD, Rose WM, Siefkes MJ. Isolation of mannose-binding C-type lectin from sea lamprey (*Petromyzon marinus*) plasma and binding to *Aeromonas salmonicida*. *Vet Immunol Immunopathol* 2008;**126**:407–12.

79. Tsutsui S, Tasumi S, Suetake H, Kikuchi K, Suzuki Y. Carbohydrate binding site of a novel mannose-specific lectin from fugu (*Takifugu rubripes*) skin mucus. *Comp Biochem Physiol* 2006;**143B**:514–9.

80. Zhang M, Hua Y, Sun L. Identification and molecular analysis of a novel C-type lectin from *Scophthalmus maximus*. *Fish Shellfish Immunol* 2010;**29**:82–8.

81. Silva CDC, Coriolano MC, Lino MAS, Melo CM, Bezerra R, Carvalho EV, et al. Purification and characterization of a mannose recognition lectin from *Oreochromis niloticus* (Tilapia Fish): cytokine production in mice splenocytes. *Appl Biochem Biotechnol* 2011;**166**:424–35.

82. Kondo H, Tzeh Y, Hirono I, Aoki T. Identification of a novel C-type lectin gene in Japanese flounder, *Paralichthys olivaceus*. *Fish Shellfish Immunol* 2007;**23**:1089–94.

83. Tasumi S, Ohira T, Kawazoe I, Suetake H, Suzuki Y, Aida K. Primary structure and characteristics of a lectin from skin mucus of the Japanese eel *Anguilla japonica*. *J Biol Chem* 2002;**277**:27305–11.

84. Tsutsui S, Iwamoto K, Nakamura O, Watanabe T. Yeast-binding C-type lectin with opsonic activity from conger eel (*Conger myriaster*) skin mucus. *Mol Immunol* 2007;**44**:691–702.

85. Hirabayashi J, Kasai K. The family of metazoan metal-independent beta-galactoside–binding lectins: structure, function and molecular evolution. *Glycobiology* 1993;**3**:304–11.

86. Nikolakopoulou K, Zarkadis IK. Molecular cloning and characterisation of two homologues of Mannose-Binding Lectin in rainbow trout. *Fish Shellfish Immunol* 2006;**21**:305–14.

87. Gonzalez SF, Buchmann K, Nielsen ME. Complement expression in common carp (*Cyprinus carpio* during infection with *Ichthyophthirius multifiliis*. *Dev Comp Immunol* 2007;**31**: 576–86.

88. Vitved L, Holmskov U, Koch C, Teisner B, Hansen S, Salomonsen J, et al. The homologue of mannose-binding lectin in the carp family Cyprinidae is expressed at high level in spleen, and the deduced primary structure predicts affinity for galactose. *Immunogenetics* 2000;**51**:955–64.

89. Tsutsui S, Okamoto M, Tasumi S, Suetake H, Kikuchi K, Suzuki Y. Novel mannose-specific lectins found in torafugu, *Takifugu rubripes*: a review. *Comp Biochem Physiol* 2006;**1D**:122–7.

90. Takahashi M, Iwaki D, Kanno K, Ishida Y, Xiong J, Matsushita M, et al. Mannose-binding lectin (MBL)-associated serine protease (MASP)-1 contributes to activation of the lectin complement pathway. *J Immunol* 2008;**180**:6132–8.

91. Eddie W, Takahashi I, Ezekowitz R, Stuart L. Mannose-binding lectin and innate immunity. *Immunol Rev* 2009;**230**:9–21.

92. Kania P, Sorensen RR, Koch C, Brandt J, Kliem A, Vitved L, et al. Evolutionary conservation of mannan-binding lectin (MBL) in bony fish: identification, characterization and expression analysis of three bona fide collectin homologues of MBL in the rainbow trout (*Onchorhynchus mykiss*). *Fish Shellfish Immunol* 2010;**29**:910–20.

93. Thongda W, Li C, Luo Y, Beck, Peatman EL. Rhamnose-binding lectins (RBLs) in channel catfish, *Ictalurus punctatus*: characterization and expression profiling in mucosal tissues. *Dev Comp Immunol* 2014;**44**:320–33.
94. Chen F, Lee Y, Jiang Y, Wang S, Peatman E, Abernathy J, et al. Identification and characterization of full length cDNAs in channel catfish (*Ictalurus punctatus*) and blue catfish (*Ictalurus furcatus*). *PLoS One* 2010;**5**:E11546.
95. Qiu L, Lin L, Yang K. Molecular cloning and expression analysis of a F-type lectin gene from Japanese sea perch (*Lateolabrax japonicus*). *Mol Biol Rep* 2011;**38**:3751–6.
96. Nitta K, Kawano T, Sugawara S, Hosono M. Regulation of globotriaosylceramide (Gb3)-mediated signal transduction by rhamnose-binding lectin. *Yakugaku Zasshi* 2007;**127**(4):553–61.

Chapter 19

Teleost Immunoglobulins

Maria R. Coscia, Stefano Giacomelli, Umberto Oreste
Institute of Protein Biochemistry, National Research Council of Italy, Naples, Italy

List of Abbreviations

AID Activation-induced deaminase
BCR B cell receptor
CDR Complementary determining region
CH Heavy chain constant region
CL Light chain constant region
D Diversity gene segment
EMPD Extracellular membrane proximal domain
Ig Immunoglobulin
IgH Immunoglobulin heavy chain
IgL Immunoglobulin light chain
J Joining gene segment
pIgR Polymeric Ig receptor
SHM Somatic hypermutation
TM Transmembrane region
V Variable gene segment
VH Heavy chain variable region
VL Light chain variable region
μ IgM heavy chain
δ IgD heavy chain
τ IgT heavy chain

INTRODUCTION

The vertebrate immune system is a complex network of cellular and chemical mediators that arose during evolution to protect the body from all potential pathogen attacks. The discrimination between self and nonself takes place at the molecular level and is mediated by specific soluble or membrane structures. In this context the antibody molecule plays a key role. The antibodies or immunoglobulins (Ig) appeared when jawed vertebrates emerged about 450 millions years ago and in the same period as the other components involved in the adaptive immunity, such as T-cell receptor, MHC, and the recombination enzymes RAGs.[1] The basic structure of the Ig molecule consists of two heavy (IgH)

Lessons in Immunity: From Single-Cell Organisms to Mammals
http://dx.doi.org/10.1016/B978-0-12-803252-7.00019-9

and two light (IgL) chains covalently linked by disulfide bridges. Igs are present in two forms: the secreted and the membrane-bound form. In most cases, a single gene encodes both forms of the IgH chain, and alternate pre-mRNA processing determines which mRNA is expressed. There are exceptions, eg, channel catfish (*Ictalurus punctatus*), in which the secreted and membrane-bound forms are encoded by different genes.[2] The membrane-bound Ig form is exposed on the cell surface of B lymphocytes in association with the CD79a–CD79b heterodimer, forming the antigen receptor complex (BCR): it is able to transduce the signal to the cell interior upon antigen binding when translocated into specific microdomains of the cell membrane named "lipid rafts."[3]

Similarly to those of mammals, teleost *IgH* genes are in the "translocon" configuration in which multiple *VH* gene segments are located upstream of many *D* and *JH* gene segments. The mechanisms used to generate the antibody diversity prior to exposure to antigens include random rearrangement of one *VH*, one *D*, and one *JH* segment, each selected from multiple sets of gene segments. Among the mechanisms that can modify the specificity of the antibody repertoire, somatic hypermutation (SHM) has been described as a distinctive feature of the affinity maturation of immune responses through activation-induced deaminase (AID). AID increases repertoire diversification by introducing point mutations in the rearranged V genes. In mice and humans, SHM occurs at such a rate (10^{-5} to 10^{-3}), which is much higher than that of mutations in most other genes. Among ectothermic vertebrates, evidence for SHM of Ig genes has been observed in cartilaginous fish, amphibians, and reptiles. Regarding teleosts, analysis of rearranged *VH/J/DH* segments in several species revealed specific features, suggesting that the hypermutational events may also occur in teleosts.[4,5]

Teleost IgH chain is present in three different isotypes, namely μ, δ, and τ, all encoded by the same gene locus. However, the structure of the IgH gene locus is different in distinct teleost species and is not strictly of the translocon type since in some species the Cτ gene is located between the *VH* and *D* genes or within the set of *VH* gene segments. A schematic representation of various gene structures is presented in Fig. 19.1. More than one gene copy is present in channel catfish, medaka (*Oryzias latipes*), and three-spined stickleback (*Gasterosteus aculeatus*) gene locus. In Atlantic salmon (*Salmo salar*) the entire gene locus is duplicated (*IgHA* and *IgHB*).[6] Many noncoding exons are scattered in the IgH locus of the majority of teleost species.

Like the Ig genes in cartilaginous fish, teleost *IgL* genes are in the "cluster" configuration, in which each cluster comprises one *VL*, one *JL*, and a single constant gene (*CL*), and the *VL–JL* rearrangement occurs exclusively within a cluster.

TELEOST IgM

IgM is probably the least "dynamic" (ie, most conserved) and best understood at the structural and functional levels of all the Ig isotypes. It is the predominant Ig found in plasma, as a tetrameric molecule of 600–850 kDa, mainly involved

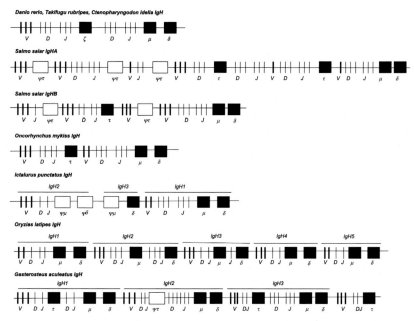

FIGURE 19.1 Schematic representation of the structure of IgH loci in different teleost species. Each species presents the typical translocon organization with *VH* gene segments (*black narrow boxes*) at the 5′ end of the locus, followed by *D* and *JH* gene segments (*narrow light and dark gray boxes*). At the 3′ end the CH exons τ/ζ, δ, and μ are indicated by the *black boxes*. The pseudogenes (Ψ) interspersed into the locus are depicted as *white boxes*. *IGHA* and *IGHB* indicate the two IgH isoloci in *Salmo salar*.

in the systemic response.[7] It is also present in secretions as bile,[8] skin, and gut mucus[9,10] and in eggs.[11] However, IgM concentration in secretions is very low compared to plasma. Teleost IgM show a number of differences if compared to mammalian IgM: they are tetrameric instead of pentameric and do not share high sequence identity with mammalian IgM. Unique to teleosts is their assembly. These molecules show high heterogeneity in their basic structure since they are found in various redox forms rather than being exclusively in the single covalently linked conformation. The redox forms differ by variation of the degree of disulfide polymerization of monomer or halfmer H–L subunits.[10] In fact, IgM are present in several teleost species studied so far such as the channel catfish, trout (*Oncorhynchus mykiss*), toadfish (*Spheroides glaber*), and sheephead (*Archosargus protocephalus*), as monomers, dimers, or trimers forming noncovalently linked tetramers as well as the entirely disulfide-linked tetramers.[12] The presence of tetramers in different oxidation states may have implications for functional diversity as done by a wide repertoire of distinct isotypes in mammals.[12]

Polymeric IgM apparently lack the J chain[13] that has a crucial role in the generation of secretory antibodies because it allows IgM to bind the polymeric Ig receptor (pIgR) and shapes the pIg structure. The pIgR mediates active transport of bound polymeric Ig from the basolateral to the apical face of epithelial cells to release secretory antibodies to the mucosal surfaces. Teleost pIgRs contain two Ig domains and are therefore smaller than those of tetrapod pIgRs, which consist of four or five Ig domains.[14]

Teleost IgM heavy chain (μ chain) consists of four constant domains and is slightly shorter than that of mammals. The invariant cysteine and tryptophan residues known to be involved in Ig folding are conserved, but the number and distribution of "extra cysteines," involved in inter-IgH chain and intersubunit bonds, vary across teleost species. Teleost Igμ chain is more glycosylated than the corresponding mammalian chain, and its carbohydrate content is about 12% of the total molecular weight.[15,16] Putatively glycosylated asparagine residues can be found in all constant domains with the exception of CH1. A particularly large number of allelic polymorphic positions have been identified in the Igμ chain of Antarctic species, mainly falling within the so-called hinge region, between the CH2 and CH3 domains, where some flexibility resides.[17]

In teleosts, the antibody repertoire is generated in a manner similar to that of mammals. A large number of germline *VH* gene segments, together with a set of *D* and *JH* segments, contribute to the synthesis of a huge number of different VH regions. *VH* gene segments are grouped into *VH* families according to the criterion that two *VH* genes belong to the same family when sharing >80% of nucleotide sequence identity.[18] Different teleost species present a variable number of *VH* families ranging from 2 in the emerald rockcod (*Trematomus bernacchii*) to 13 in the channel catfish.[19,20] Also the *JH* gene segments are variable in number and sequence, although all the encoded regions show the WGXG motif responsible for the correct structure of the VH domain.

The nucleotides at the 3′ end of the *VH* genes together with *D* and 5′ nucleotides of *JH* contribute to the somatic recombination responsible for the synthesis of the CDR3 (the third complementary region) in the VH domain, the major player in the antigen–antibody recognition. The length and the molecular flexibility of the CDR3 are remarkable features influencing the antigen binding. In teleosts, the CDR3 length varies between 5 and 18 amino acid residues.[19]

The receptor revision mechanism has been highlighted in the channel catfish[21] and in the emerald rockcod.[22]

At present, 50 sequences encoding the Igμ chain from different teleosts belonging to 11 families are available from GenBank. Based on the alignment of their deduced amino acid sequences, a tree generated by the NJ method is reported in Fig. 19.2. The topology of the tree reproduces the phylogenetic relationships among the species.

Investigations of Antarctic teleost nucleotide sequences encoding the membrane-bound form of the Igμ chain revealed an unexpected feature: unlike what was reported for other teleosts, the TM exons are spliced to the CH2 exon with the exclusion of CH3 and CH4 and inclusion of 39-nucleotide extra exons encoding an unusually long extracellular membrane-proximal domain (EMPD). Genomic DNA analysis disclosed that each 39-nucleotide extra exon falls within

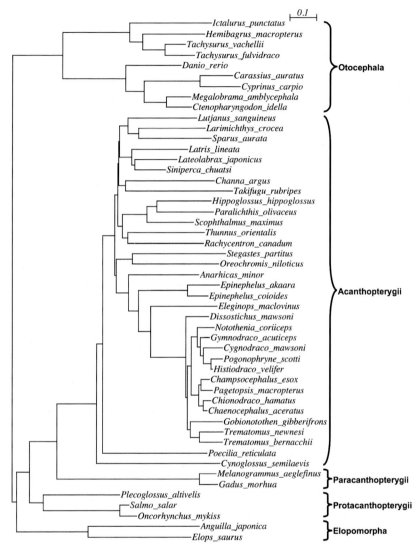

FIGURE 19.2 Phylogenetic tree of Igμ heavy chain constant domains of 50 different teleost sequences. The five superorders that the teleost species analyzed belong to are shown on the right side of the figure.

a long sequence that is the reverse complement of an upstream region of the same gene locus. Deduced amino acid sequence analysis suggested an important structural role of the EMPD resulting from the assembly of several repeats, which are composed of alternate hydrophylic and hydrophobic parts. Also the presence of additional cysteine residues in the repeats suggests that they may be required for the assembly of the two heavy chains in the absence of the CH3 domain.[23]

TELEOST IgD

IgD has been considered for a long time as a recent Ig isotype present only in primates and rodents. However, the work of Ohta and Flajnik[24] reconciled the orthology of the IgD and IgW isotypes, the latter found in cartilaginous fish that are the most ancient vertebrate group possessing an adaptive immune system. Thus it became clear that IgD is as primordial as IgM.

In contrast to IgM, which is highly structurally conserved across species, teleost IgD has long been considered an enigmatic isotype because of its chimeric structure, comprising a highly variable number of domains, and its biological role, still almost unknown.[25] However, recent studies carried out in channel catfish have highlighted that IgD, besides being expressed together with IgM as an antigen receptor on the surface of B cells, participates in the humoral immune response against some types of pathogens and is also involved in innate immunity as a mediator.[26]

To date, a large variety of IgD isoforms has been found in teleosts,[27] showing different molecular masses due to a different number of constant δ domains, arisen from duplications and deletions, occurred during evolution.

The first cDNA coding for secreted IgD was isolated in channel catfish and consisted of a rearranged *VH-D-JH* region spliced to the first constant μ exon, followed by novel constant δ exons, a transmembrane region, and a five-amino acid-long cytoplasmic tail.[28] The combination of Ig constant exons of different isotypes, initially observed in catfish, represented a novel feature shared by all the teleost IgD identified later.[29–33] A schematic representation of the IgD domain arrangement in different species is shown in Fig. 19.3.

It was suggested that the presence of $C\mu1$ exon is required to provide, at the proper position, the cysteine residue involved in the covalent binding of δ chains with L chains. None of the $Ig\delta$ genes sequenced to date have extra exons encoding a hinge. Likely, the different lengths of the Igδ chain may reflect a different function. In most species, the δ-encoding gene is located downstream of the μ-encoding gene, and these two genes are cotranscribed and expressed through RNA splicing. In channel catfish, the *IgH* locus contains multiple internal duplications and transpositions and comprises three δ genes termed $\delta1$, $\delta2$, and $\delta3$[34] (Fig. 19.1). The $\delta1$ gene is located at the 3' end of the functional $C\mu$ gene, consists of 14 exons, and encodes the membrane form of IgD. The other two δ genes are located about 500 kbp upstream of $\delta1$. $\delta3$ is almost identical to $\delta1$ except its terminal exon encodes the secretory tail. Interestingly, the secreted form of catfish IgD from IgM+/IgD+ and IgM−/IgD+ B cells lacks the VH region and begins with a leader exon spliced to $C\delta1$. This leader was shown to be functional and capable of mediating IgD secretion.[35] It is likely that this VH-less IgD functions through its Fc region, playing a role in tagging certain pathogens for destruction and in eliciting the production of proinflammatory cytokines through binding to basophils.[26] Taken together, these findings suggest that the catfish IgD Fc region, as proposed for human IgD, may act as a pattern recognition molecule.

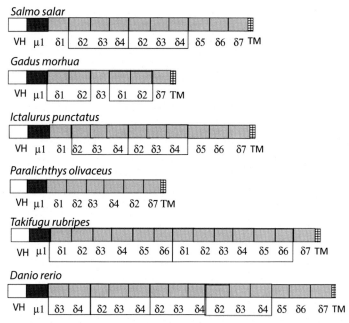

FIGURE 19.3 Schematic representation of Igδ heavy chain in six teleost species: *Salmo salar, Gadus morhua, Ictalurus punctatus, Paralichthys olivaceus, Takifugu rubripes,* and *Danio rerio.* Each species presents one VH domain, depicted as a *white box* at the N-terminus of the chain, the first constant μ domain (μ1), represented as a *dark gray box,* and a different number of δ domains (*light gray boxes*) followed by the TM domain at the C-terminus of the chain.

Different types of IgD gene duplications occur in three-spined stickle-back, Atlantic salmon, pufferfish (*Takifugu rubripes*), and Atlantic cod (*Gadus morhua*). As in channel catfish, the pufferfish membrane and secreted forms of IgD are encoded by distinct genes with variable numbers of exon duplications.[36] In three-spined stickleback, there are three sets of *IgH* genes that do not contain any exon duplication and share about 90% amino acid identity with no evidence of a functional difference between them.[37]

In salmonids, there are two *IgH* loci on different chromosomes related to their tetraploid history. Interestingly, each *IgH* locus in Atlantic salmon has multiple duplications of the Igτ gene but only one set of the *μ* and *δ* genes.[6] The corresponding seven unique δ exons in the two loci are very similar to each other, sharing 97% identity.[32] The intron between δ6 and δ7 is much longer (2240 bp) due to an insertion of a Tc1-like transposon element very frequently found in teleost genes.

Unusual IgD exon usage was characterized in zebrafish (*Danio rerio*). In this species, IgD was found to be a chimeric Ig with the third δ exon spliced to the first IgM constant exon, therefore skipping the first and second δ exons due to the presence of a stop codon in the δ2 exon. Thus the presence of different structural forms and splicing variants suggests a high plasticity of teleost IgD.

In rainbow trout, it was found that the ratio of IgD to IgM in the gills was higher than in other tissues, indicating a significant role for IgD in the gills.[38] Although the function of teleost IgD is still elusive, in light of these findings together with the detection of secreted IgD transcripts in mucosally vaccinated trout, it may be suggested that there is a role for IgD in mucosal immunity.

TELEOST IgT

The IgT isotype was identified for the first time in 2005 in teleost species belonging to different orders, under different names: "IgT" in rainbow trout (*O. mykiss*, order Salmoniformes),[39] "novel IgH" in pufferfish (order Tetraodontiformes),[40] "IgZ" in zebrafish (order Cypriniformes),[41] and referred to as "IgM-IgZ chimera" in common carp (*Cyprinus carpio*).[42] A few years later, a new IgZ variant, named "IgZ2," was identified in common carp and in zebrafish.[43,44]

Usually, IgT heavy chain (τ) has four CH domains; however, some species show a different domain number. The three-spined stickleback τ chain has three CH domains, and the pufferfish has only two, while common carp τ is a chimeric molecule since it contains a μ1 domain similar to teleost fish IgD.[45]

IgT has been recently identified in Antarctic teleosts;[46] their τ chain consists of three CH domains corresponding to τ1, τ3, and τ4 of other teleost species. Particularly, three transcript variants are synthesized in emerald rockcod, named long (L), short (S), and shortest (Sts), differing in length and deriving from different allelic sequences (L and S) or originated by the alternative splicing process (Sts). The loss, in the Antarctic fish, of almost the entire τ2 domain together with the conservation of some amino acid residues typical of hinge regions, such as proline, glycine, and cysteine, in the remaining domain more likely represents another specific and distinctive feature of the evolution of the Antarctic fish genome.

In most species, IgT share *VH* segments with IgM but, interestingly, possess their own set of *D* and *JH* gene segments that are embedded within the Ig*μ* genes (Fig. 19.3). In some other cases IgM and IgT share the same *DH* segments, whereas the *JH* gene segments are isotype specific.

At present more and more sequences from various teleost species have become available (Fig. 19.4), disclosing a wide variability in the organization of the *IgH* loci among teleosts[45] (Fig. 19.1). In rainbow trout and zebrafish, the IgH locus has been shown to present τ exons located upstream of μ and δ exons, together with their own set of *D* and *JH* gene segments.[39,41] In pufferfish, *Igτ* genes are similarly found upstream of μ and δ genes with their own *D* and *JH* segments, but the gene organization differs significantly from zebrafish and rainbow trout IgT.[40] In three-spined stickleback, τ, μ, and δ exons have been found duplicated in tandem three times and are separated by *VH*, *D*, and *JH* gene segments; moreover, a fourth τ gene exists at the 3′ end of the locus.[37,47] In Pacific blufin tuna (*Thunnus orientalis*), IgM and IgT are each composed of four CH domains. Interestingly, three *VH* gene families have been identified, shared by both IgM and IgT, and one is exclusively used by IgM. Moreover, both IgM and IgT use the same *D* segments, whereas the *JH* gene segments are isotype specific.[48] Cyprinids can also have different types of *IgH* loci.

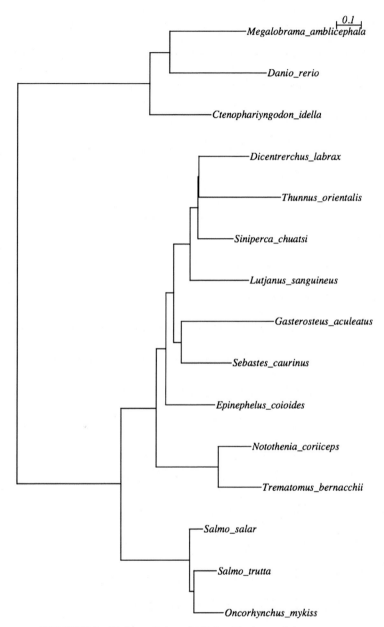

FIGURE 19.4 Phylogenetic tree of 15 teleost Igτ heavy chain sequences.

Zebrafish has only one *IgH* locus with the canonical structure[41] whereas the two common carp IgZ subisotypes are encoded by two distinct loci.[49] The two parallel *IgH* loci *IGHA* and *IGHB*, found in the family Salmonidae, have been shown to possess multiple τ genes upstream of the μ region, with three of the τ genes being functional.[6]

At present, in two well-known teleost species, medaka and channel fish, ortholog IgT genes have not yet been found.[50,51]

Serum IgT are present at low levels as monomers, whereas they are found mainly as noncovalently linked multimers in the gut, skin, and gill mucus. This multimeric form of IgT is transported into the gut lumen by means of the fish pIgR, like mammalian IgA. Moreover, IgT is present at a high level on the B cell membrane in the gut epithelium.

The proposed role of IgT is the protection of the intestinal mucosa[52] and of the skin.[53] A broad repertoire of different Ig isotypes is present in the mucosal secretions of mammals, including IgA, IgM, and IgG, with IgA being the predominant mucosal Ig playing a functional role both in homeostasis and immune response.[54] Similarly, in teleost fish, both IgT and IgM are detectable in mucosal secretions.

To date, Igs present in the gut mucus of teleosts have been poorly studied, in part due to the large amounts of proteolytic enzymes in the gut mucus, as reported for Atlantic salmon.[55] The concentration of IgT in gut mucus (0.007 mg/mL) is twice that of serum, differing from IgM, whose concentration in serum (2.5 mg/mL) is much higher than that in gut mucus (0.075 mg/mL). In olive flounder (*Paralichthys olivaceus*), a monomeric Ig was detected in the cutaneous mucus.[56] In common carp, Ig purified from cutaneous mucus has a different antigenicity, protein, and carbohydrate composition than that of serum IgM, with the majority of both Igs being tetrameric.[57] It has been hypothesized that this tetrameric cutaneous Ig in common carp may correspond to one of the two recently identified IgZ (IgZ1 and IgZ2).[42,43]

Thus far, biochemical analyses on gill mucus Ig responses have been described in a very limited number of teleost species.[58,59] The gills are an extremely important barrier for pathogens. They were defined in sea bass (*Dicentrarchus labrax*) as a major tissue for antibody secreting cell production.[60] Recent findings in rainbow trout have revealed that teleosts had already developed the nasopharynx-associated lymphoid tissue as a primary mucosal immune defense before the appearance of terrestrial vertebrates.[61] At present there are no data about which Ig isotype is mainly involved in nasal-specific immunity. However, in the absence of any antigenic stimulus, IgT is the predominant isotype similarly to what has been reported in the gut, gills, and skin. Following vaccination, both IgM and IgT proteins can be detected in the gut, gill, skin, and nasal mucosal, with IgT to IgM ratios greater than plasma in all cases.[62]

The discovery of IgT in an ancient group of vertebrates has confirmed that an Ig isotype specialized in mucosal immune responses appeared early in evolution.

TELEOST IgL CHAIN

It was previously believed that the two isotypes of human IgL chains, λ and κ, arose late in evolution, probably in the mammalian lineage. However, following studies on genomes of several vertebrate species it has been shown that these two IgL isotypes emerged in the common ancestor of all living vertebrates.

At present four IgL isotypes have been identified among teleosts: L1 (also called G), L3 or F, according to the species investigated, both considered as κ orthologs; σ (also called L2); and λ, which has been lost in several fish lineages.[63] However, the relation between the different isotypes within a species is not clear, and the presence of L1 subtypes renders this matter further complicated. After the identification of L1A and L1B subtypes in the Antarctic emerald rockcod[64] and in three-spined stickleback,[37] it has become clear that L1 subtypes arose from gene duplications, and gene divergence occurred within the superorder Acanthopterygii. Moreover, tandem Ser repeats exist within the L1 and CL-II types of orange-spotted grouper (*Epinephelus coioides*) IgL, a feature that is also present in the emerald rockcod L1A, spotted wolffish (*Anarhichas minor*) L1 and L2, and mandarin fish (*Siniperca chuatsi*) IgL.[64–66] Interestingly, these four species belong to the same order Perciformes. Several tandem repeats in eukaryote genomes have been demonstrated to form certain secondary structures that interact with specific nuclear proteins, participating in gene expression regulation.[67]

To date, *IgL* genes have been sequenced from 27 different species (Fig. 19.5). The functional significance of the presence of different IgL isotypes is still unknown; however, recent findings suggest that several structural features of the Ig molecule depend on its IgL chain isotype.[68]

The genomic organization of the *IgL* loci in teleost fish has been shown to consist of multiple clusters ($(VL–JL–CL)_n$).[69–71] This organization has been determined either directly by genomic sequencing and/or inferred from Southern blot analyses in a number of different teleost species. There are significant differences in the number of loci for each isotype among species.[72]

The combinatory mechanisms are thought to be similar to those occurring in the IgH chain synthesis although the presence of many sterile transcripts indicates that they are weakly controlled. *VL* might be in the same transcriptional orientation as *JL* and *CL*, allowing rearrangement by deletion, or opposite, permitting rearrangement by inversion. The *IgL* clusters containing *VL* segments in opposite orientations would allow increased IgL diversity. The presence of two *JL* and two or three *VL* segments in the same cluster has also been reported.[69,70] Recently, the three L chain loci of *D. rerio* have been found to be different to those of other teleosts: multiple *VL* gene segments, in the same or opposite transcriptional orientation, have been identified in two clusters.[73,74]

The presence of multiple gene segments in teleost *IgL* cluster organization functions as a reservoir of *IgL* gene segments, providing ideal conditions for receptor editing. In fact, *VL–JL* rearrangements, which are not in frame or incompatible with the H chain, and thus unwanted, can be replaced by secondary rearrangements.[75,76]

Differences in the relative expression of IgL isotypes have been documented in teleosts.

Usually, the most abundantly expressed isotype correlates with the number of genes present, according to the stochastic model.[77] The ratio of λ/L1 to σ/L2

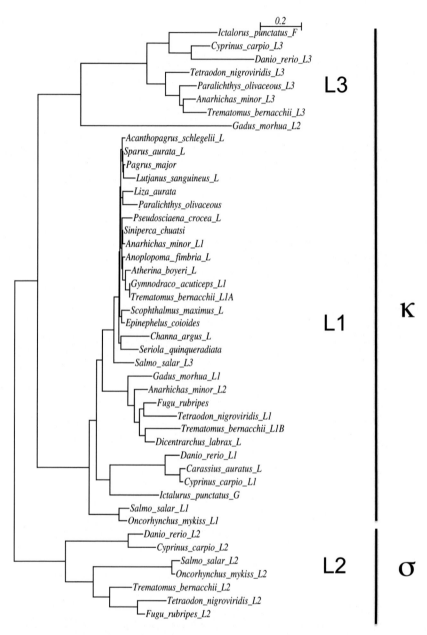

FIGURE 19.5   Phylogenetic tree of IgL chains from 27 teleost fish. The different isotypes L1 and L3 (κ orthologs), and L2 (σ orthologs) are indicated on the right side. Light chain isotypes found in *Ictalurus punctatus* are designated as F and G.

expression in trout peripheral blood leukocytes is estimated to be approximately 85:15,[69] and in emerald rockcod, the expression ratio of κ/L1A to σ/L2 in the head kidney is about 80:20.[64]

The reason why there are multiple L chains is unknown, but it might be related to particular assemblies of L chains and H chains giving rise to specific binding sites. It remains to be clarified why certain L chain isotypes preferentially combine with a particular H chain isotype, eg, in channel catfish M⁻/IgD⁺ B cells only express IgL σ.[35]

CONCLUSIONS

Igs are one of the most important molecules in adaptive immunity and are of different structures and effector functions across species. In the last two decades, many teleost Ig genes have been identified, thus contributing to our understanding of the evolutionary changes that have occurred in the *Ig* gene loci.

In the teleost fish species studied thus far three IgH chain isotypes, IgM, IgD, and IgT, and four IgL chain isotypes, L1 and L3 (κ orthologs), σ, and λ, have been identified. The translocon-type organization of *IgH* genes like that of the *IgH* loci of mammals appeared for the first time in teleost fish and represents a step forward in the evolution of isotype diversity. On the other hand, teleost *IgL* genes are organized in a cluster configuration similar to the *Ig* genes in cartilaginous fish. The discovery of IgT in teleosts has confirmed that an Ig isotype specialized in mucosal immune responses appeared early in evolution, sharing common features with mammalian mucosal immune responses. Furthermore, a recent work demonstrated a conserved defense role of the olfactory system, beyond its role as a sensory organ, not only in terrestrial vertebrates but also in fish.

The apparent structural simplicity among teleost Ig may induce one to consider teleost fish as "primitive" rather than a phylogenetically ancient vertebrate lineage. However, the increasing amount of data that have disclosed similarities between teleosts and mammals about the major players of the immune response might contribute to a better understanding of several key points such as the emergence and significance of the different IgH and L isotypes and the evolution of the Ig response, which appears to be based on evolutionarily conserved rules.

REFERENCES

1. Marchalonis JJ, Kaveri SV, Lacroix-Desmazes S, Kazatchkine M. Natural recognition repertoire and the evolutionary emergence of the combinatorial immune system. *FASEB J* 2002;**16**:842–8.
2. Bengtén E, Quiniou SM, Stuge TB, Katagiri T, Miller NW, Clem LW, et al. The IgH locus of the channel catfish, *Ictalurus punctatus*, contains multiple constant region gene sequences: different genes encode heavy chains of membrane and secreted IgD. *J Immunol* 2002;**169**:2488–97.
3. Cheng PC, Brown BK, Song W, Pierce SK. Translocation of the B cell antigen receptor into lipid rafts reveals a novel step in signaling. *J Immunol* 2001;**166**:3693–701.

4. Oreste U, Coscia M. Specific features of immunoglobulin VH genes of the Antarctic teleost *Trematomus bernacchii*. *Gene* 2002;**295**:199–204.

5. Stavnezer J, Amemiya CT. Evolution of isotype switching. *Semin Immunol* 2004;**16**:257–75.

6. Yasuike M, de Boer J, von Schalburg KR, Cooper GA, McKinnel L, Messmer A, et al. Evolution of duplicated IgH loci in Atlantic salmon, *Salmo salar*. *BMC Genomics* 2010;**11**:486. http://dx.doi.org/10.1186/1471-2164-11-486.

7. Warr GW. The immunoglobulin genes of fish. *Dev Comp Immunol* 1995;**19**:1–12.

8. Coscia MR, Oreste U. Plasma and bile antibodies of the teleost *Trematomus bernacchii* specific for the nematode *Pseudoterranova decipiens*. *Dis Aquat Organ* 2000;**41**:37–42.

9. Coscia MR, Simoniello P, Giacomelli S, Oreste U, Motta CM. Investigation of immunoglobulins in skin of the Antarctic teleost *Trematomus bernacchii*. *Fish Shellfish Immunol* 2014;**39**:206–14.

10. Guardiola FA, Cuesta A, Arizcun M, Meseguer J, Esteban MA. Comparative skin mucus and serum humoral defence mechanisms in the teleost gilthead seabream (*Sparus aurata*). *Fish Shellfish Immunol* 2014;**36**:545–51.

11. Picchietti S, Taddei AR, Scapigliati G, Buonocore F, Fausto AM, Romano N, et al. Immunoglobulin protein and gene transcripts in ovarian follicles throughout oogenesis in the teleost *Dicentrarchus labrax*. *Cell Tissue Res* 2004;**315**:259–70.

12. Kaattari S, Evans D, Klemer J. Varied redox forms of teleost IgM: an alternative to isotypic diversity? *Immunol Rev* 1998;**166**:133–42.

13. Zhang YA, Salinas I, Sunyer JO. Recent findings on the structure and function of teleost IgT. *Fish Shellfish Immunol* 2011;**31**:627–34.

14. Kaetzel CS. Coevolution of mucosal immunoglobulins and the polymeric immunoglobulin receptor: evidence that the commensal microbiota provided the driving force. *ISRN Immunol* 2014;**2014**. Article ID 541537.

15. Magnadóttir B, Gudmundsdóttir BK, Gudmundsdóttir S. The carbohydrate moiety of IgM from Atlantic Salmon (*Salmo salar* L.). *Comp Biochem Physiol* 1997;**116B**:423–30.

16. Magnadóttir B, Crispin M, Royle L, Colominas C, Harvey DJ, Dwek RA, et al. The carbohydrate moiety of serum IgM from Atlantic cod (*Gadus morhua* L.). *Fish Shellfish Immunol* 2002;**12**:209–27.

17. Coscia MR, Giacomelli S, Oreste U. Allelic polymorphism of immunoglobulin heavy chain genes in the Antarctic teleost *Trematomus bernacchii*. *Mar Genomics* 2012;**8**:43–8.

18. Brodeur PH, Riblet R. The immunoglobulin heavy chain variable region (Igh-V) locus in the mouse. I. One hundred Igh-V genes comprise seven families of homologous genes. *Eur J Immunol* 1984;**14**:922–30.

19. Coscia MR, Oreste U. Limited diversity of the immunoglobulin heavy chain variable domain of the emerald rockcod *Trematomus bernacchii*. *Fish Shellfish Immunol* 2003;**14**:71–92.

20. Yang F, Ventura-Holman T, Waldbieser GC, Lobb CJ. Structure, genomic organization, and phylogenetic implications of six new VH families in the channel catfish. *Mol Immunol* 2003;**40**:247–60.

21. Lange MD, Waldbieser GC, Lobb CJ. Patterns of receptor revision in the immunoglobulin heavy chains of a teleost fish. *J Immunol* 2009;**182**:5605–22.

22. Coscia MR, Varriale S, Giacomelli S, Oreste U. Antarctic teleost immunoglobulins: more extreme, more interesting. *Fish Shellfish Immunol* 2011;**31**:688–96.

23. Coscia MR, Varriale S, De Santi C, Giacomelli S, Oreste U. Evolution of the Antarctic teleost immunoglobulin heavy chain gene. *Mol Phylogenet Evol* 2010;**55**:226–33.

24. Ohta K, Flajnik MF. IgD, like IgM, is a primordial immunoglobulin class perpetuated in most jawed vertebrates. *Proc Natl Acad Sci USA* 2006;**103**:10723–8.

25. Sun Y, Wei Z, Hammarstrom L, Zhao Y. The immunoglobulin delta gene in jawed vertebrates: a comparative overview. *Dev Comp Immunol* 2010;**35**:975–81.

26. Chen K, Xu W, Wilson M, He B, Miller NW, Bengten E, et al. Immunoglobulin D enhances immune surveillance by activating antimicrobial, proinflammatory and B cell-stimulating programs in basophils. *Nat Immunol* 2009;**10**:889–98.

27. Quiniou SM, Wilson M, Boudinot P. Processing of fish Ig heavy chain transcripts: diverse splicing patterns and unusual nonsense mediated decay. *Dev Comp Immunol* 2011;**35**:949–58.

28. Wilson M, Bengtén E, Miller NW, Clem LW, Du Pasquier L, Warr GW. A novel chimeric Ig heavy chain from a teleost fish shares similarities to IgD. *Proc Natl Acad Sci USA* 1997;**94**:4593–7.

29. Hordvik I, Thevarajan J, Samdal I, Bastani N, Krossøy B. Molecular cloning and phylogenetic analysis of the Atlantic salmon immunoglobulin D gene. *J Virol* 1999;**73**:2136–42.

30. Stenvik J, Jørgensen TO, Immunoglobulin D. (IgD) of Atlantic cod has a unique structure. *Immunogenetics* 2000;**51**:452–61.

31. Hirono I, Nam BH, Enomoto J, Uchino K, Aoki T. Cloning and characterisation of a cDNA encoding Japanese flounder *Paralichthys olivaceus* IgD. *Fish Shellfish Immunol* 2003;**15**: 63–70.

32. Hordvik I. Identification of a novel immunoglobulin delta transcript and comparative analysis of the genes encoding IgD in Atlantic salmon and Atlantic halibut. *Mol Immunol* 2002;**39**:85–91.

33. Saha NR, Suetake H, Kikuchi K, Suzuki Y. Fugu immunoglobulin D: a highly unusual gene with unprecedented duplications in its constant region. *Immunogenetics* 2004;**56**:438–47.

34. Bengtén E, Clem LW, Miller NW, Warr GW, Wilson M. Channel catfish immunoglobulins: repertoire and expression. *Dev Comp Immunol* 2006;**30**:77–92.

35. Edholm ES, Bengten E, Stafford JL, Sahoo M, Taylor EB, Miller NW, et al. Identification of two IgD+ B cell populations in channel catfish, *Ictalurus punctatus*. *J Immunol* 2010;**185**:4082–94.

36. Aparicio S, Chapman J, Stupka E, Putnam N, Chia JM, Dehal P, et al. Whole-genome shotgun assembly and analysis of the genome of *Fugu rubripes*. *Science* 2002;**297**:1301–10.

37. Bao Y, Wang T, Guo Y, Zhao Z, Li N, Zhao Y. The immunoglobulin gene loci in the teleost *Gasterosteus aculeatus*. *Fish Shellfish Immunol* 2010;**28**:40–8.

38. Hordvik I. Immunoglobulin isotypes in Atlantic Salmon, *Salmo Salar*. *Biomolecules* 2015;**5**:166–77.

39. Hansen JD, Landis ED, Phillips RB. Discovery of a unique Ig heavy-chain isotype (IgT) in rainbow trout: implications for a distinctive B cell developmental pathway in teleost fish. *Proc Natl Acad Sci USA* 2005;**102**:6919–24.

40. Savan R, Aman A, Sato K, Yamaguchi R, Sakai M. Discovery of a new class of immunoglobulin heavy chain from fugu. *Eur J Immunol* 2005;**35**:3320–31.

41. Danilova N, Bussmann J, Jekosch K, Steiner LA. The immunoglobulin heavy-chain locus in zebrafish: identification and expression of a previously unknown isotype, immunoglobulin Z. *Nat Immunol* 2005;**6**:295–302.

42. Savan R, Aman A, Nakao M, Watanuki H, Sakai M. Discovery of a novel immunoglobulin heavy chain gene chimera from common carp (*Cyprinus carpio* L.). *Immunogenetics* 2005;**57**:458–63.

43. Ryo S, Wijdeven RH, Tyagi A, Hermsen T, Kono T, Karunasagar I, et al. Common carp have two subclasses of bonyfish specific antibody IgZ showing differential expression in response to infection. *Dev Comp Immunol* 2010;**34**:1183–90.

44. Hu YL, Xiang LX, Shao JZ. Identification and characterization of a novel immunoglobulin Z isotype in zebrafish: implications for a distinct B cell receptor in lower vertebrates. *Mol Immunol* 2010;**47**:738–46.

45. Fillatreau S, Six A, Magadan S, Castro R, Sunyer JO, Boudinot P. The astonishing diversity of Ig classes and B cell repertoires in teleost fish. *Front Immunol* 2013;**4**:28. http://dx.doi.org/10.3389/fimmu.2013.00028.

46. Giacomelli S, Buonocore F, Albanese F, Scapigliati G, Gerdol M, Oreste U, et al. New insights into evolution of IgT genes coming from Antarctic teleosts. *Mar Genomics* 2015. http://dx.doi.org/10.1016/j.margen.2015.06.009.

47. Gambón-Deza F, Sánchez-Espinel C, Magadán-Mompó S. Presence of an unique IgT on the IGH locus in three-spined stickleback fish (*Gasterosteus aculeatus*) and the very recent generation of a repertoire of VH genes. *Dev Comp Immunol* 2010;**4**:114–22.

48. Mashoof S, Pohlenz C, Chen PL, Deiss TC, Gatlin 3rd D, Buentello A, et al. Expressed IgH μ and τ transcripts share diversity segment in ranched *Thunnus orientalis*. *Dev Comp Immunol* 2014;**43**:76–86.

49. Henkel CV, Dirks RP, Jansen HJ, Forlenza M, Wiegertjes JF, Howe K, et al. Comparison of the exomes of common carp (*Cyprinus carpio*) and zebrafish (*Danio rerio*). *Zebrafish* 2012;**9**:59–67.

50. Magadán-Mompó S, Sánchez-Espinel C, Gambón-Deza F. Immunoglobulin heavy chains in medaka (*Oryzias latipes*). *BMC Evol Biol* 2011;**11**:165. http://dx.doi.org/10.1186/1471-2148-11-165.

51. Bengtén E, Quiniou S, Hikima J, Waldbieser G, Warr G, Miller N, et al. Structure of the catfish IGH locus: analysis of the region including the single functional IGHM gene. *Immunogenetics* 2006;**58**:831–44.

52. Zhang YA, Salinas I, Li J, Parra D, Bjork S, Xu Z, et al. IgT, a primitive immunoglobulin class specialized in mucosal immunity. *Nat Immunol* 2010;**11**:827–35.

53. Xu Z, Parra D, Gómez D, Salinas I, Zhang YA, von Gersdorff Jørgensen L, et al. Teleost skin, an ancient mucosal surface that elicits gut-like immune responses. *Proc Natl Acad Sci USA* 2013;**110**:13097–102.

54. Brandtzaeg P. Secretory IgA: designed for anti-microbial defense. *Front Immunol* 2013;**4**:1–17.

55. Hatten F, Fredriksen A, Hordvik I, Endresen C. Presence of IgM in cutaneous mucus, but not in gut mucus of Atlantic salmon, *Salmo salar*. Serum IgM is rapidly degraded when added to gut mucus. *Fish Shellfish Immunol* 2001;**11**:257–68.

56. Palaksha KJ, Shin GW, Kim YR, Jung TS. Evaluation of non-specific immune components from the skin mucus of olive flounder (*Paralichthys olivaceus*). *Fish Shellfish Immunol* 2008;**24**:479–88.

57. Rombout JH, Taverne N, van de Kamp M, Taverne-Thiele AJ. Differences in mucus and serum immunoglobulin of carp (*Cyprinus carpio* L.). *Dev Comp Immunol* 1993;**17**(4):309–17.

58. Lumsden JS, Ostland VE, Byrne PJ, Ferguson HW. Detection of a distinct gill-surface antibody-response following horizontal infection and bath challenge of brook trout *Salvelinus fontinalis* with *Flavobacterium branchiophilum*, the causative agent of bacterial gill disease. *Dis Aquat Org* 1993;**16**:21–7.

59. Lumsden JS, Ostland VE, MacPhee DD, Ferguson HW. Production of gill-associated and serum antibody by rainbow trout (*Oncorhynchus mykiss*) following immersion immunization with acetone-killed *Flavobacterium branchiophilum* and the relationship to protection from experimental challenge. *Fish Shellfish Immunol* 1995;**5**:151–65.

60. Nuñez Ortiz N, Gerdol M, Stocchi V, Marozzi C, Randelli E, Bernini C, et al. T cell transcripts and T cell activities in the gills of the teleost fish sea bass (*Dicentrarchus labrax*). *Dev Comp Immunol* 2014;**47**:309–18.

61. Tacchi L, Musharrafieh R, Larragoite ET, Crossey K, Erhardt EB, Martin SAM, et al. Nasal immunity is an ancient arm of the mucosal immune system of vertebrates. *Nat Commun* 2014;**5**:5205. http://dx.doi.org/10.1038/ncomms6205.

62. Salinas I. The mucosal immune system of teleost fish. *Biology* 2015;**4**:525–39. http://dx.doi.org/10.3390/biology4030525.
63. Edholm ES, Wilson M, Bengten E. Immunoglobulin light (IgL) chains in ectothermic vertebrates. *Dev Comp Immunol* 2011;**35**:906–15.
64. Coscia MR, Giacomelli S, De Santi C, Varriale S, Oreste U. Immunoglobulin light chain isotypes in the teleost *Trematomus bernacchii*. *Mol Immunol* 2008;**45**:3096–106.
65. Espelid S, Nygaard Grøntvedt R. Immunoglobulin V(H)families and light chain isotypes in the spotted wolffish (*Anarhichas minor* Olafsen). *Fish Shellfish Immunol* 2003;**15**(4):311–23.
66. Zhang YA, Nie P, Luo HY, Wang YP, Sun YH, Zhu ZY. Characterization of cDNA encoding immunoglobulin light chain of the mandarin fish (*Siniperca chuatsi*). *Vet Immunol Immunopathol* 2003;**95**(1–2):81–90.
67. Epplen JT, Kyas A, Mäueler W. Genomic simple repetitive DNAs are targets for differential binding of nuclear proteins. *FEBS Lett* 1996;**389**(1):92–5.
68. Stanfield RL, Zemla A, Wilson IA, Rupp B. Antibody elbow angles are influenced by their light chain class. *J Mol Biol* 2006;**357**(5):1566–74.
69. Timmusk S, Partula S, Pilström L. Different genomic organization and expression of immunoglobulin light-chain isotypes in the rainbow trout. *Immunogenetics* 2000;**51**(11):905–14.
70. Ghaffari SH, Lobb CJ. Structure and genomic organization of immunoglobulin light chain in the channel catfish an unusual genomic organizational pattern of segmental genes. *J Immunol* 1993;**151**:6900–12.
71. Daggfeldt A, Bengten E, Pilstrom L. A cluster type organization of the loci of the immunoglobulin light chain in Atlantic cod (*Gadus morhua* L.) and rainbow trout (*Oncorhynchus mykiss* Walbaum) indicated by nucleotide sequences of cDNAs and hybridization analysis. *Immunogenetics* 1993;**38**:199–209.
72. Edholm ES, Wilson M, Sahoo M, Miller NW, Pilstrom L, Wermenstam NE, et al. Identification of Igsigma and Iglambda in channel catfish, *Ictalurus punctatus*, and Iglambda in Atlantic cod, *Gadus morhua*. *Immunogenetics* 2009;**61**:353–70.
73. Hsu E, Criscitiello MF. Diverse immunoglobulin light chain organizations in fish retain potential to revise B cell receptor specificities. *J Immunol* 2006;**177**:2452–62.
74. Zimmerman AM, Yeo G, Howe K, Maddox BJ, Steiner LA. Immunoglobulin light chain (IgL) genes in zebrafish: genomic configurations and inversional rearrangements between (V(L)-J(L)-C(L)) gene clusters. *Dev Comp Immunol* 2008;**32**:421–34.
75. Gorman JR, Alt FW. Regulation of immunoglobulin light chain isotype expression. *Adv Immunol* 1998;**69**:113–81.
76. Klein F, Feldhahn N, Mooster JL, Sprangers M, Hofmann WK, Wernet P, et al. Tracing the pre-B to immature B cell transition in human leukemia cells reveals a coordinated sequence of primary and secondary IGK gene rearrangement IGK deletion, and IGL gene rearrangement. *J Immunol* 2005;**174**:367–75.
77. Fleurant M, Changchien L, Chen CT, Flajnik MF, Hsu E. Shark Ig light chain junctions are as diverse as in heavy chains. *J Immunol* 2004;**173**:5574–82.

Chapter 20

Immunity and Wound Healing: Regeneration or Repair?

Antonella Franchini

Modena and Reggio Emilia University, Modena, Italy

INTRODUCTION

Tissue injury triggers a highly complex and dynamic process of healing, involving several coordinated molecular and cellular events to achieve the predamage integrity and homeostasis. The response can occur in the form of regeneration or repair. Regeneration is variable and results in full replacement of any part of the body (in some invertebrates), complex structures (eg, limbs), internal organs (eg, liver), or lost/damaged tissue so that the original architecture and function are completely restored. In contrast, repair involves fibrotic reactions leading to scar formation that often impair tissue functionality. The capacity to perfectly regrow lost appendages or injured tissues varies widely among animal species. It shows a general gradual loss during ontogenesis and, although the mechanisms underlying regenerative ability have been largely investigated, the reasons for the variable potentials remain unclear.[1–3] Among adult vertebrates, regenerative phenotypes are maintained in complex structures of several species, ie, fins in fish, tails, or limbs in some lizards and amphibians.[3–6] In particular, urodeles (newt, axolotl) are champions of regeneration that is retained throughout their lives and therefore have been considered for a long time to be suitable models for providing insights into the molecular signals and cellular events modulating vertebrate perfect tissue repair.[7–9] The epimorphic regeneration of amputated limbs has been extensively studied; it involves cellular dedifferentiation, formation of a blastema, and an environment for a redevelopment phase that shares similarities with what is observed during embryogenesis.[7] In contrast, this capacity is restricted to larval stages in anuran amphibians, and species, such as *Xenopus laevis*, have become ideal systems for regeneration research and to investigate the progressive loss of the competence.[10–15] Interestingly, tadpoles are not transiently able to perfectly restore amputated tails at particular developmental stages, the so-called *refractory period*, but are helpful in examining mechanisms and signaling networks acting in regeneration

Lessons in Immunity: From Single-Cell Organisms to Mammals
http://dx.doi.org/10.1016/B978-0-12-803252-7.00020-5

promotion.[16] Zebrafish is another recent attractive vertebrate model due to the genetic manipulability and the remarkable regenerative capability observed both in embryos and adults.[4,17] In mammals, except some strains of rodents, the injury response results in perfect tissue repair in embryos/early fetuses while, during postnatal life, this ability is very limited with scar-forming healing.[18,19] Although the causes of this decline during development are still unknown, findings from various organisms suggest and reinforce the role of the immune system and inflammatory response as critical modulators for driving the series of events affecting the response quality to injury.[15,20–25] The ongoing molecular investigations in simple animals such as *Hydra* and planarians, which can perfectly rebuild any part of their body whatever the age, provide the opportunity to explore innate immune signaling in the absence of specialized cells and adaptive immunity. Genomic analyses have demonstrated the expression of many candidate genes of the innate system activated during regeneration and have highlighted an evolutionary conservation of injury-induced immune pathways.[26–28] Although a considerable body of evidence correlates the repair success with an attenuated immune response, some data in different systems indicate not only negative but also positive roles of the immune processes in the restoration of tissue homeostasis and organ functionality.[24]

INJURY-INDUCED INFLAMMATION AND ITS REGULATION DURING TISSUE REPAIR IN DIVERSE MODEL ORGANISMS

A valuable tool for understanding tissue repair and immunological influences is the wound healing of the skin that shares similarities, such as immediate trauma-activated immune response, with the initial preparation phase of amphibian limb regeneration.[7] Skin repair is a complex process constituted by several overlapping phases like inflammation, new tissue formation, and remodeling and involves communications and dynamic interplay between resident and migratory cell types and extracellular matrix components. The inflammatory response, preceded by hemostatic events, is rapidly induced after wounding. Circulating leukocytes, primarily neutrophils, attracted from nearby vessels by a variety of chemotactic factors, release mediators that influence the gene expression and activity of cells at the damaged site. Studies in larval zebrafish suggest that the initial signaling events required for leukocyte recruitment are critical for the repair success and may influence the subsequent regeneration program. In particular, reactive oxygen species (ROS), specifically a gradient of hydrogen peroxide, waves of calcium and the release of key chemokine interleukin (IL)-8 are induced in the wound area and act as early chemoattractants.[29–32] ROS are also immediately produced and released in adult zebrafish, *Xenopus* tadpoles, *Drosophila*, and in organisms with high regenerative potentials, such as *Hydra* and planarians, suggesting an evolutionary conservation of ROS signaling to trigger the regenerative process.[28,33–35] Neutrophils and then macrophages (lymphocytes are the last cells to migrate) continue to be actively recruited to the wound bed to phagocytose and remove invading microbes, foreign particles, and damaged tissue, and these cells are crucial in influencing the repair quality outcome.[23] Neutrophils play an important part in the inflammatory response, with a main function in preventing infection; however, their excessive activity or persistence at the damaged site can have deleterious effects and contribute to the development of chronic, nonhealing wounds in mammals.[36] In zebrafish, the neutrophil function seems to be dependent on the injury context, given that the deficiency of these cells improves tail fin regeneration in larvae, while it does not affect it in adults.[37,38] Already in the 1970s, Leibovich and Ross[39] observed a significant delay of healing after macrophage depletion with antisera. Although beneficial and detrimental functions during tissue repair and regeneration have been long discussed, macrophages are emerging as supportive, with sensor and effector cells coordinating tissue damage and the healing response.[40,41] These cells orchestrate the process by playing key roles in all stages; different functional phenotypes, M1 (classically activated) and M2 (alternatively activated), are stimulated in relation to a changing injury microenvironment.[42,43] Macrophages modulate the local wound milieu, producing a variety of active molecules that regulate fibrosis and scarring, release active proteases as well as pro- and antiinflammatory mediators, synthesize numerous growth factors, induce migration and activation of additional leukocytes, and clear apoptotic cells (including neutrophils) thus promoting inflammation resolution and transition to the proliferative phase.[23] Studies in adult zebrafish, using transgenic cell tracking and genetic ablation technology, highlight stage-dependent functional roles for macrophages in tail fin regeneration, and Wnt/β-catenin has been identified as a signaling pathway that regulates the injury microenvironment, inflammatory cell migration, and macrophage phenotype.[38] The live imaging analyses in transgenic larvae suggest that even neutrophils contribute to inflammation resolution by their reverse migration from wound into vasculature.[44]

It is generally believed that while inflammation is a required event preceding both scarring and regeneration, the early signals and differences in immune response can influence direct healing in the direction of regeneration or scar formation, and a proper, delicate balance between leukocyte cell subsets and inflammatory mediators is essential for a successful repair.[23,25,45,46] In axolotls, the perfect reconstitution of excisional skin wounds occurs with an attenuated immune response and few neutrophils detected.[47] However, the macrophage depletion before the limb amputation or after blastema formation blocks or delays regeneration with the production of fibrotic tissue, indicating that these cells are required to orchestrate the early response to injury and the activation of subsequent events.[48] In contrast, in zebrafish larvae the loss of *PU.1*, essential for myeloid cell development, prevents inflammation but does not affect caudal fin regeneration, suggesting that the acute response mediated by neutrophils and macrophages is not absolutely essential to initiate the process.[49] Similarly, skin repair is scar-free in neonatal *PU.1*-defective mice that lack macrophages and functional neutrophils.[50,51] Gene expression and proteomic analyses in *Xenopus* tadpoles during the complete (premetamorphic) and incomplete limb regeneration stages demonstrate differences in the expression of several immune response genes as well as in levels of immune-related proteins and highlight the importance of local inflammation and its resolution for the progression of a perfect repair.[6,25,52–54] The relevance of a continuous modulation of these activities also emerges from investigations of the effects induced by immune-stimulants (eg, beryllium, a potent agonist of inflammation that inhibits the process) or antiinflammatory agents. The events required to initiate regeneration immediately after amputation are sensitive to the glucocorticoid immunosuppression, while the treatment with specific nonsteroidal antiinflammatory agents, such as cyclooxygenase-2 inhibitors, improves the (incomplete) regeneration in larval limbs as well as reduces scarring in adult mammal skin wounds.[15,25,55] During the *refractory period*, distinct immune responses (prolonged or delayed) are activated in tadpole tail stumps compared to the regeneration period, and both the treatment with immunosuppressants or immune cell depletion by knockdown of *PU.1* significantly restore the lost capacity.[16] It has been proposed that few auto-reactive immune cells transiently infiltrate the wounded area to attack the blastema cells as "nonself," so impairing the repair.[16,56] *Xenopus* age-dependent decline in efficiency to form a new and correctly patterned tail is not only correlated with different local inflammatory responses induced after amputation but also with modifications that occur in the thymus.[14,57] In regeneration-competent larval stages, the injury provokes transient structural changes that affect the cells of the medullary microenvironment, and molecules, ie, TNF-α, critical for the organ constitutive processes are induced. A higher number of lymphocytes are also found in tail regenerates, compared to nonoperated controls, thus suggesting a stimulation in thymic function. In contrast, in the regrowing of defective tails of older larvae, severe alterations are detected in the thymus, including a significant reduction in size, and are indicative of an impairment in its activities.[57] Further studies demonstrate that young froglets, soon after metamorphosis, can perfectly heal skin wounds without scarring, resembling epimorphic regeneration,[58] while the growth to more mature adult stages leads to decreased repair efficiency.[59] In 15 month–old frogs, the inflammatory phase gets activated after the damage persists when the new granulation tissue (provisional wound matrix) is organized and matures, its resolution is delayed, and a scarlike tissue is formed. Moreover, the expression patterns of genes involved in immune responses and healing, ie, *Xenopus suppressor of cytokine signaling 3* (*XSOCS-3*) and *transforming growth factor-beta2* (*XTGF-β2*), are upregulated after wounding compared with control skin, and peak levels are detected when a large number of inflammatory cells are present in granulation tissue.[59] SOCS-3 proteins are negative-feedback regulators of cytokine signaling and also act in the fine-tuning of both innate and adaptive immune responses and inflammation.[60,61] In *Xenopus* larvae, a continued *SOCS-3* expression, probably finalized to negatively regulate the extensive cytokine-induced inflammation, is observed after limb amputation in the regeneration-incomplete stage.[53] This gene is also upregulated in murine models of impaired skin repair, and its epithelial overexpression in transgenic mice augmented the inflammatory response.[62,63] TGF-β factors are main pleiotropic mediators in all phases of the healing process, are expressed transiently (TGF-β1), or are not regulated (TGF-β2) in axolotl scarless repair[47,64]; different isoform profiles are present in mammal prenatal and adult wounds, with high levels of antifibrotic TGF-β3 in embryos.[18,65]

In postnatal mammals (including humans), the switch from a regenerative response to scarring is also accompanied by massive inflammation. In embryo/early fetus wounds, it does not occur or is minimal, with the recruitment of a low number of less differentiated cells and different (qualitatively, quantitatively, and temporally) cytokine and growth factor profiles as compared with adults.[18,22,66,67] There are findings that support the "cytokine hypothesis": relatively high levels of antiinflammatory cytokine expression as compared with proinflammatory cytokines lead to an antiinflammatory wound milieu that makes fetal tissue permissive of regenerative repair. The deficiency of IL-10 results in an exaggerated response with increased leukocyte recruitment and scar formation in mice fetal wounds (usually regenerative), while its overexpression recapitulates fetal-like scarless healing in postnatal mice, thus supporting an essential regulatory role of this cytokine in the regenerative phenotype.[68] Transgenic and knockout mouse models have been generated to better define the involvement of the various inflammatory cells and of the complex network of immune modulators. Mice deficient of specific leukocytes or inflammatory genes display enhanced healing.[69,70] For instance, neonatal *PU.1*-null mice repair without scarring, with minimal inflammation and with different cytokine and growth factor profiles, ie, reduced levels of profibrotic TGF-β1, compared to wild-type wounds. It has been suggested that neutrophils and macrophages are somewhat inhibitory but not absolutely essential and, even though inflammation is not required for efficient repair, may be causal of fibrosis.[51,66,70] However, it should be underlined that there are adult tissues, such as oral mucosa, that retain the repair efficiency observed in embryos.[71] The mechanisms of response to injury vary not only according to animal species but also factors such as environment, tissue specificity, wound size, and genetic predisposition, which may influence the quality outcome.[3,72] Interestingly, investigations in some strains of rodents capable of tissue regeneration, such as nude mice, and in African spiny mice, the only wild-type adults able to heal severe skin wounds in a scar-free manner, point out that even adult mammals maintain the molecular machinery for regeneration.[19,73]

INFLAMMATION IS NOT ALL BAD FOR REPAIR

There is also evidence for another viewpoint: inflammation has positive, or no, effects on repair. In adult zebrafish, cutaneous wounds heal with minimal scar despite the massive inflammatory response, and the loss of *PU.1* gene prevents the inflammation but does not affect fin regeneration.[17,49] A further example is provided by studies in naturally autoimmune Murphy Roths Large (MRL) mice, another unexpected mouse strain, whose adults retain an unusual healing capacity in several organ systems and regenerate holes punched into the ears. In the MRL mice, an increased number of inflammatory cell populations are found after wounding compared to control nonregenerating strains, and the treatment with an inflammation inhibitor blocks the regenerative healing. Moreover, the inflammatory gene expression and cell distribution patterns suggest that a novel population of mast cells, with markers found in both immature and mature cells, may be a major player in the inflammatory and regenerative response.[74]

THE RELATIONSHIP BETWEEN IMMUNE SYSTEM DEVELOPMENT AND REGENERATIVE CAPACITY

Another point of view underlines a phylogenetic correlative link between the development of a functional immune system and the progressive loss of regenerative ability. In *Xenopus*, two distinct immune systems are sequentially developed: the ancestral one with inefficient effector mechanisms in the larval stage and the adult one fundamentally similar to that of mammals.[75,76] The age-dependent decrease of the capability to heal skin in a scar-free manner is associated with the progressive complexity of frog immune responses; in mammals, the switch from regeneration to scarring during the fetal period is concomitant with an increased inflammatory response and maturation of adaptive immunity.[59,76,77] Conversely, urodeles, capable of perfect repair, have a well-developed innate immunity but are considered relatively "immunodeficient" with weak responses and have less efficient adaptive immunity compared to that of anurans.[20,21] However, there are also evidences indicating that immune competence and regenerative/scar-free mechanisms are not mutually exclusive: examples are provided by the perfect repair of fin in adult zebrafish or fingertips in postnatal mammals and the regeneration of lens in adult news that requires the trafficking of dendritic cells to the spleen and is abrogated by splenectomy.[24,78]

ROLE OF LYMPHOCYTES IN REPAIR MECHANISMS

The patterns of leukocyte subsets change, both spatially and temporally, during the inflammatory response to wounding, and the lymphocytes, especially T cells, are the last cells attracted to the injury site. The precise contribution of adaptive response cells to the healing process has not been studied extensively; the results produced are rather conflicting, and T-lymphocyte involvement in a successful repair remains unclear and requires further studies. In *Xenopus*, the restoration of regenerative potential in the larval postrefractory period overlaps the emergence of T-regulatory cells that transiently infiltrate the amputated tail stumps. These cells are suggested to suppress the function of a few unregulated immune cells that interfere with the functional process.[16] Moreover, in adult frogs, T-lymphocytes, immunoreactive to anti-XT1 (*Xenopus* specific T-cell marker) and anti-CD3ε antibodies, are detected in skin wounded areas during the tissue maturation phase, and their infiltration is associated with stimulation of the thymus activity.[79] Evidences from mammals have pointed out a modulatory role of T-lymphocytes that might influence tissue remodeling by secreting distinct lymphokines and by direct cell–cell interactions with resident and nonresident cells at the damaged site.[24,80,81] The global T-cell depletion before injury impairs mice wound healing with a severe reduction in mechanical strength and collagen deposition.[82] Adult athymic nude mice have initially attracted some attention as models for examining the contribution of T-lymphocytes: the skin repairs without scarring, and regeneration in the external ears occurs with the formation of a blastema.[19,73,83] Nevertheless, investigations in several immunodeficient mice indicate that the lack of thymus and/or T cells could not support the regenerative capacity.[84] Experiments of selective cell depletions have highlighted different and opposing actions of individual T subsets on repair mechanisms, ie, upregulatory for CD4- and downregulatory for CD8-lymphocytes.[81,85] Gawronska-Kozak et al.[84] show that scarless healing in athymic nude-*nu* mice differs from other immunologically compromised animals for the absence of CD8-cells. A recent study demonstrates that deficiency of CD4- or CD8-cells significantly changes the inflammatory cell infiltration and profiles of cytokine expression in skin wounds; however, healing is not impaired, suggesting that, despite being present and involved, the influence of both cell subtypes is not critical.[86] Epidermal resident T-cells, a source of key cytokines and growth factors, are also considered important mediators in several aspects of repair with immunoregulatory activities.[87] Regarding B-lymphocytes, although they are detected within injured adult tissue,[88,89] little is known about their function. Evidence of the involvement of these cells in the process is provided by experiments performed in splenectomized mice: in these animals the wound healing is delayed, the binding of IgG1 antibodies to damaged tissues is reduced, and the transfer of B-cells restores the repair ability.[90] A mechanism to explain how B-cells regulate cutaneous healing has been proposed: B-lymphocytes, which infiltrate injury sites, are stimulated, through Toll-like receptor-4 signaling in a CD19-dependent manner, to produce various cytokines and growth factors that cooperatively promote repair, in part by activating other immune cells.[91]

CONCLUSION

In summary, although extensive research to investigate variable repair efficiency among animal species has been conducted, further investigations are required for a deeper understanding of the mechanisms by which the immune system directs the response to tissue/organ injury and the transition from regeneration to scar formation.

REFERENCES

1. Gurtner GC, Werner S, Barrandon Y, Longaker MT. Wound repair and regeneration. *Nature* 2008;**453**:314–21.
2. Murawala P, Tanaka EM, Currie JD. Regeneration: the ultimate example of wound healing. *Semin Cell Dev Biol* 2012;**23**:954–62.
3. Ud-Din S, Volk SW, Bayat A. Regenerative healing, scar-free healing and scar formation across the species: current concepts and future perspectives. *Exp Dermatol* 2014;**23**:615–9.
4. Gemberling M, Bailey TJ, Hyde DR, Poss KD. The zebrafish as a model for complex tissue regeneration. *Trends Genet* 2013;**29**:611–20.
5. Alibardi L. Histochemical, biochemical and cell biological aspects of tail regeneration in lizard, an amniote model for studies on tissue regeneration. *Prog Histochem Cytochem* 2014;**48**: 143–244.
6. Godwin JW, Rosenthal N. Scar-free wound healing and regeneration in amphibians: immunological influences on regenerative success. *Differentiation* 2014;**87**:66–75.
7. Roy S, Lévesque M. Limb regeneration in axolotl: is it superhealing? *TSW Dev Embryol* 2006;**6**:12–25.
8. Roy S, Gatien S. Regeneration in axolotls: a model to aim for! *Exp Gerontol* 2008;**43**:968–73.
9. Seifert AW, Monaghan JR, Voss SR, Maden M. Skin regeneration in adult axolotls: a blueprint for scar-free healing in vertebrates. *PLoS One* 2012;**7**:e32875.
10. Slack JM, Beck CW, Gargioli C, Christen B. Cellular and molecular mechanisms of regeneration in *Xenopus. Philos Trans R Soc Lond B Biol Sci* 2004;**359**:745–51. http://www.ncbi.nlm. nih.gov/pubmed/15293801.
11. Slack JM, Lin G, Chen Y. The *Xenopus* tadpole: a new model for regeneration research. *Cell Mol Life Sci* 2008;**65**:54–63.
12. Tseng AS, Levin M. Tail regeneration in *Xenopus laevis* as a model for understanding tissue repair. *J Dent Res* 2008;**87**:806–16.
13. Beck CW, Izpisúa Belmonte JC, Christen B. Beyond early development: *Xenopus* as an emerging model for the study of regenerative mechanisms. *Dev Dyn* 2009;**238**:1226–48. http://www. ncbi.nlm.nih.gov/pubmed/19280606.
14. Franchini A, Bertolotti E. Tail regenerative capacity and iNOS immunolocalization in *Xenopus laevis* tadpoles. *Cell Tissue Res* 2011;**344**:261–9.
15. Mescher AL, Neff AW, King MW. Changes in the inflammatory response to injury and its resolution during the loss of regenerative capacity in developing *Xenopus* limbs. *PLoS One* 2013;**8**:e80477.
16. Fukazawa T, Naora Y, Kunieda T, Kubo T. Suppression of the immune response potentiates tadpole tail regeneration during the refractory period. *Development* 2009;**136**:2323–7.
17. Richardson R, Slanchev K, Kraus C, Knyphausen P, Eming S, Hammerschmidt M. Adult zebrafish as a model system for cutaneous wound healing research. *J Invest Dermatol* 2013;**133**:1655–65.
18. Ferguson MW, O'Kane S. Scar-free healing: from embryonic mechanisms to adult therapeutic intervention. *Philos Trans R Soc Lond B Biol Sci* 2004;**359**:839–50.
19. Gawronska-Kozak B, Grabowska A, Kopcewicz M, Kur A. Animal models of skin regeneration. *Reprod Biol* 2014;**14**:61–7.
20. Harty M, Neff AW, King MW, Mescher AL. Regeneration or scarring: an immunologic perspective. *Dev Dyn* 2003;**226**:268–79.
21. Mescher AL, Neff AW. Limb regeneration in amphibians: immunological considerations. *TSW Dev Embryol* 2006;**6**:1–11.

22. Stramer BM, Mori R, Martin P. The inflammation-fibrosis link? A Jekyll and Hyde role for blood cells during wound repair. *J Invest Dermatol* 2007;**127**:1009–17.

23. Eming SA, Krieg T, Davidson JM. Inflammation in wound repair: molecular and cellular mechanisms. *J Invest Dermatol* 2007;**127**:514–25.

24. Eming SA, Hammerschmidt M, Krieg T, Roers A. Interrelation of immunity and tissue repair or regeneration. *Semin Cell Dev Biol* 2009;**20**:517–27.

25. King MW, Neff AW, Mescher AL. The developing *Xenopus* limb as a model for studies on the balance between inflammation and regeneration. *Anat Rec* 2012;**295**:1552–61.

26. Sandmann T, Vogg MC, Owlarn S, Boutros M, Bartscherer K. The head-regeneration transcriptome of the planarian *Schmidtea mediterranea*. *Genome Biol* 2011;**12**:R76.

27. Peiris TH, Hoyer KK, Oviedo NJ. Innate immune system and tissue regeneration in planarians: an area ripe for exploration. *Semin Immunol* 2014;**26**:295–302.

28. Wenger Y, Buzgariu W, Reiter S, Galliot B. Injury-induced immune responses in *Hydra*. *Semin Immunol* 2014;**26**:277–94.

29. Niethammer P, Grabher C, Look AT, Mitchison TJ. A tissue-scale gradient of hydrogen peroxide mediates rapid wound detection in zebrafish. *Nature* 2009;**459**:996–9.

30. Yoo SK, Starnes TW, Deng Q, Huttenlocher A. Lyn is a redox sensor that mediates leukocyte wound attraction in vivo. *Nature* 2011;**480**:109–12.

31. Yoo SK, Freisinger CM, LeBert DC, Huttenlocher A. Early redox, Src family kinase, and calcium signaling integrate wound responses and tissue regeneration in zebrafish. *J Cell Biol* 2012;**199**:225–34.

32. De Oliveira S, Reyes-Aldasoro CC, Candel S, Renshaw SA, Mulero V, Calado A. Cxcl8 (Interleukin-8) mediates neutrophil recruitment behavior in the zebrafish inflammatory response. *J Immunol* 2013;**190**:4349–59.

33. Gauron C, Rampon C, Bouzaffour M, Ipendey E, Teillon J, Volovitch M, et al. Sustained production of ROS triggers compensatory proliferation and is required for regeneration to proceed. *Sci Rep* 2013;**3**:2084.

34. Love NR, Chen Y, Ishibashi S, Kritsiligkou P, Lea R, Koh Y, et al. Amputation-induced reactive oxygen species are required for successful *Xenopus* tadpole tail regeneration. *Nat Cell Biol* 2013;**15**:222–8.

35. Vriz S, Reiter S, Galliot B. Cell death: a program to regenerate. *Curr Top Dev Biol* 2014;**108**: 121–51.

36. Wilgus TA, Roy S, McDaniel JC. Neutrophils and wound repair: positive actions and negative reactions. *Adv Wound Care* 2013;**2**:379–88.

37. Li L, Yan B, Shi YQ, Zhang WQ, Wen ZL. Live imaging reveals differing roles of macrophages and neutrophils during zebrafish tail fin regeneration. *J Biol Chem* 2012;**287**:25353–60.

38. Petrie TA, Strand NS, Tsung-Yang C, Rabinowitz JS, Moon RT. Macrophages modulate adult zebrafish tail fin regeneration. *Development* 2014;**141**:2581–91.

39. Leibovich SJ, Ross R. The role of the macrophage in wound repair. A study with hydrocortisone and anti-macrophage serum. *Am J Pathol* 1975;**78**:1–100.

40. Chazaud B. Macrophages: supportive cells for tissue repair and regeneration. *Immunobiology* 2014;**219**:172–8.

41. Willenborg S, Eming SA. Macrophages - sensors and effectors coordinating skin damage and repair. *J Dtsch Dermatol Ges* 2014;**12**:214–21.

42. Brancato SK, Albina JE. Wound macrophages as key regulators of repair. Origin, phenotype, and function. *Am J Pathol* 2011;**178**:19–25.

43. Mahdavian Delavary B, van der Veer WM, van Egmond M, Niessen FB, Beelen RH. Macrophages in skin injury and repair. *Immunobiology* 2011;**216**:753–62.

44. Yoo SK, Huttenlocher A. Spatiotemporal photolabeling of neutrophil trafficking during inflammation in live zebrafish. *J Leukoc Biol* 2011;**89**:661–7.

45. LeBert DC, Huttenlocher A. Inflammation and wound repair. *Semin Immunol* 2014;**26**:315–20.

46. Seifert AW, Maden M. New insights into vertebrate skin regeneration. *Int Rev Cell Mol Biol* 2014;**310**:129–69. http://www.ncbi.nlm.nih.gov/pubmed/14673598.

47. Lévesque M, Villiard E, Roy S. Skin wound healing in axolotls: a scarless process. *J Exp Zool B Mol Dev Evol* 2010;**314**:684–97.

48. Godwin JW, Pinto AR, Rosenthal NA. Macrophages are required for adult salamander limb regeneration. *Proc Natl Acad Sci USA* 2013;**110**:9415–20.

49. Mathew LK, Sengupta S, Kawakami A, Andreasen EA, Löhr CV, Loynes CA, et al. Unraveling tissue regeneration pathways using chemical genetics. *J Biol Chem* 2007;**282**:35202–10.

50. McKercher SR, Torbett BE, Anderson KL, Henkel GW, Vestal DJ, Baribault H, et al. Targeted disruption of the *PU.1* gene results in multiple hematopoietic abnormalities. *EMBO J* 1996;**15**:5647–58.

51. Martin P, D'Souza D, Martin J, Grose R, Cooper L, Maki R, et al. Wound healing in the PU.1 null mouse - tissue repair is not dependent on inflammatory cells. *Curr Biol* 2003;**13**:1122–8.

52. King MW, Neff AW, Mescher AL. Proteomics analysis of regenerating amphibian limbs: changes during the onset of regeneration. *Int J Dev Biol* 2009;**53**:955–69.

53. Grow M, Neff AW, Mescher AL, King MW. Global analysis of gene expression in *Xenopus* hindlimbs during stage-dependent complete and incomplete regeneration. *Dev Dyn* 2006;**235**:2667–85.

54. Pearl EJ, Barker D, Day RC, Beck CW. Identification of genes associated with regenerative success of *Xenopus laevis* hindlimbs. *BMC Dev Biol* 2008;**8**:66.

55. Wilgus TA, Vodovotz Y, Vittadini E, Clubbs EA, Oberyszyn TM. Reduction of scar formation in full-thickness wounds with topical celecoxib treatment. *Wound Repair Regen* 2003;**11**: 25–34.

56. Naora Y, Hishida Y, Fukazawa T, Kunieda T, Kubo T. Expression analysis of *XPhyH-like* during development and tail regeneration in *Xenopus* tadpoles: possible role of *XPhyH-like* expressing immune cells in impaired tail regenerative ability. *Biochem Biophys Res Commun* 2013;**431**: 152–7.

57. Franchini A, Bertolotti E. The thymus and tail regenerative capacity in *Xenopus laevis* tadpoles. *Acta Histochem* 2012;**114**:334–41.

58. Yokoyama H, Maruoka T, Aruga A, Amano T, Ohgo S, Shiroishi T, et al. *Prx-1* expression in *Xenopus laevis* scarless skin-wound healing and its resemblance to epimorphic regeneration. *J Invest Dermatol* 2011;**131**:2477–85.

59. Bertolotti E, Malagoli D, Franchini A. Skin wound healing in different aged *Xenopus laevis*. *J Morphol* 2013;**274**:956–64.

60. Tamiya T, Kashiwagi I, Takahashi R, Yasukawa H, Yoshimura A. Suppressors of cytokine signaling (SOCS) proteins and JAK/STAT pathways: regulation of T-cell inflammation by SOCS1 and SOCS3. *Arterioscler Thromb Vasc Biol* 2011;**31**:980–5.

61. Yoshimura A, Suzuki M, Sakaguchi R, Hanada T, Yasukawa H. SOCS, inflammation, and autoimmunity. *Front Immunol* 2012;**3**:20.

62. Goren I, Linke A, Muller E, Pfeilschifter J, Frank S. The suppressor of cytokine signaling-3 is upregulated in impaired skin repair: implications for keratinocyte proliferation. *J Invest Dermatol* 2006;**126**:477–85.

63. Linke A, Goren I, Bosl MR, Pfeilschifter J, Frank S. Epithelial overexpression of SOCS-3 in transgenic mice exacerbates wound inflammation in the presence of elevated TGF-β1. *J Invest Dermatol* 2010;**30**:866–75.

64. Denis JF, Lévesque M, Tran SD, Camarda AJ, Roy S. Axolotl as a model to study scarless wound healing in vertebrates: role of the transforming growth factor beta signaling pathway. *Adv Wound Care* 2013;**2**:250–60.

65. Behm B, Babilas P, Landthaler M, Schreml S. Cytokines, chemokines and growth factors in wound healing. *J Eur Acad Dermatol Venereol* 2011;**26**:812–20.

66. Redd MJ, Cooper L, Wood W, Stramer B, Martin P. Wound healing and inflammation: embryos reveal the way to perfect repair. *Philos Trans R Soc Lond B Biol Sci* 2004;**359**:777–84.

67. Kishi K, Okabe K, Shimizu R, Kubota Y. Fetal skin possesses the ability to regenerate completely: complete regeneration of skin. *Keio J Med* 2012;**61**:101–8.

68. King A, Balaji S, Le LD, Crombleholme TM, Keswani SG. Regenerative wound healing: the role of interleukin-10. *Adv Wound Care* 2014;**3**:315–23.

69. Grose R, Werner S. Wound-healing studies in transgenic and knockout mice. *Mol Biotechnol* 2004;**28**:147–66.

70. Martin P, Leibovich SJ. Inflammatory cells during wound repair: the good, the bad and the ugly. *Trends Cell Biol* 2005;**15**:599–607.

71. Glim JE, van Egmond M, Niessen FB, Everts V, Beelen RH. Detrimental dermal wound healing: what can we learn from the oral mucosa? *Wound Repair Regen* 2013;**21**:648–60.

72. Brown JJ, Bayat A. Genetic susceptibility to raised dermal scarring. *Br J Dermatol* 2009;**161**:8–18.

73. Barbul A, Shawe T, Rotter SM, Efron JE, Wasserkrug HL, Badawy SB. Wound healing in nude mice: a study on the regulatory role of lymphocytes in fibroplasia. *Surgery* 1989;**105**:764–9.

74. Gourevitch D, Kossenkov AV, Zhang Y, Clark L, Chang C, Showe LC, et al. Inflammation and its correlates in regenerative wound healing: an alternate perspective. *Adv Wound Care* 2014;**3**:592–603.

75. Du Pasquier L, Schwager J, Flajnik MF. The immune system of *Xenopus*. *Annu Rev Immunol* 1989;**7**:251–75.

76. Robert J, Ohta Y. Comparative and developmental study of the immune system in *Xenopus*. *Dev Dyn* 2009;**238**:1249–70.

77. Yannas IY. Similarities and differences between induced organ regeneration in adults and early foetal regeneration. *J R Soc Interface* 2005;**2**:403–17.

78. Godwin JW, Brockes JP. Regeneration, tissue injury and the immune response. *J Anat* 2006;**209**:423–32.

79. Franchini A, Bertolotti E. The thymus and skin wound healing in *Xenopus laevis* adults. *Acta Histochem* 2014;**116**:1141–7.

80. Schäffer M, Barbul A. Lymphocyte function in wound healing and following injury. *Br J Surg* 1998;**85**:444–60.

81. Park JE, Barbul A. Understanding the role of immune regulation in wound healing. *Am J Surg* 2004;**187**:11S–6S.

82. Efron JE, Frankel HL, Lazarou SA, Wasserkrug HL, Barbul A. Wound healing and T-lymphocytes. *J Surg Res* 1990;**48**:460–3.

83. Gawronska-Kozak B. Regeneration in the ears of immunodeficient mice: identification and lineage analysis of mesenchymal stem cells. *Tissue Eng* 2004;**10**:1251–65.

84. Gawronska-Kozak B, Bogacki M, Rim JS, Monroe WT, Manuel JA. Scarless skin repair in immunodeficient mice. *Wound Repair Regen* 2006;**14**:265–76.

85. Davis PA, Corless DJ, Aspinall R, Wastell C. Effect of CD4(+) and CD8(+) cell depletion on wound healing. *Br J Surg* 2001;**88**:298–304.

86. Chen L, Mehta ND, Zhao Y, DiPietro LA. Absence of CD4 or CD8 lymphocytes changes inflammatory cells and profiles of cytokine wounds, but does not impair healing. *Exp Dermatol* 2014;**23**:189–94.

87. Havran WL, Jameson JM. Epidermal T cells and wound healing. *J Immunol* 2010;**184**:5423–8.

88. Cowin AJ, Brosnan MP, Holmes TM, Ferguson MW. Endogenous inflammatory response to dermal wound healing in the fetal and adult mouse. *Dev Dyn* 1998;**212**:385–93.

89. Boyce DE, Jones WD, Ruge F, Harding KG, Moore K. The role of lymphocytes in human dermal wound healing. *Br J Dermatol* 2000;**143**:59–65.

90. Nishio N, Ito S, Suzuki H, Isobe K. Antibodies to wounded tissue enhance cutaneous wound healing. *Immunology* 2009;**128**:369–80.

91. Iwata Y, Yoshizaki A, Komura K, Shimizu K, Ogawa F, Hara T, et al. CD19, a response regulator of B lymphocytes, regulates wound healing through hyaluronan-induced TLR4 signaling. *Am J Pathol* 2009;**175**:649–60.

Chapter 21

Marine Mammal Immunity Toward Environmental Challenges

Annalaura Mancia
University of Ferrara, Ferrara, Italy

ADAPTATION OF MAMMALS TO THE MARINE ENVIRONMENT

Mammals reentered the oceans on at least seven separate occasions. The five extant clades belong to one of three orders: Cetartiodactyla (cetaceans: whales, dolphins, and porpoises), Sirenia (dugongs and manatees), or Carnivora (pinnipeds: seals, sea lions, fur seals, and walruses; sea otters and polar bears). Cetaceans and sirenians emerged during the Eocene epoch. Pinnipeds emerged approximately 20 million years later during the Miocene from within the Carnivora. While maintaining the basic characteristics of all other mammals, they have adapted to living all or part of their lives in the ocean. Despite their independent evolutionary origins and the diversity in morphology seen among groups, improving feeding proficiency has been the main driver in the evolution of these lineages, and that is why pinnipeds, sirenians, and cetaceans share a number of phenotypic adaptations to the thermal, locomotory, hypoxic, sensory, and pathogenic challenges of an aquatic existence.[1]

The International Union for the Conservation of Nature Red List currently classifies 32 of 128 species of marine mammals (25%) as threatened with extinction. Examination of the threats on the basis of the Red List shows that nearly half of all species are threatened by two or more human impacts, with pollution being the most pervasive, followed by fishing, invasive species, industrial development, hunting, and climate change.

MARINE MAMMALS, SENTINELS FOR THE HEALTH OF THE ECOSYSTEM

The increasing number of humans inhabiting the coast and the increasing consumption (and destruction) of resources place enormous pressures on the environment. The effects can be found in every ecosystem, but the major

Lessons in Immunity: From Single-Cell Organisms to Mammals
http://dx.doi.org/10.1016/B978-0-12-803252-7.00021-7
287

impact is observed in the ocean, which covers 79% of the Earth's surface. The effects can be direct, such as alteration in the abundance of fish or shellfish and the prevalence of infectious/toxic agents, or indirect, through the effects of runoff and climate change. Oceans facilitate the distribution of toxic contaminants such as heavy metals and organochlorine chemicals (eg, polychlorinated biphenyls (PCBs), and chlorinated pesticides, like DDT), which tend to be stable and lipophilic. Runoff from urban, industrial, and agricultural activities bioaccumulate up the food chain, with the greatest concentrations in animals at the highest trophic levels, such as marine mammals. Numerous studies have shown that marine mammals can accumulate anthropogenic contaminants such as organohalogens and heavy metal contaminants.[2]

Marine mammals are also subject to the stress posed by biotoxins (eg, brevetoxins, ciguatoxin/maitotoxin, saxitoxins, domoic acid, and okadaic acid) produced by harmful algal blooms (HABs). HABs are periodically experienced by coastal waters around the world and have been increasing over the last 25 years, affecting dolphins, sea lions, southern sea otters, Florida manatees, Mediterranean monk seals, gray whales, and humpback whales.[2]

Emerging disease agents have been reported in marine mammals, including various papillomaviruses, morbillivirus, dolphin poxvirus, and other viral infections, lobomycosis, toxoplasmosis, leptospirosis, and various neoplastic diseases (urogenital cancer, lingual and genital papillomas, squamous cell carcinomas) that may be direct or indirect consequences of pathological infections.[2] In some instances, they are caused by new species-specific pathogens, like the dolphin papillomavirus, the etiologic agent of several benign and malignant tumors. In other cases, they are caused by agents pathogenic to man as well; an example is the fungus *Lacazia loboi*, which causes lobomycosis, resulting in dermal and subcutaneous granulomas, which have been described only in humans and dolphins.[3]

Thus marine mammals can be informative of the status of the marine ecosystem in which they live, and for this reason they have been proposed as sentinel organisms for the health of the marine environment. Assessing the health status of marine mammals can provide valuable information for evaluating the relationship between exposure to biological and chemical agents and health effects even on humans.[2]

Marine mammals have long life spans, feed at a high trophic level, and have extensive fat stores that can serve as accumulation beds for anthropogenic toxins. They live most (if not all) of their entire lives in the aquatic environment where they are directly and constantly exposed to a variety of pathogens and other stressors of natural and anthropogenic origin. Their blubber—which plays a major role in nutrition, buoyancy, and thermoregulation—is also an ideal repository for some contaminants. Lipophilic contaminants may remain stored in the blubber until the animal dies, but others can be metabolized in times of physiological challenges (illness, nutritional compromise, pregnancy, etc.). The first to propose the use of marine mammals as environmental sentinels was Holden, in 1972. In 1998, the Marine Mammal Commission identified the California sea lion (*Zalophus californianus*), the harbor seal (*Phoca vitulina*), the beluga whale (*Delphinapterus leucas*), and the bottlenose dolphin (*Tursiops truncatus*) as model species for investigation into the effects of environmental contaminants on marine mammals.

IMMUNOTOXIC EFFECTS OF ENVIRONMENTAL CHALLENGES

Climate change and the variation in ocean temperature are predicted to stimulate the migration of marine organisms based on their temperature tolerance, with heat-tolerant species expanding their range to the poles and those less-tolerant species retreating. This, of course, has implications on the entire trophic web. The real challenge is that modifications resulting from climate change are being superimposed on a marine environment already stressed from direct and indirect anthropogenic hits associated with overfishing and improper fishing practices, coastal development, sedimentation, land-based sources of pollution, and marine pollution. Thus marine mammals are exposed to a worrying cocktail of potentially immunotoxic compounds and life-threatening conditions. Moreover, confounding factors such as age, gender, and hormonal and nutritional status can be involved in intake and in the bioaccumulation of different environmental contaminants, which also strongly affect the immune response.[4,5] Furthermore, the establishment of the link between environmental challenges and the real effects on marine mammal immunity is complicated by logistical, technical, and ethical issues.

It is estimated that over 70,000 chemicals are currently in common use as industrial compounds, pesticides, pharmaceuticals, food additives, and other purposes, and that this number is increasing by approximately 1000 each year (http://www.epa.gov). Of particular concern to the health of marine mammal populations are the halogenated hydrocarbons (PCBs, DDT, chlordane, dioxins and furans, and the chlorinated and brominated diphenyl ethers), trace metals (mercury and cadmium), and polycyclic aromatic hydrocarbons. The environmental impact can lead to dramatic events, such as the death of the animals, but can also be less evident, affecting their health, reproductive, and immune functions; this can be the cause of cancer, behavioral changes, immune and nervous dysfunction, damage to the kidney, liver and other organs, and alteration of hormone levels.[6–8] Harbor porpoises (*Phocoena phocoena*) from the North and Baltic seas, contaminated with xenobiotics, such as PCBs and methylmercury, are more frequently affected by bacterial infections and parasitism than specimens from less-polluted waters around Norway, Iceland, and Greenland.[9–12] Bottlenose dolphins inhabiting a site in Georgia (USA) showed anemia, hypothyroidism, and immune suppression associated with PCB exposure.[5] The combination of stress induced by chemical pollutants and others (natural and human derived) makes it increasingly difficult for an animal to cope with changing environmental conditions.

The Marine Mammal Protection Act of 1972 defines marine mammals as all members of the orders Cetacea (whales, dolphins, and porpoises) and Sirenia (manatees and the dugong); all members of the three Carnivora families Phocidae (true or earless seals), Otariidae (fur seals and sea lions), and Odobenidae (the walrus); two members of the Carnivora family Mustelidae (the sea otter and marine otter); and one member of the Carnivora family Ursidae (the polar bear). This arbitrarily defined group of animals lives in a large variety of habitats and pursues diverse strategies for feeding, reproduction, and other vital activities. Thus they are exposed to many kinds and levels of contaminants. Feeding strategies, in particular, influence the nature and degree of exposure to contaminants. The planktivorous baleen whales tend to have lower concentrations of organochlorines in their tissues than the more piscivorous toothed whales.[13] In general, coastal populations of dolphins, seals, and sea lions tend to have higher contaminant levels than the more pelagic populations, probably because their food webs are more exposed to concentrated terrestrial runoff. Many species, such as manatees, gray whales, and walruses, are benthic feeders. By feeding in or near bottom sediments, they risk exposure to concentrations and types of contaminants that may differ from those to which the more pelagic-feeding species are exposed. It is important to bear in mind that some aquatic mammals (eg, river dolphins, manatees, freshwater seals) inhabit river and lake systems deep within continental land masses and far removed from marine environments. Final consequences of today's new conditions are changes in the natural habitat, food supply, and ocean chemistry and increases in noise and disturbance: these are affecting marine organisms, which must adapt very quickly to survive.

MOLECULAR EFFECTS OF ENVIRONMENTAL CHANGES ON MARINE MAMMAL IMMUNITY

A healthy and comprehensive immune system is critical to the survival of all animals because they are all hosts to pathogens and parasites. The mammalian immune system is extremely complex, and there is often duplication and redundancy in specific functions. In general, no clear differences have been revealed so far comparing the immune systems of terrestrial and marine mammals, even though specific information regarding these latter is still scant, also due to sporadic sampling. However, both physical examination and assessment of the size and state of the lymphoid organs (thymus, spleen, and lymph nodes) can be useful in detecting the primary immunodeficiency state. Useful information can be gathered from routine hematological examinations and clinical serum chemistry analysis, which should be carried out repeatedly and compared with information from healthy, age-matched individuals.[17] Marine mammals' immune systems, as for all mammals, are characterized by both innate and adaptive responses, and the morphology of their lymphoid organs is similar to that of terrestrial mammals.[14-16] The cloning of the major cytokines supported their likely roles in the immune response, and a similar approach was directed toward immunoglobulins, antigen-specific effector molecules of the adaptive arm. Nonetheless, as with many other aspects of marine mammal physiology, the immune system should have uniquely adapted to the marine ecosystem. Dolphins and sea lions are incredibly good at masking illness until they are really sick and stop eating. By then, veterinarians have to take an aggressive treatment approach. The evaluation of the health status can be carried out using the exhaled breath, which contains both volatile small molecules and fine liquid droplets filled with macromolecules such as peptides and antibodies: some of those compounds could be biomarkers for disease. For example, dolphins with inflamed lungs exhale an increased amount of nitric oxide, although the finding is not exactly indicative of a certain pulmonary disease.[18]

A better understanding of the marine mammal immune system has been the result of the development of novel assays for measuring dolphin-specific antibodies and cellular responses and of the production of monoclonal antibodies for dolphin lymphocyte subpopulations, or other cell markers.[19]

In the postgenomic era, there is an intensification of the research efforts on the exploration of gene function, both individually and collectively, at the molecular, cellular, organism, and population levels. Genomic technologies offer the opportunity to study molecular responses on a broad ecological scale through the deployment of gene microarrays as transcriptomic biosensors.[20,21] Transcript profiling yields a snapshot of an entire expressed genome and is now an established technique in the biomedical models of human physiology and disease. The use of whole-genome scale transcriptomics with animal samples obtained in a minimally invasive manner is an approach that shows promise for health assessment. Neither genomes nor transcriptomes are still available for many nonmodel organisms; however, today's new instruments and the advancement of computational biology techniques allow functional genomics tools developed for other species to be applied in evolutionary-related organisms. The California sea lion, a protected marine mammal inhabiting the western coast of North America, is an animal of particular interest due to its ability to act as a sentinel species for coastal habitats. In 2009 alone, over 600 stranded sea lions were admitted to The Marine Mammal Center, in Sausalito, CA, for rehabilitation. With no availability of a California sea lion genome, a custom microarray developed from the commercially available dog (*Canis familiaris*) microarray was used to interrogate blood samples from sea lions in rehabilitation. Not only did differentially expressed genes within animal groups reflect an activation of the immune response, with many being indicative of illness, but also groups of genes could be used as the signature of a specific disease status and as a classifier, primarily distinguishing between leptospirosis infection and domoic acid exposure.[22]

The development and application of a comprehensive species-specific (*T. truncatus*) gene microarray of 24,418 unigene sequences to monitor the global gene expression of wild dolphins' blood has been very useful in the identification of geographical locations, which can reflect the high level of contamination of a specific site.[23,24] Genes involved in xenobiotic metabolism, development/differentiation, and oncogenic pathways were found to be differentially expressed in dolphins inhabiting the Georgia coast, known to be heavily contaminated by an uncommon PCB mixture. Since contaminants persist in the environment, this information can be important to understand the long-term effects of exposure for mammals residing in coastal areas. With this sensitive tool, it is possible to detect the buildup of contaminants on the coasts and spare inhabitants of all types from toxic exposure to legacy chemicals.

Finally, reduced costs and higher throughput have made next-generation sequencing more accessible to allow comparative analysis of full genomes. Foote at al[25] sequenced and performed de novo assembly of the genomes of three species of marine mammals (the killer whale, walrus, and manatee) from three mammalian orders that share independently evolved phenotypic adaptations to a marine existence. The comparative genomic analyses of those three species and a fourth represented by a previously sequenced dolphin genome found that convergent amino acid substitutions were widespread throughout the genome and that a subset of these substitutions were in genes evolving under positive selection and putatively associated with a marine phenotype. Convergent phenotypic evolution can result from convergent molecular evolution: mammals that have reentered the water about 50 million years ago have developed a series of common adaptations to the new environment. But now it is the marine environment that is changing: is the new environmental challenge affecting marine mammals to the point where they will have to adapt in order to survive? And to what level will their immune systems adapt to cope? The absence of infection in dolphins' open wounds continuously exposed to seawater is remarkable: the rate of wound healing and the apparent indifference to pain bring some questions about how they are constantly adapting to a new environment. Zasloff[26] suggested that the organohalogens accumulating in dolphin blubber are known to exhibit antimicrobial properties under certain circumstances; for example, as the blubber tissue undergoes "decomposition" following trauma, it could be released locally and could provide antimicrobial protection to the tissues within the immediate wound environment. Dolphins' accumulation of such a heavy concentration of these contaminants in their blubber, rather than metabolization and excretion, could be part of the animal's natural defense against pathogens: it could be an adaptive mechanism designed to permit the animal to concentrate and store protective compounds for its own use.[26] Marine mammal immune systems appear to be similar to that of terrestrial mammals, but when seriously wounded, they do not die of infections (novel antimicrobial agents?), apparently do not manifest overt pain-related behavior (novel analgesic compounds?), and do not bleed to death. How things are changing to enable survival in such a challenging environment is probably registered in marine mammal genomes, and it will be understood only when the relationship between genotype and phenotype is fully deciphered.

REFERENCES

1. Uhen MD. Evolution of marine mammals: back to the sea after 300 million years. *Anat Rec* 2007;**290**:514–22.
2. Bossart GD. Marine mammals as sentinel species for oceans and human health. *Vet Pathol* 2011;**48**:676–90.
3. Rotstein DS, Burdett LG, McLellan W, et al. Lobomycosis in offshore bottlenose dolphins (*Tursiops truncatus*), North Carolina. *Emerg Infect Dis* 2009;**15**:588–90.
4. Hall AJ, Kalantzi OI, Thomas GO. Polybrominated diphenyl ethers (PBDEs) in grey seals during their first year of life–are they thyroid hormone endocrine disrupters? *Environ Pollut* 2003;**126**:29–37.
5. Schwacke LH, Zolman ES, Balmer BC, et al. Anaemia, hypothyroidism and immune suppression associated with polychlorinated biphenyl exposure in bottlenose dolphins (*Tursiops truncatus*). *Proc Biol Sci* 2012;**279**:48–57.
6. Hickie BE, Ross PS, Macdonald RW, Ford JK. Killer whales (*Orcinus orca*) face protracted health risks associated with lifetime exposure to PCBs. *Environ Sci Technol* 2007;**41**:6613–9.
7. Wells DE, Campbell LA, Ross HM, Thompson PM, Lockyer CH. Organochlorine residues in harbour porpoise and bottlenose dolphins stranded on the coast of Scotland, 1988–1991. *Sci Total Environ* 1994;**151**:77–99.
8. Jessup DA, Miller MA, Kreuder-Johnson C, et al. Sea otters in a dirty ocean. *J Am Vet Med Assoc* 2007;**231**:1648–52.
9. Jepson PD, Bennett PM, Allchin CR, et al. Investigating potential associations between chronic exposure to polychlorinated biphenyls and infectious disease mortality in harbour porpoises from England and Wales. *Sci Total Environ* 1999;**243–244**:339–48.
10. Wunschmann A, Siebert U, Frese K, et al. Evidence of infectious diseases in harbour porpoises (*Phocoena phocoena*) hunted in the waters of Greenland and by-caught in the German North Sea and Baltic Sea. *Vet Rec* 2001;**148**:715–20.
11. Siebert U, Prenger-Berninghoff E, Weiss R. Regional differences in bacterial flora in harbour porpoises from the North Atlantic: environmental effects? *J Appl Microbiol* 2009;**106**:329–37.
12. Siebert U, Tolley K, Vikingsson GA, et al. Pathological findings in harbour porpoises (*Phocoena phocoena*) from Norwegian and Icelandic waters. *J Comp Pathol* 2006;**134**:134–42.
13. O'Shea TJ, Brownell Jr RL. Organochlorine and metal contaminants in baleen whales: a review and evaluation of conservation implications. *Sci Total Environ* 1994;**154**:179–200.
14. Romano TA, Felten SY, Olschowka JA, Felten DL. A microscopic investigation of the lymphoid organs of the beluga, *Delphinapterus leucas*. *J Morphol* 1993;**215**:261–87.
15. Romano TA, Felten SY, Olschowka JA, Felten DL. Noradrenergic and peptidergic innervation of lymphoid organs in the beluga, *Delphinapterus leucas*: an anatomical link between the nervous and immune systems. *J Morphol* 1994;**221**:243–59.
16. Cowan DF, Smith TL. Morphology of the lymphoid organs of the bottlenose dolphin, *Tursiops truncatus*. *J Anat* 1999;**194**(Pt 4):505–17.
17. Dierauf L, Gulland FMD. *CRC handbook of marine mammals medicine*. Boca Raton (FL): Taylor & Francis Group; 2001.
18. Yeates LC, Carlin KP, Baird M, Venn-Watson S, Ridgway S. Nitric oxide in the breath of bottlenose dolphins: effects of breath hold duration, feeding, and lung disease. *Mar Mammal Sci* 2013;**30**:272–81.
19. Beineke A, Siebert U, Wohlsein P, Baumgartner W. Immunology of whales and dolphins. *Vet Immunol Immunopathol* 2010;**133**:81–94.

20. Almeida JS, McKillen DJ, Chen YA, Gross PS, Chapman RW, Warr G. Design and calibration of microarrays as universal transcriptomic environmental biosensors. *Comp Funct Genomics* 2005;**6**:132–7.

21. Gracey AY, Cossins AR. Application of microarray technology in environmental and comparative physiology. *Annu Rev Physiol* 2003;**65**:231–59.

22. Mancia A, Ryan JC, Chapman RW, et al. Health status, infection and disease in California sea lions (*Zalophus californianus*) studied using a canine microarray platform and machine-learning approaches. *Dev Comp Immunol* 2012;**36**:629–37.

23. Mancia A, Ryan JC, Van Dolah FM, et al. Machine learning approaches to investigate the impact of PCBs on the transcriptome of the common bottlenose dolphin (*Tursiops truncatus*). *Mar Environ Res* 2014;**100**:57–67.

24. Mancia A, Abelli L, Kucklick JR, et al. Microarray applications to understand the impact of exposure to environmental contaminants in wild dolphins (*Tursiops truncatus*). *Mar Genomics* 2015;**19**:47–57.

25. Foote AD, Liu Y, Thomas GW, et al. Convergent evolution of the genomes of marine mammals. *Nat Genet* 2015;**47**:272–5.

26. Zasloff M. Observations on the remarkable (and mysterious) wound-healing process of the bottlenose dolphin. *J Invest Dermatol* 2011;**131**:2503–5.

Index